I0410639

NIVEN'S

VETERINARY HOMOEOPATHY
VOLUME ONE

REPERTORY
AND
MATERIA MEDICA

SECOND EDITION

DR ALEX NIVEN

COPYRIGHT

DISCLAIMER

No responsibility accepted by the author, publisher, or distributors of this book for the application of any of the enclosed information in practice.

Published by Niven Family Trust April 2025

DEDICATION

Dedicated to my best friend Theresa whose constant support and faith in the power of The Lord keeps me sane.

'What good is butter if you haven't got bread?' McCartney

/

CONTENTS

INTRODUCTION

Homoeopathy works!
As a gentle complementary system of medicine, homoeopathy is forgiving.
Often lifesaving!

Justify making these powerful statements because homoeopathy engendered radical changes in my working life, and medical philosophy after three successful decades embracing the wonderful, standard, field of allopathic veterinary medicine. When delving into the field of potentised remedies, scare could believe the cures which followed.

Success.
And, as nothing succeeds like success, even before embarking on a three-year course in homoeopathy for medical practitioners impatience allowed for serious experimentation.

Yes! Until studying, then implementing art of healing with homoeopathy into the daily management of my practice, only then did the system ripen my skill.
With its encompassing drive and energy, when used either as the sole agent, or as adjunctive therapy, which declared unheard of possibilities, hopes. And yes... dreams.
Initially, major improvements in my medical management of diverse conditions such as backs, bleeders (EIPH), and coughing, proved the necessary, welcome impetus driving me on.

Doubtless homoeopathy works.
In this works companion volume, *Veterinary Homoeopathy, Theory, and Clinical Application*, I offer examples of scientific proof.

Interest in homoeopathy stems from 1986. When that doyen of the South Africa turf: Barbara Sanne told me my *drugs* might struggle to help her horse *Royal Malta* following a savage attack by two pit bull terriers.
Indefatigable, the lady declared I *must not worry*. Gracious, advised homoeopathic *Calendula officinalis* must heal.
Therapy proved remarkable: lesson learned.
While enlightened, still insufficient to divert me from standard veterinary medicine.

Years afterwards, my assistant Linda Engelbrecht complained my constant sinusitis irritated her. *Please take real medicine and start healing.*
Opened my eyes, and yet, as a scientist, resisted the temptation to experiment with homoeopathy. Until desperate, drowning in antibiotics, another severe bout of sinusitis demanded treatment with *Kali bich* in the 200CH potency.
With treatment immediate and effective, seed then planted grew at a fantastic rate.
To colleague's surprise, career expanded into homoeopathy as research unlocked for me what everyone else accepted. Its healing potential and hooked me and helped me

survive through comments such as 'So, shall we soon find you chanting incense and wearing a kaftan.' raided eyebrows.

Teachers: David Lilley and Barclay Digby revealed possibilities, while encouragement from my mentor, the late Dr {Swami} Michael Levien, a doctor of standing in South Africa for holistic healing, and passion for animal welfare, stirred my imagination.

Where the Christian philosophy of Alpha taught the importance of the LORD, homoeopathy introduced spatial dimensions in animal treatment. First, consumed works of the veterinary masters with MacLeod and Day encouraging me to implement their wisdom. Overjoyed, watched amazing healing processes daily.

During my years at the Fourways Equine Hospital in Johannesburg, considerate colleagues encouraged my practice of animal homoeopathy. Still scarcely believe how effective and gentle this form of medicine is after achieving immediate success with conditions where modern medicine struggles. These include EIPH, back, joint problems, while even the sad, common, kidney insufficiencies, surrendered to remedies.
Easy to practice with and evaluate, remedies wrought dramatic lifestyle changes. Energy, excitement, and drive for the subject led to the development of international medicines under the *ECO-VET®* label where thousands of animals benefit from affordable and effective health care.

But and sensibly, while cognisant of how much I still had to learn, found easy to empathise with the young Milton, who, when rushed into a precocious writing career, penned this incredible, erudite verse.
> *'Yet once more ye laurels and once more ye myrtles brown, I come to pluck your berries harsh and crude and with forced fingers rude, shatter your leaves before the mellowing year.'*

When lecturing to colleagues and informed public, recognised their hunger for knowledge. The growing needs of homoeopathic veterinarians deserve support. Modernised since the first edition, earnest hope is for learned colleagues to embrace and enjoy this work. *Enjoy* is a valuable word since this volume may stimulate jaded vets to again embrace the power of healing.

Our job as practitioners of the art freely offers opportunity to become the
refreshed Veterinary Healers the vocational nature of our talents demands and encourage fellow students in the *University of Life* to delve deeper into the art of homoeopathy.
Doubtless, the author sits in awe at the feet of the masters. Hahnemann, Boericke, Kent, Vithoulkas and their peers inflamed medicine with their guiding lights. Now, more radiant than ever, agree with Milton, and together, *refresh their laurels*.
Warning: Because of the fact increasing numbers of veterinary colleagues show interest in homoeopathy, worth repeating.

Three additional points require notice.
First. Admit that with some signs; anxiety and others in the Mind section, and also diarrhoea and in the skin sections, allowed myself to slip into the practice of loading remedies in often large numbers.

Make no excuses for this as these conditions offer a challenging, although a stimulating challenge. As always, begin with the polycrests and mark the pages, highlight them as one does when studying the bible. Always remembering a clean bible suggests a non-believer.

Second. Important to accept this work is a consulting guide, a working tool to simplify what may at first appear a daunting prospect.
Thus, allowed plenty of space in the formatting to permit the serious student room to append their own thoughts, and successes.

Three. As this is a working guide, the Repertory contains only; and bearing in mind there are around five thousand, the major remedies; the ones likely to satisfy ninety per cent of cases.

Good luck and God bless: may the remedies be with you.

Homoeopathy works.
Homoeopathy works Naturally!

Easter Sunday 2025 Johannesburg

FOREWORD

Adapted from Dr Michael Levien: first edition.

Non-human animals have a sense of self-consciousness, to a lesser extent than humans. Their sense of awareness is far greater. Senses are more acute than ours. We cannot imagine smells thousands of times more acute than human.
Also, birds often enjoy better hearing and eyesight. The eyesight of Birds of Prey is virtually 'out of sight' of humans! Their exquisitely acute sense of awareness keeps them informed as to occurrences in their environment. But not only to environmental events but also to the demands, conditions, events within their family unit.

In their very ordered society, each animal must learn its exact position in the hierarchy. The well-known pecking order is an extensively recorded phenomenon.
The pack leader is the BOSS.
Every family member, understands and responds. They are the Alpha male or female. Species of non-human animals have a highly structured social order to match our own. Dedicated, self-sacrificing maternal care, the envy of our children.

Scientists study the involved social behaviour of primate species, and packs of canines, e.g., the hunting dogs of Africa, of families of mongooses and troops of elephants, pods of pilot whales and prides of lion. They record consistency, objective, unprejudiced observer logically declares as evidence of an important level of consciousness.

But enter the human animal...
For his own use, pleasure, protection, and status, he extracted many species from their natural habitat and environment and domestication put them, usually, into solitary confinement.
Stabled, if a horse, or maintained in human homes if a dog or cat.
Deprived of species-specific survival and social integration & education by pack-leaders and peers, they depend on human owners for training, protection, sustenance, housing, even life support.
Such alien, restricted environment demands they adapt to different modes and systems of social behaviour.

Calculating and clever, man took animals out of their natural 'bush.' He never removed the 'bush' from the animal.
The elephant, with his phenomenal memory, never forgets cruelties and indignities received during early handling and training.
Even the pimped, adorned, shampooed, and perfumed lap dog retains the instinct to bite, if frustrated beyond the limits of learned submission. Often a mere growl, the cause of which the owner is blissfully unaware of or indifferent to.
    Particularly the dog, but not excluding other species of animal, this affects even the normally aloof and independent feline, subjected to intense, systematic domestication for centuries. With dogs, we supplanted the natural pack leader with ourselves, the owner and, if the dog is incredibly lucky, sometimes our own family have become the dog's pack.

By nature, dogs are pack-dependent and gregariously orientated. They need the company, example, training, and security of their pack. It is their ingrained nature. Deprived of their natural and essential environment they stress, become unnaturally aggressive, or cowed to a degree dependent on the intelligent thought or understanding of their human owner, and to the degree owners incorporate them into the owner's household as a family (pack) member.

When left at home, or tied, or confined in a limited space, we subject dogs to emotional stress beyond the understanding of most humans.

In his pre-domesticated life as a wild animal, he was wont to roam vast distances and experience a vast array of stimulations and experiences. They enjoy the essentials of physical unconstrained activities natural to the specie.

Social animals are skilled in reading and responding to body language. Smile at my dog, and he wags his tail. As I shake my fist or glower, down goes his tail, and he slinks under the bed.

When depressed, he sits in front of me, looks into my eyes, and wags his tail. Or he lies with his head on my feet.

Having to leave home for a few days, I put the luggage bag on my bed and as fast as I put clothes into it, he tries to remove them.

Self-employed, I take three of my dogs (rescued strays) to work.

One sits on a chair at the front door. She watches to make sure I cannot slip out without her noticing. She always gets to the car before me. Flew my plane countrywide to see patients.

Dogs loved flying and on arriving at the hanger entrance each had a wee and a poo before rushing into the hanger, finding their plane, and barking at me to open the sliding canopy, lift them on to the wing whereupon they grabbed a vantage point at the opened canopy. Tongues lolled excitedly, and I swear, they grinned rapturously.

When they cannot go with me, they wait expectantly at the front door. Shake my head show the palm and they turn and walk away. Body language!

Stress, inadequate stimulation, and adequate exercise are the major problems we subject dogs to. Caring owners note essential needs and may even resort to take advantage of the rewarding and valuable benefits of Training Schools.

Have you ever been to such a school and seen the excitement of the dogs and their keenness to follow orders and the love and devotion that positively flows out of them towards their caring owner. It is exciting and humbling to watch.

Such dogs are fortunate: indeed, they stress in natural, healthy manner and thrive.

Horses respond to stimuli essential to the species.

Between these two extremes are myriad conditions to which life subjects our domestic animals who experience stress to varying degrees.

Here Doctor Alex Niven as the author of this book, he finds his special niche.

His care and compassion for animals motivated him to become a veterinary surgeon. But he felt there was more to treating ailing animals than customary approach to veterinary treatments. Being a thoughtful person, he investigated wider therapies than his education.

He first accepted the fact his mind-set towards medicine must undergo a quantum leap. He saw it enter a paradigm shift. Expanding horizons evolved away from reductionist and mechanistic approach to dis-ease.

Illness, even injury lies at the door of psychosomatic origin. Increasing awareness that older systems of invasive therapies are not the only course.

Scientific circles understand healing forces as innate processes of health.

Niven accepted the Creator endowed the organism with powerful self-healing defence mechanisms capable of generating its own immunological protection. He accepted in modern-day medicine we no longer rely on only 'interference' medicines but now incorporate an increasingly wider range of therapies and medicines.

To combine with and stimulate natural defence and healing energies. He looked at the possibility of incorporating complementary or alternative systems of therapeutics into his practice. But first, he was motivated to evaluate their potentials.

Niven found roots of homoeopathy trace back to Paracelsus and Hippocrates. Their formalization as science-based therapeutics awaited the genius and intuition of Dr. Samuel Hahnemann, medical doctor, and chemist, in 1887.

Modern science recognizes the processing of a gross substance into a homoeopathic medicine complements the art of an experienced homoeopath accurately aiming the vibrational energies of his selected remedy to interact with the dis-eased vibrations characterizing the ailment of the patient. It is in this non-material realm of pure energy that the fields of force act in complementarity and resonance. This is the strength of Homoeopathy.

Also, its Achilles heel for even today when we accept Einstein's Theories and Plank's Quanta as verifiable scientific facts. Many locked in the Newtonian paradigm of the mechanistic material world, ignore the vast areas of potential that are quantum mechanics of modern science.

Schrodinger describes atoms as a system of nucleus and matter waves. Bohr considers the two pictures, particle picture, and wave picture, as two complementary descriptions of the same reality. It is primarily the wave component that is the inherent energy of the potentised homoeopathic substance, not the physiological material particles, which alone imparts the characteristic pattern of medicinal energy of the substance.

The homoeopathic medicine's potentised form is the energy of the substance.

Every organ, cell, and part of living organisms have their own individual electro- magnetic frequency or field of energy.

Similarly, every homoeopathic substance has its own individual electromagnetic frequency or field of energy. And we understand the manifestation of *Similia Similibus Curentur*.

When applying the appropriate homoeopathic medicine to the disordered organism, the electromagnetic frequency of the homoeopathic medicine matches the electromagnetic frequency of the disordered organism, stimulating the auto-immune defence system into remedial action.... and Likes cure Likes!

These patterned processes of self-organizing energies, characteristic of living organisms react to homoeopathic remedies by a process of resonance. Hahnemann's dictum of *Similia similibus curentur:* as *likes cure likes*, exemplifies how remedies act on the mind and body. The equivalent frequency of a material substance can match the electromagnetic frequency of every cell when rendered in its homoeopathic form.

Precise anamnesis allows accurate prescribing. They liken energy patterns to how stringed instruments vibrate in harmonic unison when they activate a similarly tuned string of another instrument.

We concede in today's ultra-demanding environment, practitioners, whether veterinary or medical cannot spend hours eliciting every factor that affects the ailing patient. Reality demands complex remedies in the hands of concerned, informed practitioners. Complexes, meticulously formulated, treat symptoms characteristic of specific ailments by prescribing single enhanced-energy packets of remedies combined according to their synergistic fields of action. Remember the ridicule they subjected Einstein to when he first introduced the concept of nuclear physics! Before they understood his *Theory of Relativity*. Even he was shocked when his formula of E= MC2, eventuated as nuclear fission to release the potential of the explosive power of the atom bomb.

During the process of potentisation, we force atoms against each other during each sequential step in the progressive dilution of the original substance. Gross material diminishes with each successive dilution. The quanta of energy, the actual character of the substance, is progressively released at each step of potentisation. The process, though simple, is itself dynamic and dynamic in its effectiveness. Science marched on, enlarged horizons to open new fields of therapeutics.

Practitioners better understand the art and science of healing. More veterinarians are using more of the range of the homoeopathically prepared 'Energy' medicines which function dynamically in concert with the natural healing forces of the living organism, the innate immune defence system.

Here I applaud the courage, the skilled knowledge, self-sacrificing dedication to the cause of healing through the medium of homoeopathy in the vast and difficult domain of veterinary medicine, embracing Doctor Alex Niven. He saw that underlying the traditional philosophy of the homoeopathic system of therapeutic was a potential force for healing which reached deeply into the realm of the truly scientific.

He had enough knowledge of the Theory of Quantum Physics and Mechanics to be intellectually aware of the tremendous energy contained within a single atom of, e.g., Uranium isotope 145, and that this energy is potentially present, though in lesser available degree in every other substance.

Atomic electrons bear the same characteristics. Even in water. Remember the tremendous efforts made by the allied forces during World War 11 to destroy the Heavy Water factories of Germany?

Hahnemann's remarkable intuition of the essentials of health and dis-ease
meant he did not succumb to the antagonism and scepticism within the traditional orthodox medical practice of his day. With colleagues seeking a more efficient system of healing, they courageously experimented with an increasingly wide range of substances by a process of systematized and scrupulously recorded provings of the effects of the homoeopathic substances on healthy volunteers, mostly themselves. These recorded provings formed the basis of the original Materia Medica and later repertories.

Today duly registered pharmaceutical companies produce and develop complementary medicines in strict observance of Good Manufacturing Procedures and complying with the prerequisites of Quality Efficacy and Stability as demanded by the Medicines Control Council.

Well, over four thousand substances are available as single remedies. When synergistically combined, formulations embrace most ailments to which human and non-human are liable.

In homoeopathic practice since 1960 have accumulated many volumes of Homoeopathic Materia Medica and Homoeopathic Repertories, many authored by acknowledged masters in the art and science of homoeopathy.

Until I received a draft copy of Doctor Niven's work, I had not found a single user-friendly, comprehensive work for treating animals holistically. The more perceptive and detailed the taking of a patient's case history, the more clearly will the most appropriate homoeopathic drug become clear.

Realizing and accepting that the determination of symptom pictures is mostly subjective and not readily accessible when seeking the ideal matching homoeopathic substance, Doctor Niven paid attention to the more readily accessible organotrophic, functional signs and dis-ease phenomena that may be immediate and observable in the animal patient.

Doctor Niven's Veterinary Materia Medica and Repertory realistically present the essential rubrics, both objective and subjective, to enable vets to select homoeopathic drugs whose immune / healing stimulus may most effectively match to the pathology of the patient. *Similia Similibus Curentur.*

Dr Michael Levien Pretoria 2003

REMEDIES: SCIENTIFIC NAME FIRST

Abelmoschus	Abel	Musk mallow
Abies canadensis	Abies-c	Spruce: hemlock
Abies nigra	Abies-n	Spruce: black
Abies pectinata (alba)	Abies-p	Fir tree: European silver
Abrus precatorius	Abr	Jequirty
Acalyphya indica	Acal	Nettle: indian
Achillea millefolium	Mill	Yarrow, Millefolium.
Achyranthes calea	Achy	Fever herb
Acidum aceticum	Acid-acet	Acid: acetic, glacial
Acidum benzoicum	Acid-benz	Acid: benzoic
Acidum boracicum	Acid-bor	Acid: boracic
Acidum butyricum	Acid-but	Acid: butyric
Acidum carbolicum	Acid-carb	Acid: carbolic
Acidum fluoricum	Acid-fl	Acid: fluoric
Acidum hydrocyanic	Acid-hydr	Acid: prussic
Acidum nitricum	Acid-nit	Acid: nitric
Acidum oxalicum	Acid-oxal	Acid: oxalic
Acidum phosphoricum	Acid-phos	Acid: phosphoric
Acidum picricum	Acid-pic	Acid: picric
Acidum sulphuricum	Acid-sul	Acid: sulphuric
Aconitum napellus	Acon	Aconite. Monk's hood
Actea spicata	Act-sp	Baneberry
Adonis vernalis	Adon	Pheasant's eye
Aesculus glabra	Aesc-g	Ohio buckeye
Aesculus hippocastanum	Aesc	Chestnut: horse
Aethusa cynapium	Aeth	Parsley: fools
Agaricus muscarius	Agar	Fly agaric. Toadstool
Ailanthus glandulosa	Ail	Chinese sumach
Aletris farinosa	Alet	Grass: star
Alfalfa	Alf	Lucerne
Allium cepa	All-c	Onion: red
Allium sativum	All-s	Garlic
Alloxanum	Allox	Alloxan
Aloe	Aloe	Aloe socotrina
Alumen	Alumn	Potash
Alumina	Alum	Alluminium oxide
Ambra grisea	Ambr	Ambergris. Sperm whale
Ammonium benzoicum	Am-be	Ammonium benzoate
Ammonium carbonicum	Am-c	Ammonium carbonate.
Ammonium causticum	Am-caust	Ammonium hydrate
Ammonium muriaticum	Am-m	Ammonium chloride
Anacardium orientale	Anac	Marking nut
Anagallis arvensis	Anag	Scarlet pimpernel
Anhalonium lewinii	Anh	Mescal button
Anthemis nobilis	Anth	Chamomile: Roma
Anthracinum	Anthr	Anthrax: nosode
Antimonium crudum	Ant-c	Black sulphide of antimony
Antimonium tartaricum	Ant-t	Antimony tartrate

Antipyrine	Antip	Phenazone
Apis mellifica	Apis	Honeybee
Apocynum cannabinum	Apoc	Indian hemp
Apomorphinum hydrochlor	Apom	Apomorphine
Aqua marina	Aq-mar	Water: Quinton's sea
Aragallus lamberti	Arag	White loco weed
Aralia racemosa	Aral	American spikenhard
Aranea diadema	Aran	Spider: Papal cross
Areca catechu	Arec	Nut: betal
Argentum metallicum	Arg-m	Silver
Argentum nitricum	Arg-n	Silver nitrate
Aristolochia clematitis	Arist-cl	Brazilian snake root
Arnica montana	Arn	Leopard's bane
Arsenicum album	Ars	White arsenic
Arsenicum iodatum	Ars-i	Arsenious oxide
Artemisia abrotanum	Abrot	Wormwood: Southern
Artemisia absinthium	Absin	Wormwood: common
Artemisia maritima	Cina	Wormwood: Levant
Artemisia vulgaris	Art-v	Mugwort
Arum triphyllum	Arum-t	Jack in the Pulpit
Asarum europaeum	Asar	Snakeroot: European
Asclepias syriaca	Asc-c	Silkweed
Aspidosperma quebracho	Queb	Quebracho
Astacus fluviatilis	Astac	Crawfish
Asterias rubens	Aster	Starfish: red
Astragalus excapus	Astra-e	European astagalus
Atropa belladonna	Bell	Deadly nightshade
Aurum metallicum	Aur	Gold
Aurum muriaticum nat	Aur-m-n	Sodium chloroaurate
Avena sativa	Aven	Common oat
Bacillinum Burnett	Bac	Bovine TB nosode
Bacillis proteus	Prot	Bacterium nosode
Ballota foetida	Ball	Black horehound
Balsamum peruvianum	Bals-p	Peruvian balsam
Baptisia tinctoria	Bapt	Wild indigo
Baryta carbonica	Bar-c	Barium carbonate
Baryta muriatica	Bar-m	Barium chloride
BCG	Bcg	TB vaccine: bovine
Bellis perennis	Bell-p	Common clarity, daisy
Benzinum	Ben	Petroleum ether
Berberis aquifolium	Berb-a	Mahonia
Berberis vulgaris	Berb	Barberry: common
Beryllium metallicum	Beryl	Beryllium
Bismuthum metallicum	Bism	Bismuth sub nitrate
Blatta orientalis	Blatta	Cockroach: Asian
Borax veneta	Bor	Sodium borate
Bothrops lanceolatus	Both	Snake: viper, yellow
Bovista lycoperdon	Bov	Puffball: giant
Bromium	Brom	Bromium
Bryonia alba	Bry	Bryony: white
Bufo rana	Bufo	Toad: common
Bunias orientalis	Buni-o	Rocket: Turkish
Cadmium metallicum	Cadm-m	Cadmium
Cadmium sulphuratum	Cadm-s	Cadmium sulphate
Cajuputum	Caj	Cajput oil
Calcarea carbonica H	Calc	Carbonate of lime
Calcarea fluorica naturalis	Calc-fl	Fluoride of lime
Calcarea phosphorica	Calc-p	Phosphate of lime
Calcarea sulphurica	Calc-s	Plaster of Paris

Calendula officinalis	Calen	Marigold
Caltha palustris	Calth	Cowslip
Camphora	Camph	Camphor
Cannabis indica	Cann-i	Hashish
Cannabis sativa	Cann-s	Hemp: American
Cantharis vesicatoria	Canth	Spanish fly
Capsicum annuum	Caps	Pepper: cayenne
Carbo animalis	Carb-an	Charcoal: animal
Carbo vegetabilis	Carb-v	Charcoal: wood
Carboneum oxygenisatum	Carbn-o	Carbonous oxide
Carboneum sulphuratum	Carbn-s	Bisulphide of carbon
Carcinosinum Burnett	Carc	Carcinosin: nosode
Carpinus betulus	Carp-b	Hornbeam tree
Cartilago articulus	Cart-a	Cartilage: nosode
Castor equi	Cast-eq	Equine ergot
Caulophyllum thalictroides	Caul	Blue cohosh
Causticum Hahnemanni	Caust	Tinctura acris sine kali
Ceanothus americanus	Cean	Tea: New Jersey
Cedron	Cedr	Rattlesnake bean
Cenchris contortrix	Cench	Snake: copperhead
Cephaelis acuminata	Ip	Ipecacuanha
Cereus bonplandii	Cere-b	Cactus: night blooming
Chelidonium majus	Chel	Celandine: greater
Chelone glabra	Chelo	Snakehead
Chimaphila umbellata	Chim	Ivy: ground, Pipsissewa
Chininum arsenicosum	Chin-ar	Quinine: arsenite
Chininum sulphuricum	Chin-s	Quinine: sulphite
Chionanthus virginicum	Chion	Tree: fringe
Chloralum hydratum	Chlol	Chloral hydrate
Chloramphenicolum	Chloram	Antibiotic: chloramphenicol
Chloroformium	Chlf	Chloroform
Chlorpromazinum	Chlorpr	Chlorpromazine
Chlorum	Chlor	Chlorine gas in water
Cholesterinum	Chol	Cholesterol: nosode
Chrysarobinum	Chrysar	Goa powder
Cicuta virosa	Cic	Hemlock: water
Cimex lectularius	Cimx	Acanthia lectularia, Bed bug
Cimicifuga racemosa	Cimic	Actea racemosa, Cohosh
Cinchona succirubra	Chin	Peruvian bark
Cinnamomum ceylanicum	Cinnm	Cinnamon
Cistus canadensis	Cist	Rock rose: Canadian
Citrullus colocynthis	Coloc	Cucumber: bitter
Clematis erecta	Clem	Virgins bower
Cobaltum nitricum	Cob-n	Cobalt nitrate
Cocainum hydrochloricum	Cocain	Erythroxlon coca
Cocculus indicus	Cocc	Coccle: Indian
Coccus cacti	Coc-c	Cochineal
Coffea cruda	Coff	Coffea arabica
Colchicum autumnale	Colch	Meadow saffron
Collinsonia canadensis	Coll	Stoneroot
Colostrum bovis	Colos	Colostrum: bovine
Conium maculatum	Con	Poison hemlock
Convallaria majalis	Conv	Lily of the valley
Copaiva	Cop	Balsalm: Peruvian
Corallium rubrum	Cor-r	Coral: red
Cornus circinata	Corn	Dog wood: round leaved
Corticotrophinum	Cortico	ACTH
Cortisonum	Cortiso	Hydrocortisone

Corylus avellana	Coryl-a	Hazelnut
Corynanthe yohimbe	Yohim	Yohimbine
Crataegus oxyacantha	Crat	Hawthorn. Mayflower
Cresolum	Kres	Kreosote BP 88
Crocus sativus	Croc	Saffron
Crotalus horridus	Crot-h	Snake: rattlesnake
Croton tiglium	Crot-t	Croton: purging
Cubeba officinalis	Cub	Piper cubeba
Cucurbita pepo	Cuc-p	Pumpkin
Cundurango	Cund	Condor plant
Cuprum arsenicosum	Cupr-ars	Copper: arsenite
Cuprum metallicum	Cupr	Copper
Curare	Cur	Poison: arrow
Curcuma longa	Curc	Turmeric
Cusparia febrifuga	Ang	Angustura vera
Cyclamen europaeum	Cycl	Sow bread
Cypripedium pubescens	Cypr	Yellow lady's slipper
Cytisus laburnum	Cyt-l	Laburnum
Daphne indica	Daph	Spurge laurel
Daphne mezereum	Mez	Spurge olive
Datura stramonium	Stram	Thorn apple. Stramonium
Delphinium staphysagria	Staph	Housewort. Stavesacre
Deoxyribonucleic acid	Dna	DNA
Diesel oil	Dies	Diesel oil
Digitalis purpurea	Dig	Foxglove, purple
Dioscorea villosa	Dios	Wild yam
Diosma lincaris	Diosm	Buku
Diptherinum	Dipth	Diphtheria: nosode
Drosera rotundifolia	Dros	Sundew: round-leaved
Duboisinum	Dub	Corkwood elm
Echinacea angustifolia	Echi	Cone flower, narrow-leaved
Echinacea purpurea	Echi-p	Coneflower, purple
Elaps corallinus	Elaps	Snake: coral
Elaterium officinarum	Elat	Cucumber: squirting
Eleutherococcus senticosus	Eleuth	Ginseng: Siberian
Epihysterinum	Epih	Uterine fibroid
Equisetum hiemale	Equis	Horsetail: rough
Ergotinum	Ergot	Ergot: alkaloid
Erigeron canadensis	Erig	Fleabane
Erythroxylum coca	Coca	Divine plant of the Incas
Eserinum	Esin	Calabar bean
Eucalyptus globulus	Eucal	Blue gum: Tasmanian
Eugenia jambosa	Eug	Rose-apple
Euonymus europaea	Euon	Spindle tree: Wahoo
Eupatorium perfoliatum	Eup-per	Boneset. Thoroughwort
Eupatorium purpureum	Eup-pur	Queen of the meadow
Euphorbia lathyris	Euph-l	Gopher plant
Euphorbia resinifera	Euph-r	Wood spurge
Euphrasia officinalis	Euphr	Eyebright
Ferrum arsenicosum	Ferr-ars	Iron arsenate
Ferrum metallicum	Ferr	Iron
Ferrum phosphoricum	Ferr-p	Iron phosphate
Ferrum picricum	Ferr-pic	Iron picrate
Ficus religiosa	Fic	Pakur
Flavus	Flav	Bacterium: Neisseria flava
Flor de piedra	Flor-p	Lopophytum leandri
Folliculinum	Foll	Ovarian follicle, ripe
Formicicum acidum	Form-ac	Acid: formic
Fragaria vesca	Frag	Strawberry: wild

Fucus vesiculosus	Fuc	Sea kelp
Fuligo ligni	Fuli	Soot
Galium aparine	Gali	Grass: goose
Galphimia glauca	Galph	Thyrallis glauca
Gaultheria procumbens	Gaul	Wintergreen
Gelsemium sempervirens	Gels	Jasmine: yellow
Geranium maculatum	Ger	Cranesbill: wild
Gingko biloba	Gink-b	Tree: maidenhair
Glonoinum	Glon	Nitro glycerine
Granatum	Gran	Pomegranate
Graphites	Graph	Lead: black
Gratiola officinalis	Grat	Hyssop: hedge
Guaco	Gua	Weed, climbing hemp
Guaiacum officinale	Guai	Lignum vitae: resin
Gunpowder	Gunp	Gunpowder: black
Haloperidol	Halo	Butyrophenol
Hamamelis virginiana	Ham	Witch hazel: Virginian
Harpagophytum procumbens	Harp	Devil's claw
Hedeoma pulegoides	Hedeo	Penny royal
Hedera helix	Hed	Ivy: European
Hekla lava	Hekla	Lava scoriae
Helleborus niger	Hell	Rose: Christmas
Heloderma suspectum	Helo	Gila monster
Helonias dioica	Helon	Unicon root: false
Hepar sulphuris H.	Hep	Calcium sulphide
Hippomanes	Hipp	Equine allantoic deposit
Hippozaeninum	Hippoz	Glanders disease: nosode
Hirudo medicinalis	Hir	Leech: medicinal
Histaminum muriaticum	Hist	Histamine
Hoitzia coccinea	Hoit	Colibri flower
Hydrangea arborescens	Hydrang	Seven barks
Hydrastis canadensis	Hydr	Golden seal
Hydrocotyl asiatica	Hydrc	Pennywort: Indian
Hydrophis cyanocinctus	Hydroph	Snake: sea Snake
Hyoscyamus niger	Hyos	Henbane: black
Hypericum perforatum	Hyper	St. John's Wort
Hypophysis posterior	Pitu	Pituitary gland, posterior
Iberis amara	Iber	Candytuft: bitter
Ignatia amara	Ign	Bean: St Ignatia's
Indigo tinctoria	Indg	Indigo: dye
Influenzinum	Infl	Influenza nosode: human
Insulinum	Ins	Insulin
Iodum purum	Iod	Iodine
Iris versicolor	Iris	Blue flag
Jacaranda caroba	Jac-c	Tree: carab tree, Brazilian
Jalapa	Jal	Exogonium purga
Juglans regia	Jug-r	Walnut: GB
Juniperus communis	Juni-c	Juniper
Kalium arsenicosum	Kali-ars	Fowler's solution
Kalium bichromicum	Kali-bi	Potassium bichromate
Kalium bromatum	Kali-br	Bromide of potash
Kalium carbonicum	Kali-c	Potassium carbonate
Kalium chlorosum	Kali-chls	Potassium chlorate
Kalium iodatum	Kali-i	Potassium iodide
Kalium muriaticum	Kali-m	Potassium chloride
Kalium phosphoricum	Kali-p	Potassium phosphate
Kalium sulphuricum	Kali-s	Potassium sulphate
Kalmia latifolia	Kalm	Mountain laurel

Karwinskia humboldtiana	Karw-h	Wild capuli
Kigelia africana	Kig	Tree: sausage
Kousso	Kou	Brayera anthelmintica
Lac caninum	Lac-c	Milk: canine
Lachesis muta	Lach	Snake: bushmaster
Lapis albus	Lap-a	Silico-fluoride of calcium
Lappa arctium	Lappa	Burdock
Lathyrus sativus aut cicera	Lath	Chickpea
Latrodectus mactans	Lat-m	Spider: black widow
Ledum palustre	Led	Tea: marsh
Lemna minor	Lem-m	Duckweed
Leptandra virginica	Lept	Root: Culver's
Levomepromazine	Levo	Nozenan
Liatris spicata	Liat	Root: colic
Lilium tigrinum	Lil-t	Lilly: Tiger
Lithium carbonicum	Lith-c	Carbonate of lithium
Lobelia inflata	Lob	Tobacco: Indian
Lobelia purpurascens	Lob-p	Lobelia: purple
Lolium temulentum	Lol	Darnel
Luffa operculata	Luf-op	Esponjilla
Lycopodium clavatum	Lyc	Moss: club
Lycopus virginicus	Lycps	Weed: bugle
Lyssinum	Lyss	Hydrophobinum
Magnesia carbonica	Mag-c	Carbonate of magnesium
Magnesia fluorata	Mag-f	Magnesium fluoride
Magnesia muriatica	Mag-m	Magnesium chloride
Magnesia phosphorica	Mag-p	Magnesium phosphate
Magnesia sulphurica	Mag-s	Epsom salts
Magnolia grandiflora	Magn-gr	Magnolia: Southern
Malandrinum	Maland	Grease: equine nosode
Mancinella	Manc	Apple: Manganeel
Mandragora officinarum	Mand	Mandrake
Manganum aceticum	Mang	Manganese acetate
Medorrhinum	Med	Gonorrhea: nosode
Medusa	Medus	Jelly fish
Meliliotus officinalis	Meli	Clover: sweet
Mercurius corrosivus	Merc-c	Mercuric chloride
Mercurius solubilis	Merc	Mercury
Morbillinum	Morb	Measles
Morphinum	Morph	Morphine: opium poppy
Moschus	Mosch	Musk gland
Mucuna pruriens	Dol	Cowhage. Dolichos
Murex purpureus	Murx	Fish: purple
Myrica cerifera	Myric	Bayberry
Myristica sebifera	Myris	Brazilian ucuba
Naja tripudians	Naja	Snake: cobra
Natrum carbonicum	Nat-c	Sodium carbonate
Natrum hypochlorosum	Nat-hchls	Sodium hypochlorite
Natrum muriaticum	Nat-m	Sodium chloride
Natrum phosphoricum	Nat-p	Sodium phosphate
Natrum sulphuricum	Nat-s	Sodium sulphate
Nepenthe distillatoria	Nep	Plant: pitcher
Nerium odorum	Ner	Laurel: rose
Nux moschata	Nux-m	Nutmeg
Nux vomica	Nux-v	Poison: nut
Ocimum canum	Oci	Alfavaca: Brazilian
Oenanthe crocata	Oena	Dropwart: water
Onosmodium virginianum	Onos	Cromwell: false
Orchitinum	Orchi	Testes nosode

Orchitinum canis	Orchi-c	Testes nosode: canine
Orchitinum equus	Orchi-e	Testes nosode: equine
Ornithogalum umbellatum	Orni	Star of Bethlehem
Osmium metallicum	Osm	Osmium
Osteo nosodum	Osteo-N	Bone nosode
Ovininum	Ov	Ovarian extract
Oxytropis lamberti	Oxyt	Loco weed
Paeonia officinalis	Paeon	Peony: tree
Palladium metallicum	Pall	Palladium
Panax quinquefolia	Gins	Ginseng
Pancreatinum	Pancr	Pancreas
Papaver somniferum	Op	Poppy: opium
Parathyroid hormone	Parathyr	Parathormone
Pareira brava	Pareir	Virgin vine
Paris quadrifolia	Par	One berry
Paronychia illecebrum	Paro-i	Sanguinaria: Cuba
Parotidinum	Parot	Parotid nosode
Passiflora incarnata	Passi	Flower: Passion
Penicillinum	Penic	Antibiotic: benzylpenicillin
Perhexilin	Perh	Perhexiline maleate
Petroleum	Petr	Petrol
Phenobarbitalum	Phenob	Phenylethylmalonurea
Phosphorus	Phos	Phosphorus
Physostigma venosum	Phys	Bean: calabar
Phytolacca decandra	Phyt	Pokeroot
Pilocarpus pennatifolius	Pilo	Jaborandi
Pinus montana	Pin-mo	Pine: mountain
Pinus sylvestris	Pin-s	Scots Pine
Placenta equinus	Plac-e	Placenta: equine
Platinum metallicum	Plat	Platinum
Plectranthus fruticosus	Plect	Pink spur flower
Plumbum metallicum	Plb	Lead
Podophyllum peltatum	Podo	Apple: May
Populus tremula	Pop	Aspen: American
Primula obconica	Prim-o	Primrose
Prunus laurocerasus	Laur	Laurel: cherry
Prunus spinosa	Prun	Thorn: black
Psorinum	Psor	Scabies mite: nosode
Ptelea trifoliata	Ptel	Ash: wafer
Pulex irritans	Pulx	Flea: human
Pulsatilla vulgaris	Puls	Flower: Passion
Pyrogenium	Pyrog	Meat: rotting meat
Quercus e glandibus	Querc	Kernal: acorn
Radium	Rad	Radium bromide
Rajania subsamarata	Raj-s	Raison seed
Ranunculus bulbosus	Ran-b	Buttercup: bulbous
Raphanus sativus	Raph	Radish: black
Ratanhia peruviana	Rat	Mapato
Rauwolphia serpentina	Rauw	Rauwolphia
Reserpinum	Reser	Rauwolphia: alkaloid
Rhamnus californica	Rham-cal	Tree: Californian, coffee
Rheum palmatum	Rheum	Rhubarb
Rhododendron chrysanthum	Rhod	Snow rose
Rhus toxicodendron	Rhus-t	Ivy: poison
Rhus venenata	Rhus-v	Poison: elder
Ribes nigrum	Ribes-n	Black currant
Ribonucleic acid	Rna	RNA
Rosa canina	Ros-ca	Dog rose

Rumex crispus	Rumx	Dock: yellow
Ruta graveolens	Ruta	Rue: common
Sabadilla officinalis	Sabad	Asagraea cevadilla
Sabal serrulatum	Sabal	Saw palmetto
Sabina	Sabin	Savine
Saccharum officinale	Sacch	Sucrose
Salicylicum acidum	Sal-ac	Aspirin
Salvia officinalis	Salv	Sage
Sambucus nigra	Samb	Elder: black
Sanguinaria canadensis	Sang	Blood root
Sanguinarinum nitricum	Sang-n	Nitrate of sanguinarine
Sanicula aqua	Sanic	Water: Sanicula springs
Sarcolacticum acidum	Sarcol-ac	Dextrum lacticum acidum
Sarothamnus scoparius	Saroth	Broom: Scotch
Sceletium tortuosum	Scel-t	Sceletium
Scrophularia nodosa	Scroph-n	Figwort: knotted
Scutellaria lateriflora	Scut	Skullcap
Secale cornutum	Sec	Ergot
Selenium	Sel	Selenium
Senecio aureus	Senec	Ragwort: golden
Senega	Seneg	Snakewort
Sepia succus	Sep	Cuttlefish
Sequoia gigantea	Seq-g	Giant redwood
Serum anguillae	Ser-ang	Eel Serum
Silicea terra	Sil	Flint
Silybum marianum	Card-m	Thistle: St. Mary's
Sol	Sol	Sunlight
Solanum dulcamara	Dulc	Bittersweet
Solanum nigrum	Sol-n	Nightshade: black
Solidago virgaurea	Solid	Rod: golden
Spigelia anthelmia	Spig	Pinkroot
Spongia tosta	Spong	Sponge, roasted
Stannum metallicum	Stann	Tin
Staphylococcinum	Staphyloc	Bacterium
Sticta pulmonaria	Stict	Lungwort
Streptococcinum	Streptoc	Bacterium: steptococcus
Strontium metallicum	Stront	Strontium
Strophanthus hispidus	Stroph-h	Kombe seed
Strophanthus sarmentosus	Stroph-s	Poison: arrow vine
Sulfanilamidum	Sulfa	Antibiotic: sulphanilamide
Sulfonalum	Sulfon	Coal tar: derivative of
Sulfonamidum	Sulfonam	Antibiotic: sulphonamide
Sulphur iodatum	Sulph-i	Sulphur iodide
Sulphur lotum	Sulph	Sulphur: sublimate
Symphytum officinale	Symph	Comfrey
Syphilinum	Syph	Syphilinum: nosode
Syzygium jambolanum	Syzyg	Jambol
Tabacum	Tab	Tobacco: nicotiana
Tamarix gallica	Tama-g	Tamarisk
Taraxicum officinale	Tarax	Dandelion
Tarentula cubensis	Tarent-c	Spider: tarentula, Cuban
Tarentula hispanica	Tarent	Spider: tarentula, Spanish
Tellurium metallicum	Tell	Tellurium
Terebinthiniae oleum	Tereb	Turpentine
Teucrium marum verum	Teucr	Thyme: cat
Thalamus	Thala	Thalamic nosode
Thallium aceticum	Thal	Thallium acetate
Theridion curassavicum	Ther	Spider: orange spider
Thiopentonum	Thiopen	Sodium thiopental

21

Thioproperazinum	Thiop	Majeptil
Thiosinaminum	Thiosin	Mustard seed
Thlaspi bursa pastoris	Thlas	Shepherd's purse
Thuja occidentalis	Thuj	Arbor vitae
Thymolum	Thymol	Thyme-camphor
Thyroidinum	Thyr	Thyroid: ovine, nosode
Tribulus terrestris	Trib	Ikshugandha
Trifolium pratense	Trif-p	Clover: red
Trillium pendulum	Tril	Beth root: white
Trinitrotoluenum	Tnt	TNT
Triticum repens	Tritic	Grass: couch
Tuberculinum bovinum	Tub	TB: bovine, nosode
Turnera aphrodisiaca	Dam	Damiana
Uranium nitricum	Uran-n	Uranium nitrate
Urea pura	Urea	Carbamide
Urtica urens	Urt-u	Nettle: stinging
Ustilago maydis	Ust	Corn smut
Uva ursi	Uva	Bearberry
Vaccininum	Vac	Vaccine: cowpox nosode
Vaccinum vitis idaea	Vacc-v	Cowberry
Valeriana officinalis	Valer	Valerian
Vanadium metallicum	Vanad	Vanadium metallicum
Variolinum	Variol	Smallpox: nosode
Venus mercenaria	Ven-m	Scallop: American
Veratrum album	Verat	Hellebore, white
Veratrum viride	Verat-v	Hellebore, American
Verbascum thapsus	Verb	Mullein
Verbena hastata	Verbe-h	Blue vervain
Vespa crabo	Vesp	Hornet, European
Viburnum lantana	Vib-l	Wayfaring tree
Viburnum opulus	Vib	Cranberry: high
Viburnum prunifolium	Vib-p	Black haw
Vinca minor	Vinc	Periwinkle: lesser
Viola odorata	Viol-o	Violet: blue
Viola tricolor	Viol-t	Pansy
Vipera aspis	Vip-a	Snake: viper, German
Viscum album	Visc	Mistletoe
Vitex agnus castus	Agn	Tree: chaste
Vitis vinifera	Vitis-v	Grape vine
Wyethia helenoides	Wye	Weed: poison
Xanthoxylum fraxineum	Xan	Ash: prickly
X-ray	X-ray	X-ray
Zincum metallicum	Zinc	Zinc
Zincum valerianicum	Zinc-val	Zinc Valerianate
Zingiber officinale	Zing	Ginger

REMEDIES COMMON NAME FIRST

Acanthia lectularia, Bed bug	Cimex lectularius	Cimx
Acid: acetic, glacial	Acidum aceticum	Acid-acet
Acid: benzoic	Acidum benzoicum	Acid-benz
Acid: boracic	Acidum boracicum	Acid-bor
Acid: butyric	Acidum butyricum	Acid-but
Acid: carbolic	Acidum carbolicum	Acid-carb
Acid: fluoric	Acidum fluoricum	Acid-fl
Acid: formic	Formicicum acidum	Form-ac
Acid: nitric	Acidum nitricum	Acid-nit
Acid: oxalic	Acidum oxalicum	Acid-oxal
Acid: phosphoric	Acidum phosphoricum	Acid-phos
Acid: picric	Acidum picricum	Acid-pic
Acid: prussic	Acidum hydrocyanic	Acid-hydr
Acid: sulphuric	Acidum sulphuricum	Acid-sul
Aconite. Monk's hood	Aconitum napellus	Acon
Actea racemosa, Cohosh	Cimicifuga racemosa	Cimic
ACTH	Corticotrophinum	Cortico
Alfavaca: Brazilian	Ocimum canum	Oci
Alloxan	Alloxanum	Allox
Alluminium oxide	Alumina	Alum
Aloe socotrina	Aloe	Aloe
Ambergris. Sperm whale	Ambra grisea	Ambr
American spikenhard	Aralia racemosa	Aral
Ammonium benzoate	Ammonium benzoicum	Am-be
Ammonium carbonate.	Ammonium carbonicum	Am-c
Ammonium chloride	Ammonium muriaticum	Am-m
Ammonium hydrate	Ammonium causticum	Am-caust
Angustura vera	Cusparia febrifuga	Ang
Anthrax: nosode	Anthracinum	Anthr
Antibiotic: benzylpenicillin	Penicillinum	Penic
Antibiotic: chloramphenicol	Chloramphenicolum	Chloram
Antibiotic: sulphanilamide	Sulfanilamidum	Sulfa
Antibiotic: sulphonamide	Sulfonamidum	Sulfonam
Antimony tartrate	Antimonium tartaricum	Ant-t
Apomorphine	Apomorphinum	Apom
Apple: Manganeel	Mancinella	Manc
Apple: May	Podophyllum peltatum	Podo
Arbor vitae	Thuja occidentalis	Thuj
Arsenic, white	Arsenicum album	Ars
Arsenious oxide	Arsenicum iodatum	Ars-i
Asagraea cevadilla	Sabadilla officinalis	Sabad
Ash: prickly	Xanthoxylum fraxineum	Xan
Ash: wafer	Ptelea trifoliata	Ptel
Aspen: American	Populus tremula	Pop
Aspirin	Salicylicum acidum	Sal-ac
Bacterium nosode	Bacillis proteus	Prot
Bacterium: Neisseria flava	Flavus	Flav
Bacterium: staphylococci spp	Staphylococcinum	Staphyloc
Bacterium: steptococcus	Streptococcinum	Streptoc
Balsalm: Peruvian	Copaiva	Cop
Baneberry	Actea spicata	Act-sp
Barberry: common	Berberis vulgaris	Berb

23

Barium carbonate	Baryta carbonica	Bar-c
Barium chloride	Baryta muriatica	Bar-m
Bayberry	Myrica cerifera	Myric
Bean: calabar	Physostigma venosum	Phys
Bean: St Ignatia's	Ignatia amara	Ign
Bearberry	Uva ursi	Uva
Beryllium	Beryllium metallicum	Beryl
Beth root: white	Trillium pendulum	Tril
Bismuth sub nitrate	Bismuthum metallicum	Bism
Bisulphide of carbon	Carboneum sulphuratum	Carbn-s
Bittersweet	Solanum dulcamara	Dulc
Black horehound	Ballota foetida	Ball
Black currant	Ribes nigrum	Ribes-n
Black haw	Viburnum prunifolium	Vib-p
Black sulphide of antimony	Antimonium crudum	Ant-c
Blood root	Sanguinaria canadensis	Sang
Blue cohosh	Caulophyllum thalictroides	Caul
Blue flag	Iris versicolor	Iris
Blue gum: Tasmanian	Eucalyptus globulus	Eucal
Blue vervain	Verbena hastata	Verbe-h
Bone nosode	Osteo nosodum	Osteo-N
Boneset. Thoroughwort	Eupatorium perfoliatum	Eup-per
Bovine TB nosode	Bacillinum Burnett	Bac
Brayera anthelmintica	Kousso	Kou
Brazilian carob tree	Jacaranda caroba	Jac-c
Brazilian snake root	Aristolochia clematitis	Arist-cl
Brazilian ucuba	Myristica sebifera	Myris
Bromide of potash	Kalium bromatum	Kali-br
Bromium	Bromium	Brom
Broom: Scotch	Sarothamnus scoparius	Saroth
Bryony: white	Bryonia alba	Bry
Buku	Diosma lincaris	Diosm
Burdock	Lappa arctium	Lappa
Buttercup: bulbous	Ranunculus bulbosus	Ran-b
Butyrophenol	Haloperidol	Halo
Cactus: night blooming	Cereus bonplandii	Cere-b
Cadmium	Cadmium metallicum	Cadm-m
Cadmium sulphate	Cadmium sulphuratum	Cadm-s
Cajput oil	Cajuputum	Caj
Calabar bean	Eserinum	Esin
Calcium sulphide	Hepar sulphuris calc H.	Hep
Californian coffee tree	Rhamnus californica	Rham-cal
Camphor	Camphora	Camph
Candytuft: bitter	Iberis amara	Iber
Carbamide	Urea pura	Urea
Carbonate of lime	Calcarea carbonica H.	Calc
Carbonate of lithium	Lithium carbonicum	Lith-c
Carbonate of magnesium	Magnesia carbonica	Mag-c
Carbonous oxide	Carboneum oxygenisatum	Carbn-o
Carcinosin: nosode	Carcinosinum Burnett	Carc
Carpinus betulus	Hornbeam tree	Carp-b
Cartilage: nosode	Cartilago articulus	Cart-a
Celandine: greater	Chelidonium majus	Chel
Chamomile: Roma	Anthemis nobilis	Anth
Charcoal: animal	Carbo animalis	Carb-an
Charcoal: wood	Carbo vegetabilis	Carb-v
Chaste tree	Vitex agnus castus	Agn
Chestnut: horse	Aesculus hippocastanum	Aesc

Chickpea	Lathyrus sativus cicera	Lath
Chinese sumach	Ailanthus glandulosa	Ail
Chloral hydrate	Chloralum hydratum	Chlol
Chlorine gas in water	Chlorum	Chlor
Chloroform	Chloroformium	Chlf
Chlorpromazine	Chlorpromazinum	Chlorpr
Cholesterol: nosode	Cholesterinum	Chol
Cinnamon	Cinnamomum ceylanicum	Cinnm
Clover: red	Trifolium pratense	Trif-p
Clover: sweet	Meliliotus officinalis	Meli
Coal tar: derivative of	Sulfonalum	Sulfon
Cobalt nitrate	Cobaltum nitricum	Cob-n
Coccle: Indian	Cocculus indicus	Cocc
Cochineal	Coccus cacti	Coc-c
Cockroach: Asian	Blatta orientalis	Blatta
Coffea arabica	Coffea cruda	Coff
Colibri flower	Hoitzia coccinea	Hoit
Colostrum: bovine	Colostrum bovis	Colos
Comfrey	Symphytum officinale	Symph
Common clarity, daisy	Bellis perennis	Bell-p
Common oat	Avena sativa	Aven
Condor plant	Cundurango	Cund
Cone flower, narrow leaved	Echinacea purpurea	Echi-p
Cone flower, purple	Echinacea angustifolia	Echi
Copper	Cuprum metallicum	Cupr
Copper: arsenite	Cuprum arsenicosum	Cupr-ars
Coral: red	Corallium rubrum	Cor-r
Corkwood elm	Duboisinum	Dub
Corn smut	Ustilago maydis	Ust
Cowhage. Dolichos	Mucuna pruriens	Dol
Cowberry	Vaccinum vitis idaea	Vacc-v
Cowslip	Caltha palustris	Calth
Cranberry: high	Viburnum opulus	Vib
Cranesbill: wild	Geranium maculatum	Ger
Crawfish	Astacus fluviatilis	Astac
Cromwell: false	Onosmodium virginia	Onos
Croton: purging	Croton tiglium	Crot-t
Cucumber: bitter	Citrullus colocynthis	Coloc
Cucumber: squirting	Elaterium officinarum	Elat
Cuttlefish	Sepia succus	Sep
Damiana	Turnera aphrodisiaca	Dam
Dandelion	Taraxicum officinale	Tarax
Darnel	Lolium temulentum	Lol
Deadly nightshade	Atropa belladonna	Bell
Dextrum lacticum acidum	Sarcolacticum acidum	Sarcol-ac
Devil's claw	Harpagophytum	Harp
Diesel oil	Diesel oil	Dies
Diphtheria: nosode	Diptherinum	Dipth
Divine plant of the Incas	Erythroxylum coca	Coca
DNA	Deoxyribonucleic acid	Dna
Dock: yellow	Rumex crispus	Rumx
Dog wood: round leaved	Cornus circinata	Corn
Dog rose	Rosa canina	Ros-ca
Dropwart: water	Oenanthe crocata	Oena
Duckweed	Lemna minor	Lem-m
Eel Serum	Serum anguillae	Ser-ang
Elder: black	Sambucus nigra	Samb
Epsom salts	Magnesia sulphurica	Mag-s
Equine allantoic deposit	Hippomanes	Hipp

25

Equine ergot	Castor equi	Cast-eq
Ergot	Secale cornutum	Sec
Ergot: alkaloid	Ergotinum	Ergot
Erythroxlon coca	Cocainum hydrochloricum	Cocain
Esponjilla	Luffa operculata	Luf-op
European astagalus	Astragalus excapus	Astra-e
European silver fir	Abies alba	Abies-a
Exogonium purga	Jalapa	Jal
Eyebright	Euphrasia officinalis	Euphr
Fever herb	Achyranthes calea	Achy
Figwort: knotted	Scrophularia nodosa	Scroph-n
Fish: purple	Murex purpureus	Murx
Flea: human	Pulex irritans	Pulx
Fleabane	Erigeron canadensis	Erig
Flint	Silicea terra	Sil
Flower: Passion	Passiflora incarnata	Passi
Flower: Passion	Pulsatilla vulgaris	Puls
Fluoride of lime	Calcarea fluorica nat	Calc-fl
Fly agaric. Toadstool	Agaricus muscarius	Agar
Fowler's solution	Kalium arsenicosum	Kali-ars
Foxglove, purple	Digitalis purpurea	Dig
Fringe tree	Chionanthus virginicum	Chion
Garlic	Allium sativum	All-s
Gila monster	Heloderma suspectum	Helo
Ginger	Zingiber officinale	Zing
Ginseng	Panax quinquefolia	Gins
Ginseng: Siberian	Eleutherococcus senticosus	Eleuth
Glanders disease: nosode	Hippozaeninum	Hippoz
Goa powder	Chrysarobinum	Chrysar
Gold	Aurum metallicum	Aur
Golden seal	Hydrastis canadensis	Hydr
Golondrina	Euphorbia polycarpa	Euph-po
Gonorrhea: nosode	Medorrhinum	Med
Gopher plant	Euphorbia lathyris	Euph-l
Grape vine	Vitis vinifera	Vitis-v
Grass: couch	Triticum repens	Tritic
Grass: goose	Galium aparine	Gali
Grass: star	Aletris farinosa	Alet
Grease: equine nosode	Malandrinum	Maland
Gunpowder: black	Gunpowder	Gunp
Hashish	Cannabis indica	Cann-i
Hawthorn. Mayflower	Crataegus oxyacantha	Crat
Hazelnut	Corylus avellana	Coryl-a
Hellebore, American	Veratrum viride	Verat-v
Hellebore, white	Veratrum album	Verat
Hemlock: water	Cicuta virosa	Cic
Hemp: American	Cannabis sativa	Cann-s
Henbane: black	Hyoscyamus niger	Hyos
Histamine	Histaminum muriaticum	Hist
Honeybee	Apis mellifica	Apis
Hornbeam	Carpinus betulus	Carp-b
Hornet, European	Vespa crabo	Vesp
Horsetail: rough	Equisetum hiemale	Equis
Housewort. Stavesacre	Delphinium staphysagria	Staph
Hydrocortisone	Cortisonum	Cortiso
Hydrophobinum	Lyssinum	Lyss
Hyssop: hedge	Gratiola officinalis	Grat
Ikshugandha	Tribulus terrestris	Trib

Indian hemp	Apocynum cannabinum	Apoc
Indigo: dye	Indigo tinctoria	Indg
Influenza nosode: human	Influenzinum	Infl
Insulin	Insulinum	Ins
Iodine	Iodum purum	Iod
Ipecacuanha	Cephaelis acuminata	Ip
Iron	Ferrum metallicum	Ferr
Iron arsenate	Ferrum arsenicosum	Ferr-ars
Iron phosphate	Ferrum phosphoricum	Ferr-p
Iron picrate	Ferrum picricum	Ferr-pic
Ivy: European	Hedera helix	Hed
Ivy: ground, Pipsissewa	Chimaphila umbellata	Chim
Ivy: poison	Rhus toxicodendron	Rhus-t
Jaborandi	Pilocarpus pennatifolius	Pilo
Jack in the Pulpit	Arum triphyllum	Arum-t
Jambol	Syzygium jambolanum	Syzyg
Jasmine: yellow	Gelsemium sempervirens	Gels
Jelly fish	Medusa	Medus
Jequirty	Abrus precatorius	Abr
Juniper	Juniperus communis	Juni-c
Kernal: acorn	Quercus e glandibus	Querc
Kombe seed	Strophanthus hispidus	Stroph-h
Kreosote BP 88	Cresolum	Kres
Laburnum	Cytisus laburnum	Cyt-l
Laurel: cherry	Prunus laurocerasus	Laur
Laurel: rose	Nerium odorum	Ner
Lava scoriae	Hekla lava	Hekla
Lead	Plumbum metallicum	Plb
Lead: black	Graphites	Graph
Leech: medicinal	Hirudo medicinalis	Hir
Leopard's bane	Arnica montana	Arn
Lignum vitae: resin	Guaiacum officinale	Guai
Lilly: Tiger	Lilium tigrinum	Lil-t
Lily of the valley	Convallaria majalis	Conv
Lobelia: purple	Lobelia purpurascens	Lob-p
Loco weed	Oxytropis lamberti	Oxyt
Lopophytum leandri	Flor de piedra	Flor-p
Lucerne	Alfalfa	Alf
Lungwort	Sticta pulmonaria	Stict
Maidenhair tree	Gingko biloba	Gink-b
Magnesium chloride	Magnesia muriatica	Mag-m
Magnesium fluoride	Magnesia fluorata	Mag-f
Magnesium phosphate	Magnesia phosphorica	Mag-p
Magnolia: Southern	Magnolia grandiflora	Magn-gr
Mahonia	Berberis aquifolium	Berb-a
Majeptil	Thioproperazinum	Thiop
Mandrake	Mandragora officinarum	Mand
Manganese acetate	Manganum aceticum	Mang
Mapato	Ratanhia peruviana	Rat
Marigold	Calendula officinalis	Calen
Marking nut	Anacardium orientale	Anac
Meadow saffron	Colchicum autumnale	Colch
Measles	Morbillinum	Morb
Meat: rotting meat	Pyrogenium	Pyrog
Mercuric chloride	Mercurius corrosivus	Merc-c
Mercury	Mercurius solubilis	Merc
Mescal button	Anhalonium lewinii	Anh
Milk: canine	Lac caninum	Lac-c
Mistletoe	Viscum album	Visc

27

Morphine: opium poppy	Morphinum	Morph
Moss: club	Lycopodium clavatum	Lyc
Mountain laurel	Kalmia latifolia	Kalm
Mountain pine	Pinus montana	Pin-mo
Mugwort	Artemisia vulgaris	Art-v
Mullein	Verbascum thapsus	Verb
Musk gland	Moschus	Mosch
Musk mallow	Abelmoschus	Abel
Mustard seed	Thiosinaminum	Thiosin
Nettle: indian	Acalyphya indica	Acal
Nettle: stinging	Urtica urens	Urt-u
Nightshade: black	Solanum nigrum	Sol-n
Nightshade: deadly	Atropa belladonna	Bell
Nitrate of sanguinarine	Sanguinarinum nitricum	Sang-n
Nitro glycerine	Glonoinum	Glon
Nozenan	Levomepromazine	Levo
Nut: betal	Areca catechu	Arec
Nutmeg	Nux moschata	Nux-m
Ohio buckeye	Aesculus glabra	Aesc-g
One berry	Paris quadrifolia	Par
Onion: red	Allium cepa	All-c
Osmium	Osmium metallicum	Osm
Ovarian extract	Ovininum	Ov
Ovarian follicle, ripe	Folliculinum	Foll
Pakur	Ficus religiosa	Fic
Palladium	Palladium metallicum	Pall
Pancreas	Pancreatinum	Pancr
Pansy	Viola tricolor	Viol-t
Parathormone	Parathyroid hormone	Parathyr
Parotid nosode	Parotidinum	Parot
Parsley: fools	Aethusa cynapium	Aeth
Penny royal	Hedeoma pulegoides	Hedeo
Pennywort: Indian	Hydrocotyl asiatica	Hydrc
Peony: tree	Paeonia officinalis	Paeon
Pepper: cayenne	Capsicum annuum	Caps
Perhexiline maleate	Perhexilin	Perh
Periwinkle: lesser	Vinca minor	Vinc
Peruvian balsam	Balsamum peruvianum	Bals-p
Peruvian bark	Cinchona succirubra	Chin
Petrol	Petroleum	Petr
Petroleum ether	Benzinum	Ben
Pheasant's eye	Adonis vernalis	Adon
Phenazone	Antipyrine	Antip
Phenylethylmalonurea	Phenobarbitalum	Phenob
Phosphate of lime	Calcarea phosphorica	Calc-p
Phosphorus	Phosphorus	Phos
Pinkroot	Spigelia anthelmia	Spig
Piper cubeba	Cubeba officinalis	Cub
Pituitary gland, posterior lobe	Hypophysis posterior	Pitu
Placenta: equine	Placenta equinus	Plac-e
Plant: pitcher	Nepenthe distillatoria	Nep
Plaster of Paris	Calcarea sulphurica	Calc-s
Platinum	Platinum metallicum	Plat
Poison hemlock	Conium maculatum	Con
Poison: arrow	Curare	Cur
Poison: arrow vine	Strophanthus sarmentosus	Stroph-s
Poison: elder	Rhus venenata	Rhus-v
Poison: nut	Nux vomica	Nux-v

Pokeroot	Phytolacca decandra	Phyt
Pomegranate	Granatum	Gran
Poppy: opium	Papaver somniferum	Op
Potash	Alumen	Alumn
Potassium bichromate	Kalium bichromicum	Kali-bi
Potassium carbonate	Kalium carbonicum	Kali-c
Potassium chlorate	Kalium chlorosum	Kali-chls
Potassium chloride	Kalium muriaticum	Kali-m
Potassium iodide	Kalium iodatum	Kali-i
Potassium phosphate	Kalium phosphoricum	Kali-p
Potassium sulphate	Kalium sulphuricum	Kali-s
Primrose	Primula obconica	Prim-o
Puffball: giant	Bovista lycoperdon	Bov
Pumpkin	Cucurbita pepo	Cuc-p
Quebracho	Aspidosperma quebracho	Queb
Queen of the meadow	Eupatorium purpureum	Eup-pur
Quinine: arsenite	Chininum arsenicosum	Chin-ar
Quinine: sulphite	Chininum sulphuricum	Chin-s
Radish: black	Raphanus sativus	Raph
Radium bromide	Radium	Rad
Ragwort: golden	Senecio aureus	Senec
Raison seed	Rajania subsamarata	Raj-s
Rattlesnake bean	Cedron	Cedr
Rauwolphia	Rauwolphia serpentina	Rauw
Rauwolphia: alkaloid	Reserpinum	Reser
Redwood tree: giant	Sequoia gigantea	Seq-g
Rhubarb	Rheum palmatum	Rheum
RNA	Ribonucleic acid	Rna
Rock rose: Canadian	Cistus canadensis	Cist
Rocket: Turkish	Bunias orientalis	Buni-o
Rod: golden	Solidago virgaurea	Solid
Root: colic	Liatris spicata	Liat
Root: Culver's	Leptandra virginica	Lept
Rose: Christmas	Helleborus niger	Hell
Rose-apple	Eugenia jambosa	Eug
Rue: common	Ruta graveolens	Ruta
Saffron	Crocus sativus	Croc
Sage	Salvia officinalis	Sage
Sanguinaria: Cuba	Paronychia illecebrum	Paro-i
Sausage tree	Kigelia africana	Kig
Savine	Sabina	Sabin
Saw palmetto	Sabal serrulatum	Sabal
Scabies mite: nosode	Psorinum	Psor
Scallop: American	Venus mercenaria	Ven-m
Scarlet pimpernel	Anagallis arvensis	Anag
Sceletium	Sceletium tortuosum	Scel-t
Scots Pine	Pinus sylvestris	Pin-s
Sea kelp	Fucus vesiculosus	Fuc
Selenium	Selenium	Sel
Seven barks	Hydrangea arborescens	Hydrang
Shepherd's purse	Thlaspi bursa pastoris	Thlas
Silico-fluoride of calcium	Lapis albus	Lap-a
Silkweed	Asclepias syriaca	Asc-c
Silver	Argentum metallicum	Arg-m
Silver nitrate	Argentum nitricum	Arg-n
Skullcap	Scutellaria lateriflora	Scut
Smallpox: nosode	Variolinum	Variol
Snake: bushmaster	Lachesis muta	Lach
Snake: cobra	Naja tripudians	Naja

Snake: copperhead	Cenchris contortrix	Cench
Snake: coral	Elaps corallinus	Elaps
Snake: rattlesnake	Crotalus horridus	Crot-h
Snake: sea Snake	Hydrophis cyanocinctus	Hydroph
Snake: viper, German	Vipera aspis	Vip-a
Snake: viper, yellow	Bothrops lanceolatus	Both
Snakehead	Chelone glabra	Chelo
Snakeroot: European	Asarum europaeum	Asar
Snakewort	Senega	Seneg
Snow rose	Rhododendron	Rhod
Sodium borate	Borax veneta	Bor
Sodium carbonate	Natrum carbonicum	Nat-c
Sodium chloride	Natrum muriaticum	Nat-m
Sodium chloroaurate	Aurum muriaticum nat	Aur-m-n
Sodium hypochlorite	Natrum hypochlorosum	Nat-hchls
Sodium phosphate	Natrum phosphoricum	Nat-p
Sodium sulphate	Natrum sulphuricum	Nat-s
Sodium thiopental	Thiopentonum	Thiopen
Soot	Fuligo ligni	Fuli
Sow bread	Cyclamen europaeum	Cycl
Spanish fly	Cantharis vesicatoria	Canth
Spider: black widow	Latrodectus mactans	Lat-m
Spider: orange spider	Theridion curassavicum	Ther
Spider: Papal cross	Aranea diadema	Aran
Spider: tarentula, Cuban	Tarentula cubensis	Tarent-c
Spider: tarentula, Spanish	Tarentula hispanica	Tarent
Spindle tree: Wahoo	Euonymus europaea	Euon
Sponge, roasted	Spongia tosta	Spong
Spruce: black	Abies nigra	Abies-n
Spruce: hemlock	Abies canadensis	Abies-c
Spruce: silver fir	Abies pectinata (alba)	Abies-a
Spur flower: pink	Plectranthus fruticosus	Plect
Spurge laurel	Daphne indica	Daph
Spurge olive	Daphne mezereum	Mez
St. John's Wort	Hypericum perforatum	Hyper
Star of Bethlehem	Ornithogalum umbellata	Orni
Starfish: red	Asterias rubens	Aster
Stoneroot	Collinsonia canadensis	Coll
Strawberry: wild	Fragaria vesca	Frag
Strontium	Strontium metallicum	Stront
Sucrose	Saccharum officinale	Sacch
Sulphur iodide	Sulphur iodatum	Sulph-i
Sulphur: sublimate	Sulphur lotum	Sulph
Sundew: round-leaved sundew	Drosera rotundifolia	Dros
Sunlight	Sol	Sol
Syphilinum: nosode	Syphilinum	Syph
Tamarisk	Tamarix gallica	Tama-g
TB: bovine, nosode	TB bovinum Kent	Tub
Tea: marsh	Ledum palustre	Led
Tea: New Jersey	Ceanothus americanus	Cean
Tellurium	Tellurium metallicum	Tell
Testes nosode	Orchitinum	Orchi
Testes nosode: canine	Orchitinum canis	Orchi-c
Testes nosode: equine	Orchitinum equus	Orchi-e
Thalamic nosode	Thalamus	Thala
Thallium acetate	Thallium aceticum	Thal
Thistle: St. Mary's	Silybum marianum	Card-m
Thorn apple. Stramonium	Datura stramonium	Stram

Thorn: black	Prunus spinosa	Prun
Thyme: cat	Teucrium marum verum	Teucr
Thyme-camphor	Thymolum	Thymol
Thyrallis glauca	Galphimia glauca	Galph
Thyroid: ovine, nosode	Thyroidinum	Thyr
Tin	Stannum metallicum	Stann
Tinctura acris sine kali	Causticum Hahnemanni	Caust
TNT	Trinitrotoluenum	Tnt
Toad: common	Bufo rana	Bufo
Tobacco: Indian	Lobelia inflata	Lob
Tobacco: nicotiana	Tabacum	Tab
Tuberculosis vaccine: bovine	BCG	Bcg
Turmeric	Curcuma longa	Curc
Turpentine	Terebinthiniae oleum	Tereb
Unicon root: false	Helonias dioica	Helon
Uranium nitrate	Uranium nitricum	Uran-n
Uterine fibroid	Epihysterinum	Epih
Vaccine: cowpox nosode	Vaccininum	Vac
Valerian	Valeriana officinalis	Valer
Vanadium metallicum	Vanadium metallicum	Vanad
Viburnum	Viburnum lantana	Vib-l
Violet: blue	Viola odorata	Viol-o
Virgin vine	Pareira brava	Pareir
Virgins bower	Clematis erecta	Clem
Wayfaring tree	Viburnum lantana	Vib-l
Walnut: GB	Juglans regia	Jug-r
Water: Quinton's sea	Aqua marina	Aq-mar
Water: Sanicula springs	Sanicula aqua	Sanic
Weed: bugle	Lycopus virginicus	Lycps
Weed, climbing hemp	Guaco	Gua
Weed: poison	Wyethia helenoides	Wye
White loco weed	Aragallus lamberti	Arag
Wild capuli	Karwinskia humboldtiana	Karw-h
Wild indigo	Baptisia tinctoria	Bapt
Wild yam	Dioscorea villosa	Dios
Wintergreen	Gaultheria procumbens	Gaul
Witch hazel: Virginian	Hamamelis virginiana	Ham
Wood spurge	Euphorbia resinifera	Euph-r
Wormwood: common	Artemisia absinthium	Absin
Wormwood: Levant	Artemisia maritima	Cina
Wormwood: Southern	Artemisia abrotanum	Abrot
X-ray	X-ray	X-ray
Yarrow, common. Millefolium.	Achillea millefolium	Mill
Yellow lady's slipper	Cypripedium pubescens	Cypr
Yohimbine	Corynanthe yohimbe	Yohim
Zinc	Zincum metallicum	Zinc
Zinc Valerianate	Zincum valerianicum	Zinc-val

REMEDIES: ABBREVIATION FIRST

Abel	Abelmoschus	Musk mallow
Abies-a	Abies pectinata (alba)	Fir: Silver spruce
Abies-c	Abies canadensis	Spruce: hemlock
Abies-n	Abies nigra	Spruce: black
Abr	Abrus precatorius	Jequirty
Abrot	Artemisia abrotanum	Wormwood: Southern
Absin	Artemisia absinthium	Wormwood: common
Acal	Acalyphya indica	Nettle: indian
Achy	Achyranthes calea	Fever herb
Acid-acet	Acidum aceticum	Acid: acetic, glacial
Acid-benz	Acidum benzoicum	Acid: benzoic
Acid-bor	Acidum boracicum	Acid: boracic
Acid-but	Acidum butyricum	Acid: butyric
Acid-carb	Acidum carbolicum	Acid: carbolic
Acid-fl	Acidum fluoricum	Acid: fluoric
Acid-hydr	Acidum hydrocyanic	Acid: prussic
Acid-nit	Acidum nitricum	Acid: nitric
Acid-oxal	Acidum oxalicum	Acid: oxalic
Acid-phos	Acidum phosphoricum	Acid: phosphoric
Acid-pic	Acidum picricum	Acid: picric
Acid-sul	Acidum sulphuricum	Acid: sulphuric
Acon	Aconitum napellus	Aconite. Monk's hood
Act-sp	Actea spicata	Baneberry
Adon	Adonis vernalis	Pheasant's eye
Aesc	Aesculus hippocastanum	Chestnut: horse
Aesc-g	Aesculus glabra	Ohio buckeye
Aeth	Aethusa cynapium	parsley: fools
Agar	Agaricus muscarius	Fly agaric. Toadstool
Agn	Vitex agnus castus	Tree: chaste
Ail	Ailanthus glandulosa	Chinese sumach
Alet	Aletris farinosa	Grass: star
Alf	Alfalfa	Lucerne
All-c	Allium cepa	Onion: red
Allox	Alloxanum	Alloxan
All-s	Allium sativum	Garlic
Aloe	Aloe	Aloe socotrina
Alum	Alumina	Alluminium oxide
Alumn	Alumen	Potash
Am-be	Ammonium benzoicum	Ammonium benzoate
Ambr	Ambra grisea	Ambergris. Sperm whale
Am-c	Ammonium carbonicum	Ammonium carbonate.
Am-caust	Ammonium causticum	Ammonium hydrate
Am-m	Ammonium muriaticum	Ammonium chloride
Anac	Anacardium orientale	Marking nut
Anag	Anagallis arvensis	Scarlet pimpernel
Ang	Cusparia febrifuga	Angustura vera
Anh	Anhalonium lewinii	Mescal button
Ant-c	Antimonium crudum	Black antimony
Anth	Anthemis nobilis	Chamomile: Roma
Anthr	Anthracinum	Anthrax: nosode
Antip	Antipyrine	Phenazone
Ant-t	Antimonium tartaricum	Antimony tartrate
Apis	Apis mellifica	Honeybee

Apoc	Apocynum cannabinum	Indian hemp
Apom	Apomorphinum hydrochlor	Apomorphine
Aq-mar	Aqua marina	Water: Quinton's sea
Arag	Aragallus lamberti	White locoweed
Aral	Aralia racemosa	American spikenhard
Aran	Aranea diadema	Spider: Papal cross
Arec	Areca catechu	Nut: betal
Arg-m	Argentum metallicum	Silver
Arg-n	Argentum nitricum	Silver nitrate
Arist-cl	Aristolochia clematitis	Brazilian snake root
Arn	Arnica montana	Leopard's bane
Ars	Arsenicum album	Arsenic, white
Ars-i	Arsenicum iodatum	Arsenious oxide
Art-v	Artemisia vulgaris	Mugwort
Arum-t	Arum triphyllum	Jack in the Pulpit
Asar	Asarum europaeum	Snakeroot: European
Asc-c	Asclepias syriaca	Silkweed
Astac	Astacus fluviatilis	Crawfish
Aster	Asterias rubens	Starfish: red
Astra-e	Astragalus excapus	European astagalus
Aur	Aurum metallicum	Gold
Aur-m-n	Aurum muriaticum nat	Sodium chloroaurate
Aven	Avena sativa	Common oat
Bac	Bacillinum Burnett	Bovine TB nosode
Ball	Ballota foetida	Black horehound
Bals-p	Balsamum peruvianum	Peruvian balsam
Bapt	Baptisia tinctoria	Wild indigo
Bar-c	Baryta carbonica	Barium carbonate
Bar-m	Baryta muriatica	Barium chloride
Bcg	BCG	TB vaccine: bovine
Bell	Atropa belladonna	Deadly nightshade
Bell-p	Bellis perennis	Common clarity, daisy
Ben	Benzinum	Petroleum ether
Berb	Berberis vulgaris	Barberry: common
Berb-a	Berberis aquifolium	Mahonia
Beryl	Beryllium metallicum	Beryllium
Bism	Bismuthum metallicum	Bismuth sub nitrate
Blatta	Blatta orientalis	Cockroach: Asian
Bor	Borax veneta	Sodium borate
Both	Bothrops lanceolatus	Snake: viper, yellow
Bov	Bovista lycoperdon	Puffball: giant
Brom	Bromium	Bromium
Bry	Bryonia alba	Bryony: white
Bufo	Bufo rana	Toad: common
Buni-o	Bunias orientalis	Rocket: Turkish
Cadm-m	Cadmium metallicum	Cadmium
Cadm-s	Cadmium sulphuratum	Cadmium sulphate
Caj	Cajuputum	Cajput oil
Calc	Calcarea carbonica H	Carbonate of lime
Calc-fl	Calcarea fluorica naturalis	Fluoride of lime
Calc-p	Calcarea phosphorica	Phosphate of lime
Calc-s	Calcarea sulphurica	Plaster of Paris
Calen	Calendula officinalis	Marigold
Calth	Caltha palustris	Cowslip
Camph	Camphora	Camphor
Cann-i	Cannabis indica	Hashish
Cann-s	Cannabis sativa	Hemp: American
Canth	Cantharis vesicatoria	Spanish fly
Caps	Capsicum annuum	Pepper: cayenne

Carb-an	Carbo animalis	Charcoal: animal
Carbn-o	Carboneum oxygenisatum	Carbonous oxide
Carbn-s	Carboneum sulphuratum	Bisulphide of carbon
Carb-v	Carbo vegetabilis	Charcoal: wood
Carc	Carcinosinum Burnett	Carcinosin: nosode
Card-m	Silybum marianum	Thistle: St. Mary's
Carp-b	Carpinus betulus	Hornbeam
Cart-a	Cartilago articulus	Cartilage: nosode
Cast-eq	Castor equi	Equine ergot
Caul	Caulophyllum thalictroides	Blue cohosh
Caust	Causticum H	Tinctura acris sine kali
Cean	Ceanothus americanus	Tea: New Jersey
Cedr	Cedron	Rattlesnake bean
Cench	Cenchris contortrix	Snake: copperhead
Cere-b	Cereus bonplandii	Cactus: night
Chel	Chelidonium majus	Celandine: greater
Chelo	Chelone glabra	Snakehead
Chim	Chimaphila umbellata	Ivy. Pipsissewa
Chin	Cinchona succirubra	Peruvian bark
Chin-ar	Chininum arsenicosum	Quinine: arsenite
Chin-s	Chininum sulphuricum	Quinine: sulphite
Chion	Chionanthus virginicum	Tree: fringe
Chlf	Chloroformium	Chloroform
Chlol	Chloralum hydratum	Chloral hydrate
Chlor	Chlorum	Chlorine gas in water
Chloram	Chloramphenicolum	Chloramphenicol
Chlorpr	Chlorpromazinum	Chlorpromazine
Chol	Cholesterinum	Cholesterol: nosode
Chrysar	Chrysarobinum	Goa powder
Cic	Cicuta virosa	Hemlock: water
Cimic	Cimicifuga racemosa	Actea racemosa
Cimx	Cimex lectularius	Acanthia lectularia
Cina	Artemisia maritima	Wormwood: Levant
Cinnm	Cinnamomum ceylanicum	Cinnamon
Cist	Cistus canadensis	Rock rose: Canadian
Clem	Clematis erecta	Virgins bower
Cob-n	Cobaltum nitricum	Cobalt nitrate
Coca	Erythroxylum coca	Divine plant of Incas
Cocain	Cocainum hydrochloricum	Erythroxlon coca
Cocc	Cocculus indicus	Coccle: Indian
Coc-c	Coccus cacti	Cochineal
Coff	Coffea cruda	Coffea arabica
Colch	Colchicum autumnale	Meadow saffron
Coll	Collinsonia canadensis	Stoneroot
Coloc	Citrullus colocynthis	Cucumber: bitter
Colos	Colostrum bovis	Colostrum: bovine
Con	Conium maculatum	Poison hemlock
Conv	Convallaria majalis	Lily of the valley
Cop	Copaiva	Balsalm: Peruvian
Corn	Cornus circinata	Dog wood
Cor-r	Corallium rubrum	Coral: red
Cortico	Corticotrophinum	ACTH
Cortiso	Cortisonum	Hydrocortisone
Coryl-a	Corylus avellana	Hazelnut
Crat	Crataegus oxyacantha	Hawthorn. Mayflower
Croc	Crocus sativus	Saffron
Crot-h	Crotalus horridus	Snake: rattlesnake
Crot-t	Croton tiglium	Croton: purging

Cub	Cubeba officinalis	Piper cubeba
Cuc-p	Cucurbita pepo	Pumpkin
Cund	Cundurango	Condor plant
Cupr	Cuprum metallicum	Copper
Cupr-ars	Cuprum arsenicosum	Copper: arsenite
Cur	Curare	Poison: arrow
Curc	Curcuma longa	Turmeric
Cycl	Cyclamen europaeum	Sow bread
Cypr	Cypripedium pubescens	Yellow lady's slipper
Cyt-l	Cytisus laburnum	Laburnum
Dam	Turnera aphrodisiaca	Damiana
Daph	Daphne indica	Spurge laurel
Dies	Diesel oil	Diesel oil
Dig	Digitalis purpurea	Foxglove, purple
Dios	Dioscorea villosa	Wild yam
Diosm	Diosma lincaris	Buku
Dipth	Diptherinum	Diphtheria: nosode
Dna	Deoxyribonucleic acid	DNA
Dol	Mucuna pruriens	Cowhage. Dolichos
Dros	Drosera rotundifolia	Sundew: round-leaved
Dub	Duboisinum	Corkwood elm
Dulc	Solanum dulcamara	Bittersweet
Echi	Echinacea angustifolia	Cone flower, purple
Echi-p	Echinacea purpurea	Cone flower, narrow
Elaps	Elaps corallinus	Snake: coral
Elat	Elaterium officinarum	Cucumber: squirting
Eleuth	Eleuterococcus senticosus	Ginseng: Siberian
Epih	Epihysterinum	Uterine fibroid
Equis	Equisetum hiemale	Horsetail: rough
Ergot	Ergotinum	Ergot: alkaloid
Erig	Erigeron canadensis	Fleabane
Esin	Eserinum	Calabar bean
Eucal	Eucalyptus globulus	Blue gum: Tasmanian
Eug	Eugenia jambosa	Rose-apple
Euon	Euonymus europaea	Spindle tree: Wahoo
Euph-l	Euphorbia lathyris	Gopher plant
*Euph-po	Euphorbia polycarpa	Golondrina
Euphr	Euphrasia officinalis	Eyebright
Euph-r	Euphorbia resinifera	Wood spurge
Eup-per	Eupatorium perfoliatum	Boneset.
Eup-pur	Eupatorium purpureum	Queen of the meadow
Ferr	Ferrum metallicum	Iron
Ferr-ars	Ferrum arsenicosum	Iron arsenate
Ferr-p	Ferrum phosphoricum	Iron phosphate
Ferr-pic	Ferrum picricum	Iron picrate
Fic	Ficus religiosa	Pakur
Flav	Flavus	*Neisseria flava*
Flor-p	Flor de piedra	Lopophytum leandri
Foll	Folliculinum	Ovarian follicle, ripe
Form-ac	Formicicum acidum	Acid: formic
Frag	Fragaria vesca	Strawberry: wild
Fuc	Fucus vesiculosus	Sea kelp
Fuli	Fuligo ligni	Soot
Gali	Galium aparine	Grass: goose
Galph	Galphimia glauca	Thyrallis glauca
Gaul	Gaultheria procumbens	Wintergreen
Gels	Gelsemium sempervirens	Jasmine: yellow
Ger	Geranium maculatum	Cranesbill: wild
Gink-b	Gingko biloba	Tree: maidenhair

Gins	Panax quinquefolia	Ginseng
Glon	Glonoinum	Nitro glycerine
Gran	Granatum	Pomegranate
Graph	Graphites	Lead: black
Grat	Gratiola officinalis	Hyssop: hedge
Gua	Guaco	Weed, climbing hemp
Guai	Guaiacum officinale	Lignum vitae: resin
Gunp	Gunpowder	Gunpowder: black
Halo	Haloperidol	Butyrophenol
Ham	Hamamelis virginiana	Witch hazel: Virginian
Harp	Harpagophytum procumbens	Devil's claw
Hed	Hedera helix	Ivy: European
Hedeo	Hedeoma pulegoides	Penny royal
Hekla	Hekla lava	Lava scoriae
Hell	Helleborus niger	Rose: Christmas
Helo	Heloderma suspectum	Gila monster
Helon	Helonias dioica	Unicon root: false
Hep	Hepar sulphuris calc H.	Calcium sulphide
Hipp	Hippomanes	Equine allantois
Hippoz	Hippozaeninum	Glanders disease: N
Hir	Hirudo medicinalis	Leech: medicinal
Hist	Histaminum muriaticum	Histamine
Hoit	Hoitzia coccinea	Colibri flower
Hydr	Hydrastis canadensis	Golden seal
Hydrang	Hydrangea arborescens	Seven barks
Hydrc	Hydrocotyl asiatica	Pennywort: Indian
Hydroph	Hydrophis cyanocinctus	Snake: sea Snake
Hyos	Hyoscyamus niger	Henbane: black
Hyper	Hypericum perforatum	St. John's Wort
Iber	Iberis amara	Candytuft: bitter
Ign	Ignatia amara	Bean: St Ignatia's
Indg	Indigo tinctoria	Indigo: dye
Infl	Influenzinum	Influenza nosode H
Ins	Insulinum	Insulin
Iod	Iodum purum	Iodine
Ip	Cephaelis acuminata	Ipecacuanha
Iris	Iris versicolor	Blue flag
Jac-c	Jacaranda caroba	Tree: carab tree
Jal	Jalapa	Exogonium purga
Jug-r	Juglans regia	Walnut: GB
Juni-c	Juniperus communis	Juniper
Kali-ars	Kalium arsenicosum	Fowler's solution
Kali-bi	Kalium bichromicum	Potassium bichromate
Kali-br	Kalium bromatum	Bromide of potash
Kali-c	Kalium carbonicum	Potassium carbonate
Kali-chls	Kalium chlorosum	Potassium chlorate
Kali-i	Kalium iodatum	Potassium iodide
Kali-m	Kalium muriaticum	Potassium chloride
Kali-p	Kalium phosphoricum	Potassium phosphate
Kali-s	Kalium sulphuricum	Potassium sulphate
Kalm	Kalmia latifolia	Mountain laurel
Karw-h	Karwinskia humboldtiana	Wild capuli
Kig	Kigelia africana	Tree: sausage
Kou	Kousso	Brayera anthelmintica
Kres	Cresolum	Kreosote BP 88
Lac-c	Lac caninum	Milk: canine
Lach	Lachesis muta	Snake: bushmaster
Lap-a	Lapis albus	Silico-fluoride of calc

Lappa	Lappa arctium	Burdock
Lath	Lathyrus sativus aut cicera	Chickpea
Lat-m	Latrodectus mactans	Spider: black widow
Laur	Prunus laurocerasus	Laurel: cherry
Led	Ledum palustre	Tea: marsh
Lem-m	Lemna minor	Duckweed
Lept	Leptandra virginica	Root: Culver's
Levo	Levomepromazine	Nozenan
Liat	Liatris spicata	Root: colic
Lil-t	Lilium tigrinum	Lilly: Tiger
Lith-c	Lithium carbonicum	Carbonate of lithium
Lob	Lobelia inflata	Tobacco: Indian
Lob-p	Lobelia purpurascens	Lobelia: purple
Lol	Lolium temulentum	Darnel
Luf-op	Luffa operculata	Esponjilla
Lyc	Lycopodium clavatum	Moss: club
Lycps	Lycopus virginicus	Weed: bugle
Lyss	Lyssinum	Hydrophobinum
Mag-c	Magnesia carbonica	Magnesium carbonate
Mag-f	Magnesia fluorata	Magnesium fluoride
Mag-m	Magnesia muriatica	Magnesium chloride
Magn-gr	Magnolia grandiflora	Magnolia: Southern
Mag-p	Magnesia phosphorica	Magnesium phosphate
Mag-s	Magnesia sulphurica	Epsom salts
Maland	Malandrinum	Grease: equine nosode
Manc	Mancinella	Apple: Manganeel
Mand	Mandragora officinarum	Mandrake
Mang	Manganum aceticum	Manganese acetate
Med	Medorrhinum	Gonorrhea: nosode
Medus	Medusa	Jelly fish
Meli	Meliliotus officinalis	Clover: sweet
Merc	Mercurius solubilis	Mercury
Merc-c	Mercurius corrosivus	Mercuric chloride
Mez	Daphne mezereum	Spurge olive
Mill	Achillea millefolium	Yarrow, common.
Morb	Morbillinum	Measles
Morph	Morphinum	Opium poppy
Mosch	Moschus	Musk gland
Murx	Murex purpureus	Fish: purple
Myric	Myrica cerifera	Bayberry
Myris	Myristica sebifera	Brazilian ucuba
Naja	Naja tripudians	Snake: cobra
Nat-c	Natrum carbonicum	Sodium carbonate
Nat-hchls	Natrum hypochlorosum	Sodium hypochlorite
Nat-m	Natrum muriaticum	Sodium chloride
Nat-p	Natrum phosphoricum	Sodium phosphate
Nat-s	Natrum sulphuricum	Sodium sulphate
Nep	Nepenthe distillatoria	Plant: pitcher
Ner	Nerium odorum	Laurel: rose
Nux-m	Nux moschata	Nutmeg
Nux-v	Nux vomica	Poison: nut
Oci	Ocimum canum	Alfavaca: Brazilian
Oena	Oenanthe crocata	Dropwart: water
Onos	Onosmodium virginianum	Cromwell: false
Op	Papaver somniferum	Poppy: opium
Orchi	Orchitinum	Testes nosode
Orchi-c	Orchitinum canis	Testes nosode: canine
Orchi-e	Orchitinum equus	Testes nosode: equine
Orni	Ornithogalum umbellatum	Star of Bethlehem

Osm	Osmium metallicum	Osmium
Osteo-N	Osteo nosodum	Bone nosode
Ov	Ovininum	Ovarian extract
Oxyt	Oxytropis lamberti	Loco weed
Paeon	Paeonia officinalis	Peony: tree
Pall	Palladium metallicum	Palladium
Pancr	Pancreatinum	Pancreas
Parathyr	Parathyroid hormone	Parathormone
Pareir	Pareira brava	Virgin vine
Par	Paris quadrifolia	One berry
Paro-i	Paronychia illecebrum	Sanguinaria: Cuba
Parot	Parotidinum	Parotid nosode
Passi	Passiflora incarnata	Flower: Passion
Penic	Penicillinum	Benzylpenicillin
Perh	Perhexilin	Perhexiline maleate
Petr	Petroleum	Petrol
Phenob	Phenobarbitalum	Phenylethylmalonurea
Phos	Phosphorus	Phosphorus
Phys	Physostigma venosum	Bean: calabar
Phyt	Phytolacca decandra	Pokeroot
Pilo	Pilocarpus pennatifolius	Jaborandi
Pin-mo	Pinus montana	Pine: mountain
Pin-s	Pinus sylvestris	Scots Pine
Pitu	Hypophysis posterior	Pituitary gland, Post
Plac-e	Placenta equinus	Placenta: equine
Plat	Platinum metallicum	Platinum
Plb	Plumbum metallicum	Lead
Plect	Plectranthus fruticosus	Spur flower: pink
Plect-b	Plectranthus barbatus	Spur flower
Podo	Podophyllum peltatum	Apple: May
Pop	Populus tremula	Aspen: American
Prim-o	Primula obconica	Primrose
Prot	Bacillis proteus	Bacterium nosode
Prun	Prunus spinosa	Thorn: black
Psor	Psorinum	Scabies mite: nosode
Ptel	Ptelea trifoliata	Ash: wafer
Puls	Pulsatilla vulgaris	Flower: Passion
Pulx	Pulex irritans	Flea: human
Pyrog	Pyrogenium	Meat: rotting meat
Queb	Aspidosperma quebracho	Quebracho
Querc	Quercus e glandibus	Kernal: acorn
Rad	Radium	Radium bromide
Raj-s	Rajania subsamarata	Raison seed
Ran-b	Ranunculus bulbosus	Buttercup: bulbous
Raph	Raphanus sativus	Radish: black
Rat	Ratanhia peruviana	Mapato
Rauw	Rauwolphia serpentina	Rauwolphia
Reser	Reserpinum	Rauwolphia: alkaloid
Rham-cal	Rhamnus californica	Tree: Californian Coff
Rheum	Rheum palmatum	Rhubarb
Rhod	Rhododendron chrysanth	Snow rose
Rhus-t	Rhus toxicodendron	Ivy: poison
Rhus-v	Rhus venenata	Poison: elder
Ribes-n	Ribes nigrum	Black currant
Rna	Ribonucleic acid	RNA
Rosa ca	Rosa canina	Rose: dog
Rumx	Rumex crispus	Dock: yellow
Ruta	Ruta graveolens	Rue: common

Sabad	Sabadilla officinalis	Asagraea cevadilla
Sabal	Sabal serrulatum	Saw palmetto
Sabin	Sabina	Savine
Sacch	Saccharum officinale	Sucrose
Sage	Salvia officinalis	Salvia
Sal-ac	Salicylicum acidum	Aspirin
Samb	Sambucus nigra	Elder: black
Sang	Sanguinaria canadensis	Blood root
Sang-n	Sanguinarinum nitricum	Nitrate of sanguinarine
Sanic	Sanicula aqua	Sanicula springs
Sarcol-ac	Sarcolacticum acidum	Dextrum lacticum acid
Saroth	Sarothamnus scoparius	Broom: Scotch
Scroph-n	Scrophularia nodosa	Figwort: knotted
Scel-t	Sceletium tortuosum	Sceletium
Scut	Scutellaria lateriflora	Skullcap
Sec	Secale cornutum	Ergot
Sel	Selenium	Selenium
Senec	Senecio aureus	Ragwort: golden
Seneg	Senega	Snakewort
Sep	Sepia succus	Cuttlefish
Seq-g	Sequoia gigantea	Giant redwood tree
Ser-ang	Serum anguillae	Eel Serum
Sil	Silicea terra	Flint
Sol	Sol	Sunlight
Solid	Solidago virgaurea	Rod: golden
Sol-n	Solanum nigrum	Nightshade: black
Spig	Spigelia anthelmia	Pinkroot
Spong	Spongia tosta	Sponge, roasted
Stann	Stannum metallicum	Tin
Staph	Delphinium staphysagria	Housewort. Stavesacre
Staphyloc	Staphylococcinum	Bacterium: staphylococci
Stict	Sticta pulmonaria	Lungwort
Stram	Datura stramonium	Thorn apple. Stramonium
Streptoc	Streptococcinum	Steptococcus
Stront	Strontium metallicum	Strontium
Stroph-h	Strophanthus hispidus	Kombe seed
Stroph-s	Strophanthus sarmentosus	Poison: arrow vine
Sulfa	Sulfanilamidum	Sulphanilamide
Sulfon	Sulfonalum	Coal tar: derivative of
Sulfonam	Sulfonamidum	Antibiotic: sulphonamide
Sulph	Sulphur lotum	Sulphur: sublimate
Sulph-i	Sulphur iodatum	Sulphur iodide
Symph	Symphytum officinale	Comfrey
Syph	Syphilinum	Syphilinum: nosode
Syzyg	Syzygium jambolanum	Jambol
Tab	Tabacum	Tobacco: nicotiana
Tama-g	Tamarix gallica	Tamarisk
Tarax	Taraxicum officinale	Dandelion
Tarent	Tarentula hispanica	Spider: tarentula, Sp
Tarent-c	Tarentula cubensis	Spider: tarentula, Cub
Tell	Tellurium metallicum	Tellurium
Tereb	Terebinthiniae oleum	Turpentine
Teucr	Teucrium marum verum	Thyme: cat
Thal	Thallium aceticum	Thallium acetate
Thala	Thalamus	Thalamic nosode
Ther	Theridion curassavicum	Spider: orange spider
Thiop	Thioproperazinum	Majeptil
Thiopen	Thiopentonum	Sodium thiopental
Thiosin	Thiosinaminum	Mustard seed

39

Thlas	Thlaspi bursa pastoris	Shepherd's purse
Thuj	Thuja occidentalis	Arbor vitae
Thymol	Thymolum	Thyme-camphor
Thyr	Thyroidinum	Thyroid: ovine, nosode
Tnt	Trinitrotoluenum	TNT
Trib	Tribulus terrestris	Ikshugandha
Trif-p	Trifolium pratense	Clover: red
Tril	Trillium pendulum	Beth root: white
Tritic	Triticum repens	Grass: couch
Tub	Tuberculinum bovinum Kent	TB: bovine, nosode
Uran-n	Uranium nitricum	Uranium nitrate
Urea	Urea pura	Carbamide
Urt-u	Urtica urens	Nettle: stinging
Ust	Ustilago maydis	Corn smut
Uva	Uva ursi	Bearberry
Vac	Vaccininum	Cowpox nosode
Vacc-v	Vaccinum vitis idaea	Cowberry
Valer	Valeriana officinalis	Valerian
Vanad	Vanadium metallicum	Vanadium metallicum
Variol	Variolinum	Smallpox: nosode
Ven-m	Venus mercenaria	Scallop: American
Verat	Veratrum album	Hellebore, white
Verat-v	Veratrum viride	Hellebore, American
Verb	Verbascum thapsus	Mullein
Verbe-h	Verbena hastata	Blue vervain
Vesp	Vespa crabo	Hornet, European
Vib	Viburnum opulus	Cranberry: high
Vib-l	Viburnum lantana	Wayfaring tree
Vib-p	Viburnum prunifolium	Black haw
Vinc	Vinca minor	Periwinkle: lesser
Viol-o	Viola odorata	Violet: blue
Viol-t	Viola tricolor	Pansy
Vip-a	Vipera aspis	Snake: viper, German
Visc	Viscum album	Mistletoe
Wye	Wyethia helenoides	Weed: poison
Xan	Xanthoxylum fraxineum	Ash: prickly
X-ray	X-ray	X-ray
Yohim	Corynanthe yohimbe	Yohimbine
Zinc	Zincum metallicum	Zinc
Zinc-val	Zincum valerianicum	Zinc Valerianate
Zing	Zingiber officinale	Ginger

MATERIA MEDICA

Abel
ABELMOSCHUS
Musk mallow Plant

Diseases of eye and salivary gland.
Insomniacs often sensitive to nocturnal biting insects.

HEAD	Glaucoma: Acute, chronic.
GASTROINTESTINAL	Ranula. Stomatitis.
SKIN	Pruritus after in sect bites.
MODALITIES	Agg: night.
POTENCY	6X – 12X. 30CH.

Abies-c
ABIES CANADENSIS
Hemlock spruce Plant

Mild mannered but irritable and restless when ill.
Digestive upsets with fatigue.

GASTROINTESTINAL	Appetite: voracious. Liver: weak liver. Vomiting. Tympanitic colic: overeating.
COMPARE	Acon Am-m Chin.
POTENCY	6X – 12X.

Abies-n
ABIES NIGRA
Black spruce Plant

Mild natured, but uneasy and restless from pain.

GASTROINTESTINAL	Anorexic: morning. Appetite: good in evenings. Halitosis. Colic: mild after eating. Constipation.
RESPIRATORY	Dyspnoea. Cough: laryngitis, severe.
MODALITY	Agg: lying down.
LAMENESS	Lumbar and sacroiliac: pain, stiff.
COMPARE	Bry Chin Cupr Kali-c Nux-v Puls Sabin.
POTENCY	6X – 12X.

Abies-p
ABIES PECTINATA (alba)
Silver spruce Plant

Role in bone maintenance and metabolism.

GASTROINTESTINAL	Prevention of dental disease.
LAMENESS	Arthritis. Calcium and phosphorus imbalance. Calcium: improves absorption. Encourages healthy skeletal growth in large breed dogs. Controls dysplasia, physis.
COMPARE	Calc Phos Pin-mo Thyr.

POTENCY	6X − 12X.

ABRUS PRECATORIUS
Jequirty Crabs eye Plant

HEAD	Conjunctivitis: purulent. Infection spreads to face, neck. Keratitis, pannus. Eyelids: granular, swollen.
SKIN	Epithelioma. Lupus. Ulcer.
POTENCY	6X − 12X.

ACALYPHA INDICA
Indian nettle Plant

Depression. Severe coughing.

GASTROINTESTINAL	Colic: tympanitic. Diarrhoea: blood, flatus. Forced expulsion of faeces.
RESPIRATORY	Cough: bloody, clots, dry, hard, persistent.
MODALITIES	Agg: mornings. Amel: afternoons.
COMPARE	Acid-acet Kali-i Mill Phos.
POTENCY	6X − 12X.

ACHILLEA MILLEFOLIUM
Common yarrow Plant

Polycrest. Arterial haemorrhage from **capillary** rupture. The arterial nature ensures blood is bright red. Vertigo.

HEAD	Epistaxis.
RESPIRATORY	EIPH: arterial.
UROGENITAL	Bloody urine. Postoperative haemorrhage control.
COMPETITION	**EIPH:** arterial: anxiety, painless.
MODALITIES	Agg: exercise.
COMPARE	Arn Fic Ger Ham Ip Sec. Combines well with Arn in control of traumatic haemorrhage.
CONSIDER	The management of arterial haemorrhage: <ul><li>Bladder surgery.</li><li>EIPH. Combine with Cinnm.</li><li>Rectal and peri-anal haemorrhage and surgery.</li></ul>
POTENCY	6X − 12X. 30CH.

ACHYRANTHES CALEA
Fever herb Plant

Acute, bacterial infections. Indifferent with irrational fears.

HEAD	Encephalitis: viral. Meningitis: lymphocytic. Blepharitis. Conjunctivitis: exudate: agglutinated,

	yellow. Dacryocystitis, keratitis, iritis. Eyelids: droopy, everted, hot.
	Otitis media: congested. Sinusitis: frontal, maxillary.
GASTROINTESTINAL	Gastroenteritis: anorexia. Faecal incontinence.
	Pancreatitis: acute.
CARDIOVASCULAR	Myocarditis, pericarditis.
RESPIRATORY	Cough: hoarse. Dyspnoeic: laryngitis, pleurisy, pneumonia.
UROGENITAL	Urine: clear, hot, red. Kidney: abscess, glomerulonephritis, pyelonephritis.
	Mastitis: acute. Metritis: pruritus.
	Male: impotence. Orchi-e (c).
SKIN	Lupus: acute, painful.
LAMENESS	Osteomyelitis.
JUVENILE	Neonatal: omphalophlebitis, osteomyelitis.
MODALITIES	Agg: cold. Damp. Movement.
	Amel: firm bandaging. Calm. Rest.
COMPARE	Acon Bry Echi Hep Pyr Rhus-t.
CONSIDER	Acute and secondary bacterial infections:
	• Pneumonia.
	• Salmonellosis.
POTENCY	12X. 30CH.

Acid-acet

ACIDUM ACETICUM

Acetic acid Mineral

Severe anaemia associated with oedema, weight loss and debility. Haemorrhage. Epithelial cancer. Fear of approach. Hysterical. Irritable.

HEAD	Pupil: dilated. Nose: exudate: bloody, mucous.
ABDOMEN	Ascites. Diabetes mellitus.
GASTROINTESTINAL	Cancer: lips, stomach. Marked salivation.
	PD: absents during fever. Vomit: after eating.
	Constipation: alternates with bloody diarrhoea.
	Colic: tympanitic.
CARDIOVASCULAR	Anaemia: helminthiasis, severe.
UROGENITAL	PU: glucose and phosphates.
	Mammae: enlarged. Milk: bluish, thin.
	Uterine haemorrhage: postpartum.
LAMENESS	Extremities: oedema. Lymphangitis. *Phleg leg*.
SKIN	Erythema.
COMPARE	Arn Ars Chin Dig Liat.
CONSIDER	An underutilised remedy particularly in:
	• Anaemia of parasitism – helminths.
	• Cancer of mouth.
	• Diabetes mellitus.
	• Haemorrhage.
	• Lymphangitis.
	• Mastitis.
POTENCY	6X. 30CH.

Acid-benz

43

ACIDUM BENZOICUM
Benzoic acid Mineral

Quiet and depressed, but can become excited, even hysterical.

HEAD	Incoordination with vertigo: fall to the side.
	Nasal bones, septum: painfully pruritic.
RESPIRATORY	Cough: asthmatic: hoarse.
UROGENITAL	Cystitis. FLUTD. Nephritis. Enuresis.
	Urine: brown, dribbles, offensive. Urates.
LAMENESS	Back pain referred from kidney.
	Achilles tendon: strain.
SKIN	Eczema: red, pruritic, spots.
MODALITY	Agg: air: open. Mornings. Pressure.
COMPARE	Acid-nit Sabin.
CONSIDER	• Urates in urine.
POTENCY	4X – 8X.

Acid-bor

ACIDUM BORACICUM
Boracic acid Mineral

HEAD	Conjunctivitis with photophobia.
	Cellulitis: exfoliation of skin over oedematous eyelids.
GASTROINTESTINAL	Diabetes mellitus. Pancreatitis: acute, chronic. PD.
	Tongue: cracked, dry. Saliva: cold.
UROGENITAL	PU: glycosuria Tenesmus: painful.
SKIN	Face, upper body, limbs: cellulitis: red, swollen.
COMPARE	Acid-benz.
CONSIDER	• Acute conjunctivitis.
	• Diabetes mellitus.
	• Orbital eczema.
	• Pancreatitis.
POTENCY	4X – 8X. 30CH for acute pancreatitis.

Acid-but

ACIDUM BUTYRICUM
Butyric acid Mineral

Chronic debilitating gastroenteritis with irrational fears.

GASTROINTESTINAL	Anorexia. Gingivitis. Stomatitis: salivation: offensive, profuse.
	Colic: tympanitic: ileocecal junction. IBD: chronic, copious. Diarrhoea: great tiredness.
UROGENITAL	Cervicitis: urine: smell of asparagus. Cystitis: urates.
LAMENESS	Spondylitis: lumbar, sacroiliac joints.
COMPARE	Bapt Nux-m Verat.
CONSIDER	• IBD and other chronic gastroenteritis.
POTENCY	12X. 30CH.

Acid-carb

ACIDUM CARBOLICUM
Carbolic acid Phenol Mineral

Nephritis and other painful conditions associated with great weakness.

Apathetic creatures with poor concentration. Easily excited and irritable.

GASTROINTESTINAL	Diabetes mellitus. Diphtheria. Colic: tympanitic. Enteritis: flatus. Ulcers: oral: exudate: offensive. Vomit.
UROGENITAL	Nephritis. PU: dark green, oily, glycosuria. Postpartum metritis: offensive.
LAMENESS	Stifle and distally: joint, muscle stiffness.
SKIN	Ulcers: pruritus.
COMPARE	Ars Carb-v Kres.
CONSIDER	• Debility. • Diabetes mellitus in geriatrics. • Nephritis.
POTENCY	12X. 30CH.

Acid-fl
ACIDUM FLUORICUM
Fluoric acid Mineral

Anxiety increases as animals excite themselves. After becoming energetic and lively, may slide back into an exhausted state. Indifferent to family, and this is unusual, strangers attract strangers.

Bear in mid destructive nature of lesions.

HEAD	Lachrymal duct: fistula. Nasal septum: ulcer, chronic drip. Dental fistula: bloody saliva. Jaw: osteoporosis, osteomalacia. Cartilage: bony growths. Otitis media: exudate: acrid.
GASTROINTESTINAL	Actinomycosis. Hepatitis: painful. PD. Throat: ulcers.
RESPIRATORY	Dyspnoea: pleural effusion, pulmonary oedema.
UROGENITAL	Nephritis: chronic, progressive. Urine: dark, initially scant, but PU as disease progresses. Nymphomania. Metritis: acrid.
LAMENESS	Osteomyelitis. Sequestrum. Postoperative support. Digits: osteoarthritis. Feet / nails: brittle, crumble.
MODALITIES	Agg: morning. Warmth. Amel: cold. Walking.
COMPARE	Calc-fl Calc-p Echi Hekla Sil Thiosin.
CONSIDER	Important: • Dental fistula. • Osteomalacia. • Nephritis.
POTENCY	12X. 30CH.

Acid-hydr
ACIDUM HYDROCYANIC
Prussic acid Mineral

Severe irrational fears lead to delirium. CNS and spinal neuritis.
Collapse during lung disease.

CNS	Catalepsy, narcolepsy, paralysis.
	Epilepsy: hysterical, jaws clenched tight. Salivation: great, foaming.
HEAD	Pupils: dilated, fixed. Neuralgia: supraorbital.
GASTROINTESTINAL	Tongue: cold, cyanosis. Gastritis: worse when stomach empty.
CARDIOVASCULAR	Arrhythmia. Pulse: palpitation, weak.
RESPIRATORY	Larynx: constricted, cough: dry, spasmodic, suffocating.
	Asthma: pulmonary congestion.
COMPARE	Ars Camph Cic Laur Oena Queb Verat.
CONSIDER	• Epileptic attacks with severe pulmonary congestion in a fearful, hysterical animal on point of collapse.
POTENCY	30CH. 200CH.

Acid-nit
ACIDUM NITRICUM
Aqua fortis Nitric acid Mineral

Polycrest. Difficult even dangerous personality. **Aggressive:** may be dangerous and will bite and kick. Oversensitive to jarring, noise, pain, touch and at their worst become headstrong, hysterical with rage and even hateful. This inherent, complex personality worsens during overt disease, and may be an indicator to a developing, yet undiagnosed, subclinical condition. Painful ulceration at any mucocutaneous junctions with offensive exudates that are painful. Slow to heal.

HEAD	**Corneal ulcer**. Epiphora: constant. Lachrymal fistula. Photophobia.
	Hearing: poor, yet noise sensitive.
	Nostrils: exudate: bloody, green, painful.
ABDOMEN	Hepatitis: painfully swollen.
GASTROINTESTINAL	Gums: bloody, salivation: slimy, soft, spongy.
	Halitosis. Jaundice. Tongue: clean, central furrow: red. Teeth: loose.
	Colic: acute, chronic, ulcers: duodenal, gastric.
	Constipation. Diarrhoea: offensive, slimy.
	Rectum: fissures: chronic, painful. Haemorrhage: arterial, profuse. Prolapse. Warts.
RESPIRATORY	Cough: dry, hacking, exudate: mucous.
UROGENITAL	Urine: bloody, cloudy, dark, offensive, scant. Albuminuria, haematuria, phosphaturia.
LAMENESS	Peripheral circulation, poor.
SKIN	Ulcers: mucocutaneous junctions: bleed, healing: poor, slow.
	Warts: bleed easily, irregular shape.
	Wounds: granulation: exuberant.
MODALITIES	Agg: evening and night. Chilly weather. Hot weather. Amel: travelling.
COMPARE	Ars Calc Hep Kali-c Kres Lac-c Lach Merc-c Sep Thuj.

CONSIDER	Of major importance:
	• Anal fissures.
	• Colic related to duodenal and gastric ulcers.
	• Dysentery.
	• Ulcers at mucocutaneous junction.
	Remember these typical signs:
	• Exudates are offensive.
	• Mentally difficult, dangerous.
	• Mucocutaneous junctions.
	• Pain.
POTENCY	12X. 30CH. 200CH.

Acid-oxal

ACIDUM OXALICUM

Sorrel acid Mineral

CNS	Spinal cord irritation: ataxia, confusion, vertigo.
HEAD	Photophobia without conjunctivitis.
GASTROINTESTINAL	PD: abdomen painful.
RESPIRATORY	Larynx: paralysis. LSLH.
UROGENITAL	Cystitis, urethritis. PU: oxalates.
	Spermatic cord, testes: painful.
LAMENESS	Spine: neuralgia, left, reflexes: diminished.
	Peripheral circulation: weak.
MODALITIES	Agg: pain. Touch. 3am.
COMPARE	Acid-pic Ars Arg-m Colch.
CONSIDER	• Ataxia.
	• LSLH.
POTENCY	12X. 30CH. 200CH.

Acid-phos

ACIDUM PHOSPHORICUM

Phosphoric acid Mineral

Polycrest. Consider in all conditions affecting debilitated juveniles, particularly where mental or physical abuse has led to physical weakness. Often fast growing overtaxed mentally and physically.

Challenging to train because of weakness and deficient memory. Can be calm, gentle individuals when well, but when pressurised, show complete lack of robustness, resulting in mental or physical complaints.

Apathy. Listless. Grief and shock cause marked deterioration.

HEAD	Eyelids: cold, pruritic, swollen. Pupils dilated.
	Noise intolerance. Nostrils: bloody, pruritic.
ABDOMEN	Diabetes mellitus: juveniles.
	Splenomegaly: enlarged, painful.
GASTROINTESTINAL	PD. Gums: bleed, retract from teeth.
	Lips: cracked, dry, mucous: frothy, viscid.
	Tongue: dry. Palate: ulcers. Colic: tympanitic.
	Diarrhoea: chronic, weak malnourished juveniles, flatus. Faeces: passed involuntary, painless, watery, white.

47

RESPIRATORY	Dyspnoea with arrhythmia. Cough: hoarse.
UROGENITAL	PU: milky, nocturnal, watery. Phosphaturia. Lactation: deficient.
	Prepuce, scrotum, testes: impotence, painfully swollen.
LAMENESS	**Ataxia. Back pain.** 'Kissing spines.'
	Bone: growing pains. Periostitis: shins and splints.
	Joints of carpus and fetlocks: deviation. Dysplasias and physis.
COMPETITION	**Will improve** function in 2-Y-0 horses with 'shins.'
	Useful for 2-y-o's that do quality sharp work yet fall apart when asked to work for longer periods.
	Straightens deviated limbs.
	Overtaxed mature horse, mentally or physical tired at the end of a tough season.
JUVENILE	Regulation of growth after a difficult start.
	Tonic for large, fast-growing juveniles. Helps large breed puppies and foals develop good limbs when suspicious of early joint problems.
GERIATRIC	Tonic for overworked, **aging** talented individuals.
SKIN	Weak hair falls easily. Interdigital cysts. Juveniles: adaptive mange: pimples on abdomen.
	Ulcers: offensive pus.
MODALITIES	Agg: consolation. Exercise.
	Amel: rest. Warm treatments include bandaging and soaking.
COMPARE	Acid-sarc Acid-pic Chin Nux-v Oena Phos.
CONSIDER	Enormous clinical application in juveniles:
	• Bone deformity and weakness.
	• Debility.
	• Exercise tonic.
	• Growing pains.
	Remember the characteristic tendency to easily tire, then recover after a short rest.
POTENCY	6X twice weekly as a preventative during the juvenile period. 30CH as a tonic and for treatment.

Acid-pic
ACIDUM PICRICUM
Sorrel acid mineral

Spinal disc degeneration leads to paralysis. Shock.
Anaemia from nephritis with exhaustion.

HEAD	Conjunctivitis. Exudates: chronic, copious, thick, yellow.
UROGENITAL	Cystitis, nephritis. Anuria, bloody, casts of epithelial cells. Chronic metritis.
	Oversexed males. Prostatomegaly.
LAMENESS	Paralysis: ascending and painful. Disc degeneration. Spondylitis.

MODALITIES	Agg: least exertion including mental. After sleep. Wet weather.
	Amel: chilly air and bandaging. Massage.
COMPARE	Acid oxal Arg-m C on Gels Phos Sil.
CONSIDER	Important:

- Back pain threatens paralysis.
- Disc degeneration.
- Nephritis both Acute, chronic.
- Prostatic hyperplasia.

| POTENCY | 6X – 12X. 30CH. 200CH. |

Acid-sul
ACIDUM SULPHURICUM
Sulphuric acid Mineral

Severe physical injury that results in necrosis, even gangrene.
Hurried, impatient individuals, which are easy to irritate when true rage is possible.
Massive, painful bruising in severely distressed individuals.
Complaints often left sided.

CNS	Cerebral oedema: head pressing, tremors, great weakness.
HEAD	Neuralgia: facial: right.
	May appear blind. Chemosis. Intraocular trauma with haemorrhage.
GASTROINTESTINAL	Gingivitis, stomatitis: bloody, grind teeth, vomit. Tympanitic colic.
	Diarrhoea: black, offensive. Tenesmus.
RESPIRATORY	Bronchitis: cough in juveniles: severe.
UROGENITAL	Painful cystitis. Metritis: acrid.
	Geriatric genital ulceration.
LAMENESS	Sacroiliac: left sided. Painful with jerking and trembling muscles. Severe muscle bruising: ecchymosis. Joint haemorrhage.
SKIN	Abscess: recurrent. Severest bruising, ecchymosis.
MODALITIES	Agg: excessive cold or warmth. Afternoon and evening.
	Amel: lying on affected side. Warmth.
COMPARE	Arn Bell-p Calen Calc Led Sep.
CONSIDER	Especially important:

- Brain injury.
- All chronic injury.
- Lead poisoning.
- Muscle and joint injuries with severe bruising.
- Purpura haemorrhagica.

| POTENCY | 12X. 30CH. 200CH. |

Acon
ACONITUM NAPELLUS
Monks hood Wolfs bane Plant

49

Polycrest. Has a special place in the management of **acute** conditions associated with anxiety, fever, restlessness, and severe pain. Severe and violent attacks possible but not as marked as with Bell.

Mental trauma: including prolonged anxiety and fear, when during attacks they show marked fears: crowds, thunder, touch, making them startle, *become extremely angry*. Often juveniles cannot cope with what people involved feel are reasonable situations, as pains become intolerable with extreme restlessness. Sudden in their development, often dramatic following exposure to extremes of dry, chilly weather, and sunstroke. The juvenile dog experiencing a fresh environment which, when overheated, tires, and then faces chilling from a sudden rainstorm. Marked vocalisation with persistent howling and whining.

CNS	Vertigo: worse on rising. Unconsciousness is possible.
HEAD	Jaw: left sided neuralgia: pain or numb.
	Conjunctivitis: dry, hot, inflamed, pruritic.
	Eyelids, ears: hard, red, swollen.
	Noise sensitive. **Rhinitis: sneezing:** blocked, dry, haemorrhage: arterial, mucous.
GASTROINTESTINAL	PD. Gingivitis, stomatitis: tongue dry, white, red, swollen. Tonsils: dry, swollen. **Peritonitis.**
	Vomiting: bloody, greenish, mucous. **Colic: tympanitic.**
	Diarrhoea: frequent, scant, splurges. Tenesmus.
CARDIOVASCULAR	Arteries: hard, prominent. Pulse: fast, hard, tense.
RESPIRATORY	**Laryngitis: cough:** harsh, short, after midnight. Worse palpating throat. Pneumonia: haemoptysis.
UROGENITAL	**Acute cystitis:** anxiety, restless, screaming pain. Urine: hot, red, scant.
	Female genitalia: dry, hot, painful, pruritic.
	Orchitis: painful, swollen.
LAMENESS	**Bursitis: muscles: pain,** swollen.
COMPETITION	Management of juveniles with near panic attacks. Often worsened by the emotional state of the trainer / rider.
JUVENILE	Important in acute, dramatic, painful conditions.
SKIN	Dry. Erythema, oedema.
MODALITIES	Agg: chill. Emotion. Overheating.
	Amel: open air. Rest.
COMPARE	Anth Bell Coff Ferr-p Phos.
CONSIDER	Invaluable in these situations:
	• Acute conditions.
	• Colic is tympanitic and very painful.
	• Fevers with thirst and restless.
	• Metabolic conditions.
	• Shock, particularly surgical.
	One of the great remedies.
	Remember its acute nature:
	• Anxiety.
	• Exposure.
	• Fear.

- Irritability.
- Shock.
- Thirst.

POTENCY	12X. 30CH. 200CH.

Act-sp
ACTEA SPICATA
Baneberry Plant

Fall asleep easily. When stimulated, are fearful of being alone, dark, examination, touch. Reluctant to move. Painful bursitis.

GASTROINTESTINAL	Epigastrium is painful. Salivation excessive. Vomit.
RESPIRATORY	Short, sharp breaths in chilly air.
UROGENITAL	Cystitis, sediment: chronic, white.
LAMENESS	Digits: bursitis, DJD, synovitis: mature athletes.
COMPETITION	Maintains performance in mature athletes. May help avoid surgery for joint spurs.
MODALITIES	Agg: flexion and palpation. Initial movement. Amel: regular, controlled exercise.
COMPARE	Bry Cimic Caul Led.
CONSIDER	Synovitis:

- Bog spavin.
- DJD.
- Jumper's bump.
- Thoroughpin.
- Windgall.

Often top athletes *feeling their joints* with maturity.

POTENCY	6X – 12X.

Adon
ADONIS VERNALIS
Pheasants eye Plant

Heart disease follows viral infection. Restless and sad.

HEAD	Vertigo on rising. Pupils dilated.
GASTROINTESTINAL	Ascites. Tongue: dirty, slimy, yellow.
CARDIOVASCULAR	Arrhythmia with a fast pulse. Endocarditis, myocarditis, pericarditis. Aortic and mitral valve regurgitation. Diuresis.
RESPIRATORY	Asthma and hydrothorax.
UROGENITAL	Scant urine, initially, then PU.
LAMENESS	Pain and stiffness of back. Peripheral oedema.
COMPETITION	Effective in maintaining function if treated early after viral infections.
COMPARE	Crat Con Dig Stroph-h.
CONSIDER	Heart disease:

- Athletes.
- Later when oedema develops.

POTENCY	2X – 12X.

Aesc-g

51

AESCULUS GLABRA
Ohio buckeye Plant

Lumbar and sacroiliac pain from spinal irritation. Ataxia and paresis.

HEAD	Eyes appear blind and fixed.
GASTROINTESTINAL	Vomit. Colic: tympanitic with constipation, severe.
	Perianal cancer: dark red.
CARDIOVASCULAR	Anaemia. Hypocalcaemia.
LAMENESS	Metabolic bone disorders. Back: muscle spasm, anywhere, causing spine to twist. Contracted tendons.
COMPARE	Aesc Aloe Coll Nux-v Phyt Sulph.
CONSIDER	• Hypocalcaemia.
	• Perianal tumour.
POTENCY	2X − 6X. 30CH.

Aesc

AESCULUS HIPPOCASTANUM
Horse chestnut Plant

Debility from weak circulation.

Depressed, irritable patients with poor concentration. Fear dark.

HEAD	Jaundice with excessive salivation, and a coated tongue.
GASTROINTESTINAL	Pharyngitis: exudate: mucous, ropy, sweet.
	Throat veins: distended, tortuous.
CARDIOVASCULAR	Pulse: full, irregular. Venous varicosity.
RESPIRATORY	Cough: morning, mucous. 2-y-o pharyngitis.
	The slight inspiratory noise may be difficult to detect but often proves a valuable, diagnostic pointer to the use of Aesc in early *Roaring* cases.
UROGENITAL	Urine: dark, hot, varies from scant to PU.
	Vaginal varicosities in older mares.
LAMENESS	Muscular pain and weakness anywhere along back.
	Bog spavin and hock strain.
	Laminitis, lymphadenitis, navicular disease, oedema, phleg-leg.
FEVER	Worse evening and night.
MODALITIES	Agg: defecating. After food. Movement: early morning and evening.
	Amel: cool, open air.
COMPARE	Aesc-g Aloe Coll Nux-v Phyt Sulph.
CONSIDER	Useful in:
	• Breeding mares: vaginal varicosities.
	• Geriatric tonic.
	• Lameness: hock and sacroiliac joints.
	• Liver disease: venous congestion.
	• Pharyngitis of racing 2-y-o.
POTENCY	2X − 12X.

Aeth

AETHUSA CYNAPIUM

Fools' parsley Plant

Acute conditions of the nervous and digestive systems. Broody, dull, irritable creatures. Love people and animals when well.

CNS	Chorea, head shaking. Anxious, restless. Vertigo: agg by movement.
HEAD	Eye: globe turned downwards. Ophthalmia: photophobia, pupil: dilated. Eyelids, meibomian glands swollen.
GASTROINTESTINAL	Oral lesions: dry, aphthous, pustular, regurgitate milk as curds. Toothache. Thirstless.
CARDIOVASCULAR	Palpitation: pulse: weak pulse. Lymphadenitis: neck and axilla.
RESPIRATORY	Dyspnoeic cough.
UROGENITAL	PU: sediment: red to white. Broody pseudopregnancy. Mammae: painfully engorged.
SKIN	Eruptions: bloody, cold, oedematous, periarticular.
JUVENILE	Dentition and suckling problems related to milk intolerance. Cold, unthrifty neonates.
FEVER	High with a cold, thirstless sweat.
MODALITIES	Agg: evening. Summer. Warmth. 3-4 am. Amel: open air. Company.
COMPARE	Ant-c Ars Calc Cic.
CONSIDER	• Pseudopregnancy. • Vomiting of curds.
POTENCY	4X – 12X. 30CH.

Agar
AGARICUS MUSCARIUS
Amanita muscaria Toadstool Fungus

Severest, acute, and reversible neurological disturbances.
Apprehensive, insecure, and irritable with great fear of touch.
Often marked by huge, dramatic mood swings as patients from complete indifference to fearsome rage.

CNS	Cerebral excitement with clonic spasms: jerk, twitch, tremble. Encephalitis, meningitis. Vertigo: head in constant motion. Epilepsy: marked twitching, fall backwards.
HEAD	Facial muscles: chorea. Corneal ulcer. Inner canthi inflamed, sticky and swollen.
GASTROINTESTINAL	Gums and tongue swollen with white, aphthous ulcers. Lips: tremble, twitch, snarl. Diarrhoea; flatulent.
CARDIOVASCULAR	Arrhythmia. Pulse weak, evenings.
RESPIRATORY	Cough: dyspnoea: exudate: mucous, thick.
UROGENITAL	PU with mucous.
SKIN	Eczema: angioneurotic, miliary eczema: eruptions: oedema, swollen.
MODALITIES	Agg: after food. Before thunder. Cold, open air. Mating. Amel: moving slow. Rest.

53

COMPARE	*Amanita spp* Bell Cimic Cann-i Hyos Tarent.
CONSIDER	Widespread effectiveness:
	• CCN, encephalosis, meningitis.
	• Canine distemper with chorea.
	• Muscle cramping and weakness.
	Most effective when patients show consistent muscle twitching.
POTENCY	4X – 12X. 30CH.

Ail

AILANTHUS GLANDULOSA

Chinese sumach Plant

Low grade fevers with skin and / or throat lesions, with haemorrhage. Confused, irritable and exhausted. Great vocal whining during sleep.

HEAD	Sclera congested with photophobia and dilated pupils.
	Nasal exudate: bloody, copious, thin.
	Thyroid: enlarged, painful.
GASTROINTESTINAL	Gums bleed easily. Tartar.
	Tongue: brown, cracked, dry.
	Tonsillitis: follicular. Dysentery: severe.
	Rectum: dark, oedematous, painful, red, swollen.
CARDIOVASCULAR	Lymph glands: swollen.
RESPIRATORY	Cough: dry, hacking, tiring.
	Guttural pouch mycosis: tympany.
UROGENITAL	Metritis after foetal loss: exudate: bloody, thin.
SKIN	Facial blisters, swellings: full of bloody serum, dissipate on pressure.
	Chronic miliary eczema may periodically flare into acute conditions characterised by a marked, livid, periodic rash.
FEVER	Bacterial including Strangles.
COMPARE	Am-c Arn Bapt Lach Rhus-v.
CONSIDER	Prescribe in:
	• Dysentery from infection; parvovirus.
	• Facial eczema.
	• Guttural pouch mycosis.
	• Metritis.
POTENCY	4X – 8X. 30CH.

Alet

ALETRIS FARINOSA

Star grass Plant

Poor concentration. Easily confused. Habitual foetal loss in cats.

GASTROINTESTINAL	Anorexic with frothy, profuse salivation.
	Vomiting during pregnancy.
	Colic: constipation, impactions, tympanitic: severe pain.
	Faeces: hard, large. Diarrhoea: scant, recurrent.
CARDIOVASCULAR	Severe anaemia in females.
UROGENITAL	Dysuria, incontinence. Phosphataemia with sediment.

BREEDING	Anaemic female cats with infertility problems, including failure to conceive and habitual foetal loss.
MODALITIES	Amel: lying down.
COMPARE	Chin Hell Hydr.
CONSIDER	A useful, female remedy: • Anaemia. • Colic in mares after foaling. • Conception failure: from chronic, low-grade metritis. • Habitual foetal loss
POTENCY	4X – 8X – 12X.

Alf

ALFALFA

Lucerne Plant

Dull, stupid, and sad. Irritable. Diabetes insipidus. Stimulates appetite and digestion.
Acute inflammatory conditions of upper respiratory tract and eyes.
Exudates vary from acrid to bland. Fear of pain. Restless.

HEAD	Conjunctivitis. Epiphora; **bland,** copious, watery. Photophobia. Nasal exudate: **acrid**, copious, watery. Sneezing: worse entering warm room. Nasal polyps.
GASTROINTESTINAL	Colic: tympanitic, noisy borborygmi, severe. Diarrhoea: flatus, offensive.
RESPIRATORY	Epiglottis, larynx: cough: hacking, hoarse, sensitive.
UROGENITAL	Cystitis: urine: red, tenesmus.
LAMENESS	Digits, elbows, joints, and associated muscles: painfully stiff. Neuralgia: painful following surgery or trauma.
MODALITIES	Agg: evening. Warm room. Amel: open air. Cold room.
COMPARE	Acon Euphr Gels Kali-i Ip.
CONSIDER	• Acute upper respiratory infection. • Feline herpes. • Neuritis.
POTENCY	4X – 12X.

All-c

ALLIUM CEPA

Onion Plant

Acrid nasal secretions with bland, watery tears. Borborygmi with offensive flatus. Tired.

HEAD	The nasal and eye secretions are marked with perfe of hay fever.
GASTROINTESTINAL	Offensive flatus with marked borborygmi and c Stomach colic.
RESPIRATORY	Hoarse, hacking cough agg by cold air.
UROGENITAL	PU. Irritation.
LAMENESS	Pain in small digits with tired limbs.
MODALITIES	Agg evenings and warm room. Amel open air and cold room.

COMPARE	Acon All-s Euph Gels Kali-hydr Ipecac.
POTENCY	4-6X.

All-s
ALLIUM SATIVUM
Garlic Plant

A stimulatory action on lining of bowel and respiratory system.

Escape: desire to. Fear being alone. Oversensitive. Restless. Sad.

HEAD	Epiphora with agglutinated eyelids.
GASTROINTESTINAL	Appetite: voracious.
	Tongue: pale with pronounced papillae.
	IBD from dietary changes associated with a changing picture including constipation and colitis. Diarrhoea: parasitism.
RESPIRATORY	Laryngitis, bronchitis. Bronchiolitis: chronic, purulent.
	Cough: constant if associated with harsh, tenacious, mucous.
UROGENITAL	Urine: deep brown sediment. Mammary pain.
LAMENESS	Lumbar muscles: painfully stiff.
COMPETITION	Expectorant: chronic.
	Typically the low grade, irritating lower airway disease which prevents two-year-olds performing to their best. May be absence of frank clinical signs until endoscopy reveals the exudate.
COMPARE	Ars Caps Seneg.
CONSIDER	• Bronchitis that is chronic and intractable.
	• Diarrhoea that is chronic.
	• IBD.
	• Intestinal parasitism; coccidiosis.
POTENCY	6X – 12X.

Allox
ALLOXANUM
Alloxan Mineral

Normally quiet, pleasant individuals. Uneasy and irritable when ill.

HEAD	Conjunctivitis. Otitis externa. Rhinitis. Exudates; often clear, dry.
GASTROINTESTINAL	Lips: cracked, dry in corners. PD. Painful swallowing: right side. Aerophagy.
	Diarrhoea: acrid, bloody, mornings.
RESPIRATORY	Laryngitis: chronic, right. Exudate: clear.
UROGENITAL	Dysuria: acrid. Female genitalia with pruritus.
LAMENESS	Spondylitis including 'kissing spines.'
SKIN	Cracked, dry with pruritic pimples.
MODALITIES	Agg: late afternoon. Noise.
	Amel: mornings. Movement.
COMPARE	Acid-phos Arg-n Uran-n.
CONSIDER	• Spondylitis including kissing spines.
POTENCY	8X. 30CH.

ALOE

Aloe socotrina **Plant**

Detox after drug treatment. Apprehensive, irritable individuals resent company. Fear of crowds, noise, and men. May initially be active then tire into apathy. Work intolerance.

HEAD	Nose: crusts: exudate: bloody.
GASTROINTESTINAL	Mouth: dry with PD. Throat, pharynx: congested, prominent veins. Exudate: mucous: lumpy, tough.
	IBD: colic before, after faeces. Diarrhoea: bloody, flatulent, hot, jelly-like, mucous.
	Constipated: faeces pass unnoticed, painless.
UROGENITAL	Incontinent. Urine: discoloured, scant.
LAMENESS	Lumbar: pain referred from kidney.
GERIAT	Incontinence.
MODALITIES	Agg: after drinking or eating. Early mornings. Warm, dry summers.
	Amel: open air. Flatulence.
COMPARE	All-s Kali-bi Lyc Sulph.
CONSIDER	Useful:
	• Debility.
	• Detox.
	• Geriatric tonic.
	• Immune modulation.
	• IBD.
POTENCY	2X – 4X – 12X.

ALUMEN

Potash alum Mineral

HEAD	Purulent otitis externa.
GASTROINTESTINAL	Tongue: hard, swollen. Vomiting.
	Throat: red, swollen. Tonsils: initially red and swollen, then indurate.
	Colic: chronic, severe constipation / impaction. Tenesmus.
CARDIOVASCULAR	Lymphadenitis: acute, chronic sequelae.
RESPIRATORY	Dyspnoea: haemorrhage: mucous, ropy, tenacious.
UROGENITAL	Mammary cancer: benign, hard, lumpy.
	Vagina: Aphthous patches.
	Metritis: exudate: acrid. Chronic uterine fibrosis.
LAMENESS	Severe generalised muscle weakness with ataxia.
SKIN	Alopecia. Ulcers have indurated edges.
MODALITIES	Agg by cold.
COMPARE	Acid-carb Caul Con Graph.
CONSIDER	• Actinobacillosis of the tongue.
	• Lymphoid tumours.
	• Mammary tumours.
POTENCY	12X. 30CH.

Alum

ALUMINA
Aluminium oxide Mineral

Severe weakness and debility in slow, quiet individuals.

CNS	Involuntary jerking of the head.
HEAD	Conjunctivitis: chronic: eyelids: dry, painful.
	Lachrymation: morning: excessive, thick.
	Otitis externa: crusts, dry in and around pinnae.
	Nasal exudate: acrid, copious. Nostrils: cracked, painful, red. Atrophic rhinitis: chronic: scabs: mucous, thick, yellow.
GASTROINTESTINAL	Mouth: mucous membranes, dry, painful. Chewing difficult. Bleeding gums. Tartar. DJD: jaw. Oesophagus contracted. Pica. PD.
	Colic: constipation / impacted, left. Juveniles, geriatrics. Even defecation of soft stools may be painful with rectal bleeding: tenesmus.
RESPIRATORY	COPD: cough: hoarse, morning: exudate: excessive, mucous, ropy, thick, yellowish.
UROGENITAL	Incontinent: retention with overflow. PU.
	Metritis: exudate: acrid, clear, ropy, thick.
	Prostatitis.
JUVENILE	Retention of meconium.
GERIATRIC	Confusion and advanced senility. Tendency to constipation and urinary incontinence.
SKIN	Inadequate quality dry and cracked skin and horn. Will scratch until they bleed, particularly when warm.
MODALITIES	Agg: periodically in afternoons and awakening. Warmth. Amel: alternate days. Chilly water. Damp, open air. Evenings.
COMPARE	Bry Con Kali-bi Lath Plb.
CONSIDER	An important remedy:
	• Constipation in juveniles and the elderly.
	• Debility of geriatrics.
	• Eczema.
	• Muscular weakness.
	Debilitated with thin, wrinkled skin.
POTENCY	12X. 30CH. 200CH.

Ambr
AMBRA GRISEA
Ambergris *Physeter macrocephalus* Sperm whale Animal

Geriatrics with PD and anxiety. Fear of approach, of crowds and public places. Restless sleep.

CNS	Hysterical epilepsy. Diabetes insipidus.
CARDIOVASCULAR	Debility of anaemia.
RESPIRATORY	Asthma: cough: hacking, spasmodic, severe.
	Choke due to excessively thick mucoid exudate.
UROGENITAL	Cystitis with PU. Urine: turbid: bloody, brown sediment.
	Genitalia: painfully pruritic swollen in female and male.
	Nymphomania. Oversexed.

LAMENESS	Peri-articular muscular cramping and weakness.
GERIATRIC	Anaemia with debility in anxious individuals.
	Ataxia and arthritis.
JUVENILE	Anaemia with debility in anxious individuals.
MODALITIES	Agg: music. Noise. Unusual events.
	Amel: lying down on the affected side. Slow walking.
COMPARE	Asaf Cast-eq Croc Lil-t.
CONSIDER	• Debility with anxiety.
POTENCY	30CH.

Am-be
AMMONIUM BENZOICUM
Ammonium benzoate Mineral

HEAD	Eyelids congested and swollen.
GASTROINTESTINAL	PD. Ranula. Chronic gastritis.
UROGENITAL	Nephritis: chronic, mild, right. PU. Incontinence. Albuminuria, urates.
LAMENESS	Lumbar pain referred from kidney.
GERIATRIC	Chronic nephritis with incontinence.
COMPARE	Other Ammonium salts. Acid-benz Berb Caust Canth Helon Kalm Merc Tereb.
CONSIDER	• Mild, chronic, geriatric nephritis with incontinence.
POTENCY	6X – 12X.

Am-c
AMMONIUM CARBONICUM
Sal volatile

Angry, cowardly, and disobedient, show excessive fear of dark, evening, thunder. Lazy with restless evenings. Sad during storms. Often targets respiratory mucous membranes in weak, overweight, females.

HEAD	Conjunctivitis, photophobia: eyelids: agglutinated. Deafness develops slow.
	Nasal exudate: bloody, mucous, watery. Sinusitis. Snorting, juvenile snuffles.
GASTROINTESTINAL	Diabetes mellitus. Appetite good yet eat little.
	Mouth: cracked corners, dry, painful. PD.
	Tongue: vesicles. Diphtheria.
	Colic: constipation, impaction colic. Faeces: hard, rectum: pruritic.
CARDIOVASCULAR	Circulation: weak. Palpitation. Lymphadenitis.
RESPIRATORY	Bronchitis, COPD, emphysema.
	Cough: hoarse, worse at 3am.
	Lung oedema: acute, severe.
UROGENITAL	Cystitis: urine: bloody, offensive, sandy, tenesmus, white. Nocturnal incontinence.
	Female genitalia swollen, pruritic. Metritis: acrid and watery.
	Penis: erect without desire. Scrotum, spermatic cord: painful, pruritic.

LAMENESS	Hock: periostitis. Muscles: cramp. Painfully weak.
GERIATRIC	Debility. Diabetes mellitus. Urinary incontinence.
SKIN	Pruritic blisters on extremities, folds, and joints. Fever with rash of tiny red spots.
COMPETITION	Effective in lazy, breathless females.
LATERALITY	Right.
COMPARE	*Ammonium phosphoricum* Am-phos. Facial paralysis. Lach Rhus-v.
	Important:
	• African Horse Sickness and Fog Fever.
	• Cystitis that is chronic and severe.
	• Respiratory problems that are chronic.
	• Pulmonary oedema that is acute or chronic.
CONSIDER	Often elderly, overweight females.
POTENCY	8X – 12X. 30CH.

Am-caust
AMMONIUM CAUSTICUM
Ammonium hydrate Mineral

Heart disease in restless, timid individuals startle easily.

HEAD	Diphtheria: nasal mucosa.
GASTROINTESTINAL	Colic: tympanitic, severe pain.
RESPIRATORY	Cough: choking laryngeal spasm: exudation: excessively thick, mucous.
LAMENESS	Great muscular debility particularly of shoulders.
COMPARE	Ammonium salts.
CONSIDER	• Chronic rhinitis with heart strain.
	• Tympanitic colic.
POTENCY	6X – 12X.

Am-m
AMMONIUM MURIATICUM
Ammonium chloride Mineral

Sad, they lack confidence with consequent apprehension with fear of crowds, the dark and people. Marked mucolytic effect in lethargic, obese individuals.

CNS	Epilepsy where delirium follows fits.
HEAD	Cataracts. Rhinitis: exudate: acrid, bloody, hot, profuse, watery. Ulcers.
GASTROINTESTINAL	Liver, hepatitis, swollen. Jaundice. Tonsillitis. Throat, oesophagus congested and in spasm from thick mucoid exudate. Stomach: cancer: vomiting.
	Colic: impacted after food. Constipation: crumbling, hard, mucous, faeces. May alternate with greenish, painful, diarrhoea.
RESPIRATORY	Laryngeal cough after exercise with bloody or clear, free flowing mucous. EIPH with anxiety.
UROGENITAL	Metritis: albumin-like exudate.
LAMENESS	Lumbar pain extends to contracted hamstrings. Painful digits. Neuralgia: post injury, surgery.
SKIN	Inferior quality: blisters, dry, hair loss, pruritic.

COMPETITION	Mucolytic for horses with low grade EIPH.
MODALITIES	Agg: afternoon colic.
	Amel: eating. Open air.
COMPARE	Other Ammonium salts. Calc Caust Seneg.
	Combines well with Cinnm and Mill for EIPH.
CONSIDER	Excellent in respiratory diseases:
	• COPD.
	• EIPH.
	• Feline respiratory viruses.
	Fat, lethargic individuals often with athletic ability.
POTENCY	6X – 12X. 30CH.

Anac
ANACARDIUM ORIENTALE
Marking nut Plant

Behavioural modification in **difficult individuals** who lack confidence. Easily offended, they express fear of approach and people. When suspicious, may be oversensitive, malicious, and dangerous.

CNS	Senile dementia.
HEAD	Progressive deafness and loss of smell.
GASTROINTESTINAL	Stomatitis: offensive, painful.
	Oesophagus: choke when eating and drinking. Gastritis: vomiting.
	Constipation improves after eating. Rectal sphincter: spasmodic, painful contractions. Faeces: soft, pass with difficulty.
CARDIOVASCULAR	Palpitation. Pericarditis.
RESPIRATORY	Cough: after eating. Vomiting: worse when excited.
UROGENITAL	Pruritus of genitalia.
LAMENESS	Muscle cramping, contracted joints: stiff.
SKIN	Eruptions: acute, extensive. Urticarial blisters. Digital warts.
COMPETITION	May help difficult, nervous, and talented horses to work well if overwork has made them tired and angry.
MODALITIES	Agg: coughing. Hours after food. Hot water. Noise.
	Amel: after eating. Grooming. Lying on affected side.
COMPARE	*Anacardium orientale* Anac-oc: cashew nut. Significant effect on facial eczema and poor-quality hooves.
CONSIDER	• Behavioural modification
	• Eczema.
	Temperament must fit.
POTENCY	30CH. 200CH.

Anag
ANAGALLIS ARVENSIS
Scarlet pimpernel Plant

Happy excitable individuals with eczema.

| UROGENITAL | Urethritis: sticky, painful blockage. |
| LAMENESS | Digits, shoulder: pain, swelling. |

SKIN	May expel foreign bodies. Eczema: lesions: bran-like, pruritic, scaly. Vesicles followed by ulcers. Geriatric, sessile warts.
COMPARE	Cycl Prim-o Sil.
CONSIDER	• Widespread, severely pruritic eczema.
POTENCY	6X – 12X. 30CH.

Anh

ANHALONIUM LEWINII
Mescal button cactus Plant

Sad individuals prone to mood swings with hysteria possible. Thyroiditis.

GASTROINTESTINAL	IBD: gastritis: painful, spasmodic attacks.
RESPIRATORY	Asthma: cough: spasmodic.
UROGENITAL	Female sexuality changes. Frigidity. Nymphomania. Impotent males.
MODALITIES	Agg: light. Sun.
	Amel: dark. Rest.
COMPARE	Agar.
CONSIDER	• Thyroiditis in anxious individuals with behavioural changes.
POTENCY	6X – 12X. 30CH.

Anth

ANTHEMIS NOBILIS
Roman chamomile Matricaria chamomile **Plant**

Polycrest. The mental and emotional signs are of paramount importance.

Attention: desire for yet may also be averse to company. Typical spoiled lapdog who wishes carried, but soon becomes impatient, irritable. Oversensitive and restless, when even small problems may appear unbearable, leading to mood swings with snapping. Cannot cope with pain. Significant antibacterial effect.

HEAD	Conjunctivitis. Photophobia. Jaundice.
	Swollen eyelids often associated with excessive anxiety and distress offer useful pointers.
ABDOMEN	Hepatitis: painfully swollen.
GASTROINTESTINAL	PD. Halitosis. Hypersalivation. Teething: painful.
	Tongue twitches. Vomit bile. Colic: tympanitic after emotional upsets. Diarrhoea during dentition: green, hot, offensive, slimy, watery. Proctitis.
CARDIOVASCULAR	Lymphadenitis: parotid, sub maxillary glands.
RESPIRATORY	Dyspnoea: bronchitis, laryngitis.
	Cough: hoarse, raw.
UROGENITAL	Metritis: exudate: acrid, yellow milk. Haemorrhage: clotted, dark, profuse. Mammae and teats; juveniles painfully swollen.
BREEDING	Parturition: agitated, impatient, poor mothering. Can be difficult, dangerous to examine.
LAMENESS	Back, larger joints. Painful stiffness.
COMPETITION	Assists excitable, juvenile working animals to concentrate and work better without tranquillisation.
SLEEP	**Anxious,** fearful, vocal.

MODALITIES	Agg: anger. Heat. Night. Nursing. Open air. Parturition. Wind.
	Amel, when carried. Pampered. Warm, wet weather.
COMPARE	*Matricaria recutita* Cham. German chamomile similar, but less effective. Acon Bell Coff Ign Mag-c Puls Staph.
CONSIDER	A useful remedy:

- Acute diarrhoea and digestive upsets.
- Acute respiratory conditions with watery coryza.
- Behaviour seriously deteriorates with pain.

Conditions that respond have the classic mental attitude.

| POTENCY | 8X – 12X. 30CH. 200CH. |

Anthr

ANTHRACINUM

Anthrax nosode Animal

CARDIOVASCULAR	Severe bacterial infections: lymphangitis, septicaemia.
SKIN	Infection following insect and tick bites.
	Lesions are oedematous with a hard, black, necrotic centre, rim. Typified by the toxic bite of some ticks including *Amblyomma hebraeum*; the Bont tick. Often a nuisance for people walking in the African savanna.
COMPARE	Ars Crot Echi Hipp Lach Sil Tarent-c.
CONSIDER	Use:

- Bacterial infections.
- Lymphangitis.
- Sepsis.
- Tick bite necrosis, particularly *Amblyomma spp* Bont tick.

| POTENCY | 30CH. |

Ant-c

ANTIMONIUM CRUDUM

Black sulphide of antimony Mineral

When prescribed according to mental and gastrointestinal signs a powerful remedy.

Excessive irritability and **lack of expected** pain are important indicators.

These animals may prove difficult to examine owing to marked irritability and dislike of touch when they become aggressive and will bite and kick.

Training problems.

Overweight. Vertigo.

HEAD	Facial eczema: eruptions: boil-like, crusty, pustular, yellow.
	Conjunctivitis: blepharitis. Eyelids: agglutinated, cracked, fissured, raw in corners. Cornea: pustules.
	Eyes: dull, sunken.
	Otitis externa: moist, offensive.
	Nostrils: cracked and crusted.
GASTROINTESTINAL	Anorexia with PD. Ill from overeating.

63

	Mouth, lips dry, cracked, eructation, slimy, unpleasant mucous.
	Gums: bleed, detach from teeth. Tongue and palate: raw or thick white coat.
	Vomit curds and milk after nursing. Colic: tympanitic after food. Flatulent.
	Diarrhoea alternates with constipation. Faeces: hard lumps mixed mucous and water.
RESPIRATORY	Laryngitis: loss of voice. Cough: harsh entering a warm room. Expectorate: mucous: thick, yellow.
UROGENITAL	Nephritis: chronic. PU: turbid, offensive.
	Female genitalia; pruritic. Metritis: exudate: acrid, lumpy, watery.
	Male impotence. Eruptions on genitalia.
LAMENESS	Back and muscle problems with twitching front legs. Arthritis of digits and hock. Feet: brittle, cracked.
SKIN	Inferior quality: worse during digestive upsets.
	Pimples and pustules: begin dry, hard scales and scabs, then develop into honey-coloured vesicles.
	Horny warts on extremities.
MODALITIES	Agg: acids, heat, washing, water.
	Amel: Moist, warm weather. Open air. Rest.
COMPARE	Aeth Ant-t Graph Puls Ip Sulph.
CONSIDER	Important:

Important:
- Eczema from food sensitivity.
- Gastric dilatation.
- Gastritis from food sensitivity.
- Hoof quality poor.
- IBD.
- Nephritis.
- Warts at extremities.

The characteristic mental picture is important.

POTENCY	8X. 30CH. 200CH.

Ant-t

ANTIMONIUM TARTARICUM
Antimony tartrate Mineral

Polycrest. Apathy. Company: averse to, and fearing examination, may scream. As disease worsens, may show death-like faintness, prostration, and great sleepiness. Exudative respiratory disease with drowsiness, debility, and sweating, and notable trembling weakness.

CNS	Prostration, even unconsciousness with asphyxia.
HEAD	Face: cold, incessant quivering: chin, lower jaw.
GASTROINTESTINAL	PD, but **frequent sipping** of chilly water. Tongue: thick, white coating with red edges.
	Vomiting: after food.
	Colic: tympanitic.
	Diarrhoea: flatulent, watery.
CARDIOVASCULAR	Pulse: rapid, weak.
RESPIRATORY	COPD. Dyspnoea. Emphysema, Oedema. Rales marked,

	but only slight, thick mucoid exudate. Voice: hoarse.
UROGENITAL	**Cystitis:** last drops of urine bloody. Pain during and after urination. Orchitis. Warts on genitalia.
LAMENESS	Painful sacroiliac muscles twitch.
GERIATRIC	COPD, emphysema. Expectorate: mucous, thick.
SKIN	**Eruptions:** pustules: bluish red mark after healing. Sarcoid and genital warts. Often horny on digits.
MODALITIES	Agg: evening. Cold. Damp weather. Amel: covering. Lying down. Night.
COMPARE	Kali-s Ip.
CONSIDER	A remedy of foremost importance in: <ul><li>Pneumonia with oedema.</li><li>African Horse Sickness.</li><li>Fog Fever.</li><li>Sarcoid and warts on genitalia and extremities.</li></ul>
POTENCY	4X – 12X for sarcoid and warts. 30CH. 200CH during exudation.

Antip

ANTIPYRINE

Phenazone Mineral

Anxious, fearful individuals with angioneurotic oedema.

CNS	Epilepsy with severely contracted muscles and prostration.
HEAD	Facial oedema: eyelids. Conjunctivitis, chemosis. Rhinitis and sinusitis: mucosal oedema.
GASTROINTESTINAL	Tongue and throat: abscess, diphtheria, ulcers. Vomiting.
RESPIRATORY	Dyspnoea: pulmonary oedema.
UROGENITAL	Anuria. Penis; patchy discoloration.
SKIN	Pruritic angioneurotic oedema, pemphigus. Intermittent urticaria
COMPARE	Apis.
CONSIDER	• Urticaria with oedema.
POTENCY	6X – 12X. 30CH.

Apis

APIS MELLIFICA

Honeybee Animal

Polycrest. Fascinating remedy for variable signs including apathy and destructive tendency when ill. Great fears: alone, touch. Indifferent. Irritable. Jealous. Restless whining.

Acute oedema: of direct use even when mental picture is absent. Thus, always prescribe for acute oedematous attacks. Conditions are typically, red, or with a rosy hue and stinging pains. Intolerance of heat, of the slightest touch. Afternoon aggravation.

The oedema found in patients with vaccination reactions often demonstrate a swift response. Although Apis may always be considered, it is particularly effective when dealing with right sided conditions.

Significant antibacterial agent.

CNS	Meningitis. Unconscious. Vertigo with sneezing.
HEAD	**Conjunctivitis**: acute. Chemosis: chronic, severe, keratitis. Staphyloma: infection. Epiphora profuse. Eyelids: bright red, everted, oedematous. Facial oedema: painful, spreads from right to left. Throat: fiery red, swollen.
ABDOMEN	Ascites: painful.
GASTROINTESTINAL	Gums, lips, throat, tongue: fiery red, puffy, swollen, ulcerated. Mucosae: raw, swollen, vesicles. Ranula. Throat: constricted, swallowing difficult. Swellings may be palpable externally. Uvula: swollen, sac-like.
	Neonatal diarrhoea is watery, yellow.
	Constipation painful. Faeces: bloody, painless and may be passed involuntary on every movement as though anus fixed in a wide-open position.
CARDIOVASCULAR	Pulse: fast, feeble.
RESPIRATORY	Dyspnoea. Painful pleural oedema.
	Laryngitis: cough: dry, hoarse, painful oedema.
UROGENITAL	Nephritis, cystitis: acutely painful. Incontinent. Urine dark and scant.
	Female: genitalia: oedematous, relieved by cold application. Nymphomania. Ovaritis, right.
	Prolapse and vaginal oedema especially in Boxer-types.
LAMENESS	Referred lumbar pain. Synovitis: acute, hot, oedematous, painful. Feet: hot, oedematous, painfully stiff.
FEVER	Throat signs are the main factors. Thirstless.
SKIN	**Insect** and tick bites, stings: acute, oedematous, and painful. Dramatic urticaria, generalised, local.
MODALITIES	Agg: afternoon. From bandaging. Heat. Touch.
	Amel: open air. Cold therapy. Uncovering.
COMPARE	Anthr Ars Bar-c Canth Lach Led Nat-m. Streptoc (for chronic oedema). Vesp Zinc.
CONSIDER	The typical mental picture important in acute cases.
	• Conjunctivitis, chemosis, 'cherry eye.'
	• Cystitis, nephritis.
	• Insect bites and stings.
	• Ovarian pain.
POTENCY	6X will move even great oedema.
	Pain 30CH. 200CH.

Apoc

APOCYNUM CANNABINUM
Indian hemp Plant

Oedema including ascites and hydrothorax. Confused, restless individuals.

CNS	Diabetes insipidus and meningitis.
HEAD	Conjunctivitis: epiphora.
	Nasal blockages: exudate: mucous, thick, yellow.

GASTROINTESTINAL	PD: excessive mucous salivation. Vomit: painful after food, drink.
	Diarrhoea: drips from rectum, flatulent, painful.
CARDIOVASCULAR	Arrhythmia: bradycardia, cyanosis, low BP. Incompetent mitral and tricuspid valves. Jugular pulse.
RESPIRATORY	Cough: pleural effusion.
UROGENITAL	PU: bladder distended, urine: thin.
LAMENESS	Oedema.
MODALITIES	Agg: chilly weather.
	Amel: bandaging and wrapping.
COMPARE	Apis Ars Dig Hell Stroph-h.
CONSIDER	• Diabetes mellitus and heart failure.
POTENCY	2X – 6X.

Apom
APOMORPHINUM HYDROCHLORICUM
Apomorphine Mineral

Vomiting of travel sickness preceded by lethargy and restlessness. Vertigo.

HEAD	Pupils dilated.
GASTROINTESTINAL	Severe vomiting.
COMPARE	Ip Nux-v Phos Puls.
CONSIDER	• Vomiting during sea sickness.
POTENCY	2X – 6X. 30CH.

Aq-mar
AQUA MARINA
Sea water Mineral

Various gastrointestinal signs. Anxious restlessness, worse for company.

HEAD	Chin: pruritus. Rhinitis: left, nostril blocked yet exudate mucous, watery.
GASTROINTESTINAL	Appetite increased. Pharyngitis and stomatitis: dry, swallowing difficult. Exudate: bloody, mucous, white to yellow. PD. Right sided. Tonsillitis swollen.
	Colic; tympanitic, 11pm, improves with walking. Faeces: abundant, initially firm, then soften.
	Helminthiasis with pruritus.
RESPIRATORY	Morning cough. TB.
LAMENESS	Back with spondylitis and osteoarthritis of digits and shoulder. Severe periarticular muscle stiffness.
MODALITIES	Agg: heat. Movement. Pressure. Swimming.
	Amel: eating. Rest.
COMPARE	Nat-m Puls Tub.
CONSIDER	• Polyarthritis.
POTENCY	12X. 30CH.

Arag
ARAGALLUS LAMBERTI
White loco-weed Plant

Nervous disorders. Confused, restless, and averse to company.

CNS	Ataxia. Photophobia.

GASTROINTESTINAL	Cracked lower lip. Pharynx: dark, glazed, swollen.
RESPIRATORY	Chest pain.
LAMENESS	Ataxia: left sided sacroiliac disease.
	Muscles: weak.
COMPARE	Astra-e Oxyt.
CONSIDER	• Ataxia.
POTENCY	30CH.

Aral
ARALIA RACEMOSA
American spikenard Plant

Asthmatic coughing in apprehensive, impatient individuals.

HEAD	Rhinitis: allergic, sneezing.
RESPIRATORY	Asthma, COPD. Cough: dry, before midnight.
UROGENITAL	Metritis: offensive.
MODALITIES	Agg: 11pm.
COMPARE	Ars-i All-c Sabad.
CONSIDER	• COPD with severe cough before midnight.
POTENCY	2X – 6X–12X.

Aran
ARANEA DIADEMA
Papal cross spider Animal

Nervous signs improve near water. Confused, irritable individuals.

HEAD	Facial neuralgia: right.
GASTROINTESTINAL	Arterial haemoptysis.
	Colic: periodic, after small meal. Diarrhoea.
RESPIRATORY	Intercostal neuralgia. Arterial haemorrhage.
LAMENESS	Painful hocks.
MODALITIES	Agg: afternoon. Midnight. Damp weather.
COMPARE	*Tela araneae* Tela. Spiders web. Asthma. Cardia weak. Fever with excitement. Numbness of extremities. *Araneae scinencia* Aran-sc. Grey spider. Eyelids twitch constantly. Ars Ced Helo.
CONSIDER	• Neuralgia.
POTENCY	30CH.

Arec
ARECA CATECHU
Betel nut Plant

HEAD	Glaucoma and dilated pupils.
GASTROINTESTINAL	Helminthiasis; by increasing peristalsis.
CARDIOVASCULAR	Weak heart.
CONSIDER	• Adjunct in helminthiasis.
POTENCY	2X.

Arg-m
ARGENTUM METALLICUM

Metallic silver Mineral

Polycrest. Important signalment includes destructive, widespread arthritis from atrophy of blood vessels leading to osteoporosis. Fears: crowds, public places, and dislike control required for bandaging, dressing wounds and injections. Hurried, and because time passes slow, which makes them difficult to train.

When pressurised aggression means they will bite and kick.

CNS	Epilepsy: triggered by excitement.
HEAD	Conjunctivitis, ophthalmia: photophobia. Purulent. Eyelids: red, swollen.
GASTROINTESTINAL	Good appetite. PD. Salivation: excessive, tongue may be dry. Swallowing: difficult, jelly-like, tacky mucous.
RESPIRATORY	Laryngitis: cough: dry, hoarse, severe, unproductive.
UROGENITAL	PU: sweet, turbid.
LAMENESS	Painful stiffness of back, particularly **neck and pelvis**. **Dysplasia:** carpus, elbow, hock, physis. Insidious, progressive osteoarthritis. **Bone** problems: malnutrition, excessive mineral feeding: osteomalacia and osteomyelitis. Muscles: weak and tremble. Coffin bone and **navicular**: degeneration.
JUVENILE	**Dysplasia** and physis.
GERIATRIC	Osteoarthritis and osteoporosis.
MODALITIES	Agg: noon. Touch. Amel: open air.
COMPARE	Alum Arg-n Aur Plat Sel Stann.
CONSIDER	Especially important for bone disease: <ul><li>Dysplasia and physis.</li><li>Osteoarthritis: geriatric and juvenile.</li><li>Osteomyelitis.</li><li>Osteoporosis.</li></ul>
POTENCY	12X. 30CH. 200CH.

Arg-n
ARGENTUM NITRICUM
Silver nitrate Mineral

Polycrest. Apprehensive. Claustrophobia. Fears: alone, crowds, heights, irrational, public places, work. Hurried. Impulsive. Peculiar reactions: *will jump through a window*. The terrier mentality of being cheerful, extroverted, impulsive when well. But anxious, irritable, nervous when ill, they become sad and tremble.

Marked effect on CNS with ataxia.

Inflammation of mucous membranes including violent pharyngitis, and gastroenteritis. Free mucopurulent exudate on inflamed and ulcerated membranes.

Pains increase and develop slowly.

Anaemia from red cell destruction affects all body tissues leading to them becoming prematurely old, withered.

HEAD	Chemosis, ophthalmia: conjunctivitis: inner canthi: red, swollen. Exudate: copious, granular, purulent. Corneal opacity, ulceration. Rhinitis: pruritic coryza, septal ulceration.
GASTROINTESTINAL	Gums: bleed. Throat: raw, swollen, painful from thick

69

	mucoid exudate. Tongue: papillae prominent, tip: red, swollen. Vomiting. Colic: ulcers: gastric tympany. Gastroenteritis. IBD. Sensitivity to maize. Diarrhoea: bubbly, greenish, noisy, profuse, watery, passes easily. Proctitis.
CARDIOVASCULAR	Arrhythmia. Anaemia.
RESPIRATORY	Dyspnoea: laryngitis: cough: chronic, hoarse, suffocative.
UROGENITAL	Cystitis, urethritis. Urine: bloody, dark, scant. Tenesmus.
	Metritis: haemorrhage after oestrous. Cervix: bloody erosion. Ovaritis: left.
	Male impotence: libido poor, erection weak.
BREEDING	Improve male libido.
	Encourage mating in nervous females with back pain.
LAMENESS	Ataxia, myelitis.
COMPETITION	Performance anxiety.
SKIN	Dried up, hard and withered. Darkly pigmented.
MODALITIES	Agg: anxiety. Night. Warmth.
	Amel: chilly air. Cold. Eructation.
COMPARE	Ars Arg-m Merc Phos Puls.
CONSIDER	An important remedy with widespread action on:

- Anaemia with debility.
- Behavioural problems.
- Colic, that is tympanitic.
- Conjunctivitis and corneal ulcers.
- Diarrhoea.
- Gastric ulcers.
- IBD.

This widespread sphere is important where the mental picture fits, particularly note:

- Apprehension.
- Fears.
- Hurried.

Tired, worn-out appearance.

POTENCY	12X. 30CH. 200CH.

Arist-cl
ARISTOLOCHIA CLEMATIS
Brazilian snake-root Plant

Female infertility. Reclusive, averse to work.

HEAD	Nasal exudate: morning, watery.
GASTROINTESTINAL	Colic: mares: in oestrous: better for walking.
UROGENITAL	Cystitis: albuminuria, incontinence. Ovaritis.
	Metritis: chronic, exudate: brownish, watery. Pruritic.
LAMENESS	Lumbar pain during oestrous.
MODALITIES	Agg: oestrous: pre, during and post.
	Amel: open air. Slow exercise during oestrous.
COMPARE	Caul Puls Rhus-t.
CONSIDER	• Metritis and ovaritis.

POTENCY | 6X – 12X.

Arn
ARNICA MONTANA
Leopards' bane Fall herb Plant

Polycrest. Best known and justifiably so of remedies.

A particular influence on physical and mental problems originating from grief or trauma: recent or historical.

Agoraphobia. Dull, apathetic, and indifferent, until others trigger off their fears: **approach, touch,** vets.

Indifferent during what is perceived to be a painful situation.

Important to appreciate all conditions show **oversensitivity to pain**. Haemorrhage, bruising, strains, infection, and sepsis. Acute and chronic situations.

Significant antibacterial agent.

CNS	**Confusion.** Head injury: intra-cranial haemorrhage. Chronic vertigo. Neo-natal maladjustment syndrome in foals. Unconscious.
HEAD	Paralysis of ocular muscles.
	Retinal and sub conjunctival haemorrhage.
	Aural hematoma, Hearing poor after injury.
	Rhinitis and sinusitis: exudates: bloody, dark, purulent, watery.
GASTROINTESTINAL	Dentistry: bleeding, pain after.
	Eructation. Halitosis. Hunger great, but offensive vomiting afterwards. Tonsillitis: acute, swollen.
	Colic: severe tympany.
	Diarrhoea: bloody, brown, flatus, involuntary, offensive, putrid, tenesmus. Lies down after defecation.
CARDIOVASCULAR	Arrhythmia. Heart failure: oedema, pain. Pulse: weak. Septicaemia.
RESPIRATORY	Cough: exudate: bloody, nocturnal, paroxysmal.
UROGENITAL	Urine: brick red, retained after exertion. **Mastitis**: injury. Uterine and vaginal bleeding: after mating, post parturient. Rape.
LAMENESS	Acute painful stiffness of back muscles after exercise. Bunched up and twitch from overuse. Fractures: reduces muscle spasm.
COMPETITION	Helps with fitness by improving post exercise recovery. Prevent minor injuries and strains from worsening.
SKIN	**Bruising:** ecchymosis. Eruptions: small, pruritic, pimples. Symmetrical black and blue lesions. Purpura haemorrhagica.
FEVER	Significant antibacterial action.
	Strangles from *Streptococcal spp.* May be severe shivering.
MODALITIES	Agg: cold, damp weather. Complete rest. Movement. Touch.
	Amel: head held low. Gentle, slow movement. Lying down.
COMPARE	Acid-sul Acon Bapt Bell-p Ham Hyper Nat-s Rhus-t.
CONSIDER	A most important remedy in:

- Accident and emergency therapy.
- Exercise to improve recovery.
- Head injuries where it saves lives!
- Injuries: Acute, chronic, simple, and profound.
- Septicaemia and other bacterial infection.

Consider the mental aspects, including:

- Apathy.
- **Fear of touch.**
- **Pain:** great sensitivity to.

POTENCY	6X. 30CH. 200CH.
CAUTION	Topical use on open wounds may aggravate.
	Effective haemorrhage and wound control if administered before surgery: three times at eight hourly intervals (24-16-8). **Do not** treat for longer periods as 'proving' may lead to haemorrhage.

Ars

ARSENICUM ALBUM
White arsenic Mineral

Polycrest. Debility, great restlessness, and nightly aggravations are important. Great exhaustion after slightest exertion. **Anguish.** Courage: lacking. Carried: desire to be. Fear: alone yet malicious. Bite and kick.

Restless and oversensitive to disorder, which leads to confusion.

Constant sipping of tiny amounts of water.

Heat treatments are effective.

Right sided. Significant antibacterial agent.

CNS	Delirium tremens.
HEAD	**Scalp:** bare spots, circular patches, dirty, dry scales, rough, sensitive.
	Conjunctivitis: eyelids: acrid, granular, rough, scabby, severe. Corneal ulceration. Orbital oedema. Photophobia.
	Rhinitis. **Nasal** pruritus. Otitis externa. Exudates: acrid, offensive, raw, thin, watery. Pimples. Lupus.
ABDOMEN	Ascites. Diabetes mellitus.
	Liver and spleen: painful, swollen.
	Severe tissue destruction.
GASTROINTESTINAL	Anorexia is total, Mouth: dry, hot, ulcerated. Gums bleed.
	Thirst increased but take lesser amounts often.
	Throat: constricted, hot, oedematous. Diphtheria.
	Tongue: clean, dry, red.
	Eructation: long lasting.
	Vomit after eating or drinking: bilious, bloody, brownish, green, mucous. Dysentery. Pruritus.
CARDIOVASCULAR	Anaemia. Fatty cardiac degeneration. Palpitation. Pain. Fast morning pulse.
RESPIRATORY	**Asthma:** Dyspnoea. Bronchospasm. Cough. Haemoptysis. Wheezing.
	Agg by anxiety and after midnight.

UROGENITAL	Albuminuria, epithelial cells, hot, involuntary, urinate lesser amounts often.
	Metritis: acrid, offensive, painful, watery.
LAMENESS	Sacroiliac weakness: muscles tremble and twitch. Peripheral neuritis causes poor tissue nutrition and drying up of affected parts. Coffin bone disease, navicular disease, pedal osteitis.
JUVENILE	**Neonatal** dysentery.
GERIATRIC	Bronchitis. COPD.
SKIN	Eruptions: bloody, dry, hot, oedematous, scaly. Papules. Psoriasis. Oedematous swellings are worse for cold and scratching.
	Pruritus. Wound, gangrene, pus. Urticaria.
FEVER	**Complete exhaustion**, intermittent with great restless. High and septic at 3 a.m.
MODALITIES	Agg: anxiety. Cold. Eating. After midnight. Seaside. Wet weather.
	Amel: company. Heat. Movement. Sips of water. Warm bandaging and wrapping.
COMPARE	*Arsenicum bromatum* Ars-br. Similar with an impressive antipsoric action. Diabetes mellitus, lymphoid tumours, and locomotor ataxia.
	Arsenicum hydrogenisatum Ars-h. Anxiety. Thirst is much less. Anaemia is severe. Haemorrhage mucous membranes and urine.
	Arsenicum metallicum Ars-met. Milder acting than Ars. Distinct periodicity of two to three weeks. Tongue coated white and may show imprint of the teeth. The pathology in liver, mammae and spleen is painful.
	Carb-v Cench Chin Iod Kali-p Phos Verat.
CONSIDER	Frequently employed remedy against these diseases:

- Diarrhoea and dysentery that is bloody, offensive, and profuse.
- Dyspnoea of asthma and bronchitis.
- Eczema is dry, dirty, and itchy. Oedema.
- Pain control as death approaches.
- Wounds infected and purulent.

Worth emphasising the characteristic signs:

- Exhaustion after slightest exertion.
- Constantly sip lesser amounts of water.
- Individuals are often thin, even refined.
- Nightly aggravation.
- Oversensitive with great fear.
- Progressive weakness and debility.
- Restless.
- Tissue destruction.
- Progressive weakness, debility.

POTENCY	12X. 30CH. 200CH

Ars-i

ARSENICUM IODATUM
Arsenious oxide Mineral

Thin, anxious, excitable, and impatient, they startle easily and are difficult to examine or manage. Significant antibacterial agent. Similarities with Ars, but even more corrosive and persistent. Profound weakness, rapid pulse, recurrent fever with sweating, and diarrhoea.

HEAD	Conjunctivitis. Rhinitis. Otitis: media and externa. Exudates: acrid, chronic, dirty, offensive, purulent, yellow. Worse when sneezing. Tympanic membrane thickened
GASTROINTESTINAL	PD with frequent and immediate vomiting. Diphtheria. Pharyngitis: chronic, follicular. Tonsilitis.
CARDIOVASCULAR	Lymphadenitis.
RESPIRATORY	Laryngitis, bronchitis, pneumonia. Cough: chronic, dry, hacking. Abscess. TB.
SKIN	Eczema: dry, intense pruritus. Exfoliation of large scales leaves raw, weeping surfaces. Ichthyosis. Psoriasis.
COMPARE	*Arsenicum salts.* Aral sang.
CONSIDER	Good clinical application:
	• Eczema.
	• Otitis: media and externa.
	• Pneumonia, chronic with abscess.
	• Rhinitis is chronic.
	The severely corrosive nature of the problem points to this remedy.
	Thin individuals with a reasonable appetite.
POTENCY	8X. 30CH. 200CH.

Abrot
ARTEMISIA ABROTANUM
Southern wormwood Plant

Chronic diseases in weak, depressed individuals who are irritable and obstinate when excited.
Stimulates chronic, exudative viral infections.

HEAD	Face: cold, dry, wrinkled. Nose bleeds.
GASTROINTESTINAL	FIP ascites: painful.
	Appetite good, but weight loss.
	Gastritis: painful vomiting, fluid, offensive, profuse.
CARDIOVASCULAR	Cancer: metastases to glands.
RESPIRATORY	Hydrothorax, pleurisy. Exudation: copious. Pain.
LAMENESS	Osteoarthritis: severe weakness: large muscles of back and shoulders.
	Arthritic, deformed digits. Lameness; chronic infection.
SKIN	Falling hair with folliculitis. Dark pigmentation.
JUVENILE	Helminthiasis. Neonatal naval leaks blood.
MODALITIES	Agg chilly air. Suppressed secretions.
	Amel: slow exercise.
COMPARE	Bry Scroph Stell.
CONSIDER	Useful:
	• African Horse Sickness.

- Arthritis that is chronic and deformed.
- Cancer with metastases.
- Facial eczema.
- FIP – wet form.
- Respiratory disease: acute exudation.
- Respiratory disease: chronic with tissue destruction.

POTENCY	2X for helminthiasis. 12X. 30CH. 200CH.

Absin
ARTEMISIA ABSINTHIUM
Common wormwood Plant

CNS	Epilepsy with great excitement. Violence.
HEAD	Spasmodic facial twitching.
GASTROINTESTINAL	Jaw: clamped closed, bite tongue.
	Eructation and vomiting. Colic: tympanitic.
UROGENITAL	Urine: offensive, yellow.
COMPARE	Art-v Cina Cic.
CONSIDER	• Epilepsy.
POTENCY	30CH. 200CH.

Cina
ARTEMISIA MARITIMA
Levant wormseed

Defiant juveniles. Difficult to control, may erupt into angry, violent, and vocal attacks. Make strange gestures. Prone to digestive upsets triggered by helminthiasis.

HEAD	Dilated pupils. Pruritic rhinitis.
GASTROINTESTINAL	Hunger with vomiting after food. Anal pruritus.
RESPIRATORY	Cough: choking, morning, paroxysmal.
UROGENITAL	Nocturnal incontinence. Urine: milky, turbid.
LAMENESS	Muscles jerk and twitch.
JUVENILE	Difficult because nervous.
MODALITIES	Agg: helminthiasis. Night. Summer.
COMPARE	Anth Ign Spig Teucr.
CONSIDER	• Behavioural problems in juveniles.
POTENCY	2X for helminthiasis. 30CH.

Art-v
ARTEMISIA VULGARIS
Mugwort Plant

CNS	Epilepsy: irritable, restless juveniles. Throw head back and left. Triggers include emotion, flashing lights, fright. Irritable before fit. Unconscious afterwards.
GASTROINTESTINAL	Breath smells of garlic. Facial muscles twitch.
COMPARE	Absin Cina Cic.
CONSIDER	• Juvenile epilepsy.
POTENCY	6X. 30CH.

Arum-t

ARUM TRIPHYLLUM
Jack in the pulpit Plant

Confused, even delirious individuals. Irritable and obstinate. Escape artists.

HEAD	Left eyelid quivers.
	Rhinitis: Acute, chronic: blocked. Exudate: acrid, bloody, raw, watery.
GASTROINTESTINAL	Corners of mouth: bloody, cracked. Saliva: acrid, profuse. Tongue and pharynx: inflamed, raw.
CARDIOVASCULAR	Lymphadenitis: sub maxillary.
RESPIRATORY	Cough: choking, painful.
SKIN	Pruritus. Rash: blood red.
MODALITIES	Agg: lying down. NW wind.
COMPARE	*Arum draconitium* Arum-d. Similar action.
	Ail All-c Am-c.
CONSIDER	• Acute, chronic acrid, allergic rhinitis.
POTENCY	4X – 12X.

Asar
ASARUM EUROPAEUM
European snake-root Plant

Averse to everything with significant fear of noise and touch. Confused, excitable, and oversensitive to noise, with mental and nervous conditions including neuralgia, showing great fatigue.

HEAD	Blepharitis. Choroiditis. Conjunctivitis. Chronic glaucoma. Exudate: thin, yellow. Eyelids: spasmodic twitch. Rhinitis and sinusitis.
GASTROINTESTINAL	Aerophagy, gingivitis, stomatitis: exudate: bloody, offensive papillae. Chronic hiccough.
	PD, but swallowing difficult. Tongue coated brown or white. Better after vomiting.
	Acute right sided tympanitic colic.
	Diarrhoea: bloody to grey, mucous. Tenesmus.
RESPIRATORY	Laryngitis and pharyngitis.
	Cough: exudate: green, thick, mucous.
UROGENITAL	Painful Cystitis, nephritis. Dribble after urination.
	Habitual foetal loss.
	Pruritus of male genitalia.
LAMENESS	Muscle: lumbar: painfully stiff. Improve slow exercise.
COMPETITION	Consider in difficult nervous horses with back pains that need time to warm up for exercise.
MODALITIES	Agg: lying down on left side. Windy, storm weather.
	Amel: open air. Exercise.
COMPARE	Arist-cl Rauw Rhus-t Stict Valer.
CONSIDER	• Aerophagy.
	• Behaviour control.
	• Colic.
POTENCY	6X – 12X. 30CH.

ASCLEPIAS SYRIACA
Silkweed Plant

Immune modulation. Acute arthritis and kidney diseases with fluid retention. Mood swings.

CARDIOVASCULAR	Heart failure with oedema.
UROGENITAL	Nephritis with PU and high SG.
LAMENESS	Arthritis of hip and stifle.
COMPARE	*Asclepias incarnata* Asc-i. Swamp milkweed. Chronic gastroenteritis and metritis.
	Asclepias tuberosa Asc-t. Pleurisy root. Painful arthritis and Intercostal muscles. Mucous dysentery.
	Vincetoxicum officinale Vince. Swallow wort. Diabetes mellitus, gastroenteritis, oedema, immune system modulation.
	Periploca graeca Peri. Silk vine. Cardiac and lung tonic.
CONSIDER	Useful:
	• Cardiac weakness.
	• Gastroenteritis that is chronic.
	• Immune modulation.
	• Respiratory weakness.
POTENCY	2X – 8X – 12X.

Queb
ASPIDOSPERMA QUEBRACHO
Quebracho Plant

Often termed the *Digitalis of the lungs* for its ability to improve tissue oxygenation.

RESPIRATORY	Asthma, COPD, EIPH and oedema.
COMPETITION	Improves general fitness wherever respiratory restrictions occur.
COMPARE	Ant-t Apis Ars Coca Coff.
CONSIDER	Improve tissue oxygenation:
	• Chronic allergic lower airway disease.
	• COPD.
	• EIPH.
	• Exercise intolerance of unknown origin.
POTENCY	2X – 4X for nebulisation. 6X – 8X.

Astac
ASTACUS FLUVIATILIS
Crawfish Animal

GASTROINTESTINAL	Painful swollen hepatitis with jaundice.
CARDIOVASCULAR	Cancer in painfully swollen lymph glands.
SKIN	Widespread nettle rash.
COMPARE	Apis Nat-m Rhus-t Rhus-v.
CONSIDER	• Lymphoid cancer.
	• Urticaria.
POTENCY	4X – 12X. 30CH.

Aster

ASTERIAS RUBENS
Red starfish Animal

UROGENITAL	Indurate mammary cancer.
COMPARE	Ars Carb-v Con.
POTENCY	6X – 12X.

Astra-e

ASTRAGALUS EXCAPUS
European astragalus Plant

Ataxia. Cushings disease. Anorexia. Confused. Emaciated.

HEAD	Cancer of the jaw. Sinusitis.
RESPIRATORY	Asthma: rales. Bronchitis: cough: dry, mucous plugs.
LAMENESS	Dysplasias and physis in juveniles. Osteomalacia.
COMPARE	Arg-m Ars-i Syph Tub.
CONSIDER-	• Asthma.
	• Cancer.
	• Dysplasia and physis.
POTENCY	12X. 30CH.

Bell

ATROPA BELLADONNA
Deadly nightshade Plant

Polycrest. Conditions with signs of **great intensity**.

Profound action on every part of the nervous system causing a state of excitement and active congestion.

VIOLENCE is the hallmark.

All conditions and reactions to disease are intense. Patients may become impossible with great aggression when they **bite and kick. Rage** with wild vocal violence and delirium with a desire to escape so profound horses will run into a wall. Sensitive animals are always excitable when well, with significant fears: of being alone, animals, dark, irrational.

An incredibly significant effect on the skin, glands, and vascular system. **Pains are violent.** Significant antibacterial agent.

As with other dramatic situations, with **Bell** we see homoeopathy at its magnificent best. Have treated the most difficult colic cases; even those fearful we might not get close to them, and when injected with Bell 200CH, one minute later they change. Homoeopathy works!

CNS	Encephalitis. Equine encephalosis. Meningitis. Ataxia: fall backwards or sideways. Twitching neck and throat muscles. Epilepsy: head rolls from side to side. Vomiting.
HEAD	Head pressing by boring into corners, fences, and walls. Severe shaking and twitching. Conjunctivitis. Eye protruded from socket. Pupils dilated, fixed, stare. Photophobia.
	Otitis media and externa: great pain, minimal exudate. Nasal coryza: blood red, mucous.
ABDOMEN	Pain on palpation.
GASTROINTESTINAL	Anorexia. Fear drinking: thirst for chilly water. Tongue: papillae: red painful, strawberry-like, swollen.

	Swallowing is difficult.
	Tonsils painful, red, swollen. Colic: tympanitic: severe pain.
CARDIOVASCULAR	Pulse: palpitation, rapid, weak. Lymphadenitis.
	Vessels: hot, prominent, tense.
RESPIRATORY	Laryngitis: dyspnoea: cough: hoarse.
	Voice: lost, strained. Haemoptysis: arterial.
UROGENITAL	Cystitis: acute: urine: bloody, casts, dark, turbid. Tenesmus.
	Mastitis: acute: red streaks on skin.
	Uterus: haemorrhage: arterial, offensive.
	Orchitis: painfully swollen.
BREEDING	Postpartum haemorrhage, mastitis.
LAMENESS	Muscles: neck: excruciatingly painful and stiff.
	Bursitis: hard, hot, painful.
	Laminitis: acute, **bounding** pulse, fierce pain.
JUVENILE	Acutely painful fevers, with full, throbbing pulse
SKIN	Insect and snake bites. Profuse sweat.
	Skin: dry, hot, red. Pain on palpation.
MODALITIES	Agg: afternoon. Jarring. Lying down. Noise. Touch.
	Amel: dark. Rest.
COMPARE	Atro Calc Hyos Plat.
CONSIDER	Remarkable healing properties in:

Remarkable healing properties in:
- Colic with most painful, tympany.
- Convulsions from mineral deficiencies.
- Distemper complications.
- Eclampsia.
- Fever with a bounding pulse and excitability.
- Laminitis.
- Lymphangitis.
- Snake and insect bites and stings.

The main signs are important:
- Acute onset.
- Dry, thirstless mouth.
- Pain of the most severe kind.
- Vascular congestion is intense.
- Violent attacks.

POTENCY	12X. 30CH. 200CH.

Aur

AURUM METALLICUM
Metallic gold Mineral

Polycrest. Anger. Confidence: lacking.
Depression is so severe, animals in great pain will run away and put themselves in dangerous, even fatal situations. The closest to suicide animals get. Excitable. Grief. Hurried. Oversensitive: excitement, noise.
Profound **tissue destruction** of blood, lymphatic glands, and bone.

HEAD	Facial bones: exostoses, osteomalacia, pain.
	Dermatitis: scalp.
	Eye: conjunctivitis. Interstitial keratitis.

	Pannus with marked vascularisation.
	Otitis media, externa: exudate: chronic, purulent.
	Nasal bones and mucosa: necrosis: pain, pus.
	Ulcers: pain, swollen.
GASTROINTESTINAL	Halitosis. Constipation or Ulcerated gums.
	Diarrhoea. Nocturnal pruritus
CARDIOVASCULAR	Arrhythmia; fibrillation. High BP. Tachycardia.
	Weak pulse. Lymphadenitis.
RESPIRATORY	Dyspnoea: nocturnal.
UROGENITAL	Cystitis: retention of turbid, buttermilk-like urine.
	Uterus: enlarged, sterile. Prolapse.
	Orchitis: Acute, chronic: indurate.
LAMENESS	Osteomalacia, osteoporosis, ringbone. Bursitis.
	Peripheral oedema.
SLEEP	Insomnia: agitated.
SKIN	Sarcoid and warts on genitalia.
MODALITIES	Agg: exercise. Night. Chilly weather.
	Amel: rest. Slow walking.
COMPARE	Aurum iodatum Iodide of gold. Aur-i. Chronic pericarditis and valvular insufficiency. Lupus. Periostitis. Ovarian cysts.
	Aurum muriaticum Chloride of gold. Aur-m. Cancer of tongue is leather-like. Metritis with an acrid, yellow discharge.
COMPARE	Acid-nit Asaf Kali-i Hep Merc Mez Phos.
CONSIDER	A huge influence in:

- Behavioural abnormalities with great depression.
- Bone disease with destruction.
- Corneal disease with keratitis and pannus.
- Nasal disease with severe tissue destruction.
- Orchitis.
- Otitis media is chronic and purulent.

POTENCY	8X. 30CH. 200CH.

Aur-m-n
AURUM MURIATICUM NATRONATUM
Sodium chloroaurate Mineral

HEAD	Mandibular periostitis.
GASTROINTESTINAL	Liver: cirrhosis. Cancer: tongue: indurated.
UROGENITAL	Cervix: cancer: ulcerated.
	Sterility: ovaries indurate.
	Uterine cancer. Metritis. Chronic prolapse.
COMPARE	*Aurums.* Ars-i Con Hydr Kres Phos Sep.
CONSIDER	• Cancer of the cervix and uterus.
POTENCY	30CH. 200CH.

Aven
AVENA SATIVA

Common oat Plant

A useful tonic in debilitated animals of either sex, particularly from over breeding.

COMPARE	Acid-phos Alf Gins Orchi-e (c) Ov.
	Combines well with other remedies.
POTENCY	2X – 4X.

Bac

BACILLINUM BURNETT

Bovine TB nosode Animal

Chronic lung disease in thin, depressed, irritable individuals.

HEAD	Eyelid: eczema, ringworm.
GASTROINTESTINAL	Constipation: chronic, obstinate.
CARDIOVASCULAR	Lymphadenitis: neck glands.
RESPIRATORY	Dyspnoea: congested, rales. Exudate: mucous, purulent. TB.
SKIN	Pityriasis. Ringworm.
MODALITIES	Agg: early morning. Night.
COMPARE	Ant-t Ars-i Calc-p Kali-c Lach Psor Tub.
CONSIDER	• Chronic bacterial lung disease.
	• Ringworm.
POTENCY	30CH. 200CH.

Prot

BACILLUS PROTEUS

Bacterium Animal

IBD and hoof problems. Difficult, oversensitive dangerous animals, averse to company.

HEAD	Meibomian cyst. Rhinitis: chronic.
GASTROINTESTINAL	Aerophagy. Pharyngitis. Cracked lips. IBD: gastric ulcers. Vomit. Rectal pruritus: helminthiasis.
UROGENITAL	Cystitis, nephritis. Pyelonephritis. Metritis.
LAMENESS	Bilaterally thickened annular and carpal ligaments. Horn: defective, brittle, split. Painful.
COMPETITION	Helps maintain soundness.
SKIN	Pruritic dermatitis with persistent exudate. Ulcers.
MODALITIES	Agg: cold. Exercise at the beginning. Lying down. Morning. Overwork. Storms.
	Amel: regular, steady work.
COMPARE	Ant-c Psor Sul Tub.
CONSIDER	• Brittle feet
	• IBD.
POTENCY	12X. 30CH.

Ball

BALLOTA FOETIDA

Black horehound Plant

Anxiety. Inattentive. Restlessness.

GASTROINTESTINAL	Vomiting mucous.
RESPIRATORY	Bronchitis with a spasmodic cough.
CONSIDER	• Performance anxiety. Inattentive.
POTENCY	12X. 30C.

81

Bals-p
BALSAMUM PERUVIANUM
Balsam of Peru Plant

HEAD	Rhinitis and sinusitis. Exudate: mucopurulent, profuse, thick. Ulcer.
GASTROINTESTINAL	Vomiting mucous.
RESPIRATORY	Bronchitis: cough: exudate: loose. Rales.
UROGENITAL	Cystitis: chronic, pyelitis. Urine: mucous, scant, sediment.
	Cracked nipples.
SKIN	Indolent and raw ulceration. Topical use promotes healing of granulating wounds and ulcers.
CONSIDER	• Chronic bronchitis.
	• Wounds with excessive granulation tissue.
	• Mucopurulent exudates.
	• Rhinitis is chronic and mucopurulent.
POTENCY	Topical 2X. Combines with Calendula.
	4X − 6X. 30CH.

Bapt
BAPTISIA TINCTORIA
Wild indigo Plant

Polycrest. Fever and septicaemic conditions, involving great weakness and unpleasant exudates. May appear unconscious: initially respond to attention then lapse. Significant antibacterial agent.

ABDOMEN	Liver: enlarged, painful on palpation. Right sided pain.
GASTROINTESTINAL	Halitosis. Tongue and gums: brown to **pale,** yellow discoloration. Ulceration. Vomiting.
	Tonsils: dark red. Salivation: profuse. Swallowing: difficult.
	Oesophagus, cardia contracted. Solids immediately vomited. Ulceration.
	Diarrhoea: bloody, dark, offensive, thin. Gastroenteritis. Dysentery.
CARDIOVASCULAR	Has a direct effect on blood parasites including *Babesia spp, Erhlichia spp*. Often associated with profound anaemia from rapid rbc destruction.
UROGENITAL	Metritis and septicaemia postpartum. After foetal loss.
LAMENESS	Generalised weak and painful muscles.
SKIN	Offensive ulcers with great weakness.
MODALITIES	Agg: fog. Humid heat. Indoors. 11.00am.
COMPARE	Ail Arn Ars Bry Echi Pyr.
CONSIDER	• Fever with dark, offensive exudates and great weakness.
	• Babesiosis.
	• Metritis after abortion and parturition.
	• Salmonellosis.
POTENCY	4X − 12X. 30CH.

Bar-c

BARYTA CARBONICA
Barium carbonate Mineral

Averse to company, lacking in confidence, it is their confusion and dullness that makes them easily frightened and suspicious. Juvenile and geriatrics when physically and / or mentally backward.

CNS	Senile dementia: after cerebrovascular incident.
HEAD	Cataracts. Pupils: contracted, dilated, insensitive.
	Deafness: slowly developing.
	Nose: cracked, dry. Exudate: bloody, thick, yellow.
GASTROINTESTINAL	Anorexic. Gums and lips swollen and bleed easily. Salivate at dawn.
	Pharyngitis and tonsillitis: veins engorged.
	Oesophageal spasms when eating.
	Colic: impaction: chronic, tympany.
	Constipation: retention of meconium. Severe.
CARDIOVASCULAR	Aneurism. Palpitation. High BP. Tachycardia. Lymphadenitis: sub-maxillary, axillary and mesenteric glands. Strangles.
RESPIRATORY	Dry cough on inspiration. Bronchitis, laryngitis: geriatrics: exudate: mucous, tenacious, thick. Voice weak.
UROGENITAL	Urethritis.
	Males with premature loss of libido. Prostatomegaly.
LAMENESS	Back muscles; neck, wither, sacroiliac: painfully stiff, contracted. Digits are stiff. Sole pain.
JUVENILE	Neonatal maladjustment syndrome. Backward neonates when respiration is weak: exudate: mucous, tenacious.
GERIATRIC	Chronic respiratory weakness with tenacious mucous. Any signs of mental deterioration. Vocal separation anxiety.
MODALITIES	Agg: bathing. Lying on affected side.
	Amel: open air. Solitude.
COMPARE	*Baryta iodata* Bar-i. Powerful action on indurated lymphatic cancer.
	Arag Astra-e Bar-m Con Dig Psor Rad Sil.
CONSIDER	Important:

Important:
- Delayed neonates mentally or physically.
- Geriatric degeneration anywhere.
- Lymphoid swellings with sepsis: Strangles.
- Respiratory problems with thick, tenacious mucous.
- Cancer: fibrous or fatty, of neck and stomach.

POTENCY	4X – 12X. 30CH during sepsis.

Bar-m

BARYTA MURIATICA
Barium chloride Mineral

CNS	Convulsions from cerebral degeneration. Neonatal maladjustment syndrome.
	Senile dementia. Vertigo. Loss of muscle control.
HEAD	Otitis: externa, media: offensive, pain. Blocked eustachian tube.
GASTROINTESTINAL	Vomiting from pharyngeal paralysis.
	Cardia hypertrophy. Swallowing is difficult. Chronic tonsillitis.
CARDIOVASCULAR	Heart: hypertrophy. Vessels degenerate.
	Lymphadenitis: inguinal and others. Strangles.
RESPIRATORY	Geriatric chronic bronchitis with associated heart disease and extensive mucous accumulation.
UROGENITAL	Urates.
	Nymphomania.
JUVENILE	Equine neonatal maladjustment syndrome.
COMPARE	Aur-m-n Bar-c Plb Sec Sel.
CONSIDER	• Bronchitis that is chronic in geriatrics.
	• Hypertrophy of cardia with vomiting.
	• Neonatal maladjustment syndrome.
	• Senile dementia.
POTENCY	6X – 12X. 30CH. 200CH.

BCG
BCG
Bovine TB vaccine Animal

Chronic respiratory infections. Sad, anxious and hypersensitive to noise. Individuals are restless and weak. Exudates are mucous. Geriatrics. **Left sided**.

HEAD	Blepharitis. Conjunctivitis. Keratitis. Eyelids: eczema, swollen.
	Otitis media, externa: chronic.
	Rhinitis: chronic. Polyps.
GASTROINTESTINAL	Tonsilitis: **right.** Colic: impaction. Rectal fissures.
CARDIOVASCULAR	Chronic lymphadenitis. Strangles.
RESPIRATORY	Bronchitis, pleurisy: chronic, recurrent. Cough: rasping.
UROGENITAL	Bladder: dilated: chronic.
LAMENESS	Polyarthritis of the digits.
MODALITIES	Agg: exercise. Evening. Noise.
	Amel: eating. Lying down.
COMPARE	*Baryta salts.* Calc-p Dros Nat-m
CONSIDER	• Lymphadenitis.
	• Respiratory diseases, chronic.
	• Strangles.
POTENCY	12X. 30CH. 200CH.

Bell-p
BELLIS PERENNIS
Common clarity Daisy plant

Like Arn but mentally less intense. More effective in athletic conditions with **left sided muscle** stiffness and bruising. Excitable, irritable, and restless.

UROGENITAL	**Mammae bruised,** sensitive. Pregnancy: generalised chronic stiffness. Postpartum haemorrhage and metritis.
LAMENESS	Muscle: lumbar and gluteal: chronic, painful stiffness. Tendon, ligament: strains: annular and carpal.
SKIN	Erysipelas: exudation: purulent. Petechiation.
COMPETITION	Invaluable in maintaining athletic function.
MODALITIES	Agg: heat treatments. Before storms.
COMPARE	Arn Ars Bry Ham Staph.
CONSIDER	Almost identical to Arn.
	• Athletic muscle protection and treatment.
POTENCY	12X. 30CH. 200CH.

Ben
BENZINUM
Petroleum ether Mineral

CNS	Epilepsy in sad, lethargic dogs.
HEAD	Photophobia: pupils dilated. Eyelids: twitch. Jaundice. Mucous sneezing.
CARDIOVASCULAR	Anaemia and leukaemia.
UROGENITAL	Orchitis: right, severe. Scrotal eczema.
SKIN	Extremely pruritic, papular eczema.
MODALITIES	Agg: night.
COMPARE	TNT.
CONSIDER	• Anaemia.
	• Leukaemia.
	• Orchitis.
POTENCY	12X. 30CH.

Berb-a
BERBERIS AQUIFOLIUM
Mahonia aquifolium Plant

UROGENITAL	Lithiasis: proteinuria, tenesmus. PU.
LAMENESS	Azoturia/myositis: profound muscle pain and stiffness.
SKIN	Widespread blisters and papules.
COMPETITION	Azoturia / myositis. Muscle enzymes high in sport horses. As a preventative.
MODALITIES	Agg: evening and night. Amel: cold washing.
COMPARE	Aloe Ars Berb Psor Sulph.
CONSIDER	• Acute allergic eczemas including flea bite and veld mange.
	• Azoturia/myositis: even **better than Berb**.
	• Cystitis and lithiasis.
POTENCY	6X. 30CH.

Berb
BERBERIS VULGARIS
Common barberry Plant

Polycrest. Apathetic and listless, this worsens during bouts of kidney disease. Characteristic rapid changes in pains. Thirst or thirstless.

CNS	Vertigo. Spinal nerve irritation.
HEAD	Rhinitis: obstinate: exudate: dry, mucous, thick. Left side. Ophthalmia.
ABDOMEN	Hepatitis: Acute, chronic.
GASTROINTESTINAL	Salivation: diminished, frothy, sticky.
	Tongue with vesicles. Tonsillitis.
	Proctitis. Constipation with constant straining.
	Diarrhoea: clay-coloured, painless.
	Perineal fistula.
UROGENITAL	PU. Nephritis and cystitis with lithiasis. Azoturia/myositis. FLUTD is thick, mucoid. Proteinuria. Sediment: bright red, dark, mealy. PU.
	Female genitalia: painfully pruritic. Ovaritis.
	Scrotum, spermatic cord, testes: Painful neuralgia.
LAMENESS	Postsurgical: back and neck pain. **Painfully stiff muscles** of legs and shoulders. Azoturia/myositis. Weariness and lameness of legs after walking short distances. Sprained metatarsals and metacarpals.
COMPETITION	Prevention and treatment of azoturia /myositis and elevated muscle enzymes.
SKIN	**Eczema** of anus and extremities. Pruritus worse for scratching. Widespread pustules. Flat warts.
MODALITIES	Agg: motion. Standing.
COMPARE	*Berberis aquifolium* Berb-a. More **effective in azoturia/myositis**.
	Aloe Conv Lyc Nux-v Sars.
CONSIDER	• Azoturia / myositis.
	• Lithiasis.
	• Nephritis.
	• Pain.
POTENCY	8X. 30CH. 200CH.

Beryl
BERYLLIUM METALLICUM
Beryllium Metal

HEAD	Conjunctivitis: allergic, follicular, mucous.
	Rhinitis: acute, chronic: allergic, seasonal.
GASTROINTESTINAL	Ulceration of lips and tongue with vomiting. Pharyngitis.
RESPIRATORY	COPD. Emphysema. Pneumonia: bloody, deep, painful.
	May significantly improve athletic performance: chronic, low-grade disease.
SKIN	Sarcoid: bubbles under the skin.
MODALITIES	Agg: exercise. Heat.
	Amel: cold. Fresh air.
COMPARE	Bry Lach.
CONSIDER	• COPD of allergic origin.
POTENCY	12X. 30CH. 200CH.

Bet

BETULA ALBA

Cherry or white birch Plant

Profound immunological effects including in vitro antiproliferative effects in numerous tumour cell cultures. Increases total number of thymocytes and lymphocytes.

Antibacterial effects on *Bacillus, E. coli Heliobacteria spp*.

SKIN	Reduces growth of small tumours and scarring. Improves wound healing
POTENCY	12X. 30CH. 200CH.

Bism

BISMUTHUM METALLICUM

Bismuth subnitricum Mineral

Irritable individuals that desire company, most conditions are associated with excessive mucous production.

GASTROINTESTINAL	Gums: spongy, swollen, copious salivation. Tongue: necrotic, white, swollen. Gastritis: vomiting: painful, severe, watery. Diarrhoea: flatulent, painless.
RESPIRATORY	COPD. Emphysema. Pneumonia. Chest may auscultate clear.
UROGENITAL	PU. Orchitis.
LAMENESS	Severe muscle cramps. Coronary band pain. Laminitis.
MODALITIES	Agg: movement.
COMPARE	Ant-c Ars Bell Berb Kres.
CONSIDER	• Gastroenteritis with mucous. • COPD, emphysema, and pneumonia.
POTENCY	6X. 30CH.

Blatta

BLATTA ORIENTALIS

Asian cockroach Animal

Allergic conditions in dull, sad individuals that resent work.

RESPIRATORY	Asthma, bronchitis: cough: chronic, moist, mucopurulent.
COMPARE	*Blatta americana* Blatta-a. American cockroach. Ascites and urethritis with great tiredness.
CONSIDER	• Allergic asthma. • Bronchitis.
POTENCY	6X. 30CH. 200CH.

Bor

BORAX VENETA

Sodium borate Mineral

Confused, dull, timid, and oversensitive to noise., their inherent anxiety worsens when moving downwards, including during transport in a horse box.

CNS	Epilepsy and travel sickness.
HEAD	Entropion: pain, swollen.
	Noise: oversensitive.
	Nose: atopy: crusty, dry, swollen, ulcerated.

GASTROINTESTINAL	Ulcers: mouth: aphthous, bleed, hot, painful.
	Vomiting.
	Colic: tympanitic: after eating, severe.
	Diarrhoea: after colic: mucous, offensive.
RESPIRATORY	Laryngitis: loss of voice. Cough: hacking, paroxysmal.
UROGENITAL	Urethritis: albuminuria, haematuria.
	Female genitalia: pruritic. Metritis: chronic: exudate: albumin-like. Sterile.
LAMENESS	Joint: strain: hock and others. Interdigital ulceration, vesicles.
SKIN	Ulceration, vesicles: interdigital: pus.
	Eczema: toes, nail loss. Pruritus: dorsum of digits. Psoriasis.
MODALITIES	Agg: downward movement. Noise. Smoke. Warm weather.
	Amel: bandaging and wrapping. Chilly weather. Evening.
COMPARE	Acid-sul Bry Calc Sanic.
CONSIDER	The classic picture is Bovine Foot and Mouth Disease.
	• Eczema.
	• Gastroenteritis.
	• Travel sickness.
	• Viral ulceration.
POTENCY	6X – 12X. 30CH.

Both

BOTHROPS LANCEOLATUS

Yellow viper Animal

Disease that resembles infected bite wounds with haemorrhage. Depressed, yet noise sensitive.

HEAD	Blindness: acute: conjunctival and retinal haemorrhage.
GASTROINTESTINAL	Mouth: dry, swollen. Vomiting: bloody.
	Throat: constricted, dry, swallowing difficult.
CARDIOVASCULAR	Haemoconcentration, hyper coagulation and thrombosis.
	Lymphangitis: phleg-leg: vessels corded, enlarged and tense.
LAMENESS	Acute phleg-leg.
SKIN	Ecchymosis.
COMPARE	Lach.
CONSIDER	• Iliac thrombosis.
	• Lymphangitis.
	• Prophylactic after serious bite wounds.
	• Pulmonary haemorrhage.
	• Sepsis with haemorrhage.
	• Snake bite.
	Often a diagonal signalment, worse on right.
POTENCY	30CH. 200CH.

Bov

BOVISTA LYCOPERDON

Giant puff ball Plant

Awkward, lazy, and sensitive individuals, averse to company. Allergic, eruptive eczema.

GASTROINTESTINAL	Colic improved by food.
	Diarrhoea: chronic, geriatric. Rectal pruritus.
UROGENITAL	Haematuria. Metritis: exudate: acrid, greenish, thick. Ovaritis.
LAMENESS	Pain over lower lumbar. Tired weak joints. Oedema of fractures.
SKIN	Oedema great enough to leave impression on skin from blunt objects. Eczema: moist herpetic-like pimples form crusts.
	Sweet Itch. Pruritic urticaria with diarrhoea after excitement.
MODALITIES	Agg: night and evening. Touch. Warmth.
COMPARE	Calc Cic Sep Thuj.
CONSIDER	• Allergic dermatitis from insect bites.
	• Eczema is severe.
	• Urticaria.
POTENCY	8X. 30CH.

Brom
BROMIUM
Bromium Mineral

Angry individuals dislike work and demonstrate fears. Marked jerking and starting during sleep. Severe respiratory signs in weak juveniles.

HEAD	Rhinitis: acrid, right. Fan-like motion of alar cartilage.
GASTROINTESTINAL	Pharyngitis and tonsillitis: red with dilated blood vessels.
CARDIOVASCULAR	Cardiac hypertrophy. Lymph glands: stone hard.
RESPIRATORY	Asthma: bronchospasm, rales. Cough: Kennel Cough-like, hard, spasmodic, suffocative. Diphtheria.
UROGENITAL	Ovaritis.
	Orchitis: painfully swollen, indurate.
COMPETITION	Lung and heart protector for athletes during virus infection.
MODALITIES	Agg: evening. Lying on right side. Warm room.
	Amel: gentle exercise. Damp, warm weather. Seaside.
COMPARE	Aster Arg-n Con Dros Iod Spong.
	Combines well with Crat.
CONSIDER	• Asthma.
	• Bronchospasm.
	• COPD.
	• Kennel Cough.
POTENCY	4X – 8X – 12X.

Bry
BRYONIA ALBA
White bryony Plant

Polycrest. Angry. Always busy, great escape artists worse when excited for then they become impatient, impetuous, and irritable. Severe pains **worse** for movement. Affects dark, strong, robust types, but can affect irritable, and lean individuals. When most horsey people like to walk horses affected by colic, these, despite great pain, hate moving. Any organs, especially chest and lameness. Marked dryness of mucosae.

CNS	Vertigo.
HEAD	Glaucoma. Bloody frontal sinusitis. Tip of nose swollen.
ABDOMEN	Hepatitis: painfully swollen. Worse: deep breathing, coughing.
GASTROINTESTINAL	PD. Mouth, lips: cracked, dry, sensitive.
	PU. Tongue: dry. Vomiting.
	Colic / Impaction. Faeces: bloody, brown, dry as if burnt, hard, thick. Worse in morning and from moving.
CARDIOVASCULAR	Pericarditis. Fever: fast, full pulse
RESPIRATORY	Cough: dry, hacking, hoarse, worse entering warm room. Laryngitis, pleurisy, pneumonia: tenacious mucous. Worse outdoors. Frequent desire to take a long breath to expand lungs. Respiration is difficult, quick, worse on every movement. Appears they dislike pain induced by breathing!
UROGENITAL	Urine: beer-like, brown, hot, red, and scant.
	Ovaritis: right, sensitive to pressure over loin.
	Mastitis: acute. Mammary abscess: hard, hot, painful.
LAMENESS	Painfully stiff back muscles. Bursitis: hot, red. Legs in constant left sided motion. Feet: hot and swollen. Laminitis.
COMPETITION	**Back and joint pain** in working mares. Periodic: oestrous.
SKIN	Greasy. Seborrhoea.
MODALITIES	Agg: bandaging. Eating. Exercise. Heat. Morning. Motion. Noise.
	Amel: chilly water. Lying on painful side. Pressure. Rest.
COMPARE	Arg-n Aster Con Iod Kali-i Spong.
	Works particularly with Apis.
CONSIDER	Major importance in: • Colic. • Joint and muscle lameness. • Mastitis. • Chronic respiratory disease. The main signs are: • Aggravated by any movement. • Dark, irritable lean types. • Severe pain.
POTENCY	12X. 30CH. 200CH.

Bufo

BUFO RANA

Common toad Animal

Nervous system. Dull, sad, oversensitive, and suspicious. Averse to company.

CNS	Epilepsy: anger before fit. Fits at night when sleeping.
	Oversexed, juvenile males.
	Anxiety during ovarian disease.
HEAD	Extremely oversensitive to noise.

UROGENITAL	Ulcerated cervix.
	Mammary cancer: indurate, milk bloody.
	Ovary, uterus: sacroiliacs pain. Polyps.
	Exudates: bloody, offensive.
	Male: impotent juvenile: oversexed.
COMPETITION	May improve temperament in working mares.
SKIN	Injuries suppurate. Pemphigus: pruritic, pustules.
JUVENILE	General improvement in retarded juveniles.
MODALITIES	Agg: wakening. Warm room.
	Amel: chilly air. Water. Solitude.
COMPARE	Aster Bar-c Grat.
CONSIDER	• Epilepsy.
	• Late developers.
	• Lymphangitis.
	• Ovarian and uterine disease.
POTENCY	6X – 12X. 30CH. 200CH.

Bunio-o
BUNIAS ORIENTALIS
Turkish rocket Plant

Angry, irrational, and neurotic individuals. Emaciation. Vertigo. Arthritis and female problems.

GASTROINTESTINAL	Constipation or diarrhoea periodically: days apart.
CARDIOVASCULAR	Lymph gland: cancer.
RESPIRATORY	Dyspnoea: left sided: hoarse, wheezing.
UROGENITAL	Cystitis, nephritis. Urine: bloody with bacteriuria, indol+.
	• Female genitalia: pruritic with nausea.
	• Metritis: exudate: brown to yellow.
	• Pregnancy: bleeding.
LAMENESS	Polyarthritis. Left sided periarticular oedema.
BREEDING	Prophylactically if history of female infertility.
MODALITIES	Agg: fat. Night. Lying too long on one side.
	Amel: open air. Walk.
COMPARE	Ars Bapt Sec.
CONSIDER	• Cancer of lymphatic system.
	• Gestational abnormalities.
POTENCY	12X. 30CH.

Cadm-met
CADMIUM METALLICUM
Cadmium Mineral

Hypersensitive, irritable, lazy and enjoy company. Profound gastroenteritis.

CNS	So weak they appear unconscious. Vertigo.
HEAD	Mouth distorted from osteomyelitis. Jaw trembling. Facial paralysis: left side. Corneal opacity. Night blindness. Pupils uneven.
	Nose: blocked, bloody. Polyps.
GASTROINTESTINAL	Saliva: cold, offensive, salty, stringy. Vomit: black, green, painful. Oesophagus constricted. Stomach carcinoma. Tympanitic colic.

91

	Diarrhoea: black to green, gelatinous clots.
CARDIOVASCULAR	Heart pain with palpitation.
RESPIRATORY	Laryngitis: gagging cough.
UROGENITAL	Urethritis, nephritis. Haematuria, pus.
MODALITIES	Agg: open air. Exercise. Morning.
	Amel: food. Rest.
COMPARE	*Cadmium bromatum* Cadm-br. Violent vomiting.
	Cadmium iodatum Cadm-i. Tympanitic colic pruritic constipation.
	Ars Bry Cadm-s.
CONSIDER	• Carcinoma of the stomach.
	• Dysentery with prostration.
	• IBD.
	• Poisoning from heavy metals.
POTENCY	8X. 30CH. 200CH.

Cadm-s
CADMIUM SULPHURATUM
Cadmium sulphate Mineral

Restless. Dislike company. Role in patients undergoing extensive drug therapy to reduce side effects, without interfering with curative chemotherapy. Often left sided.

GASTROINTESTINAL	Always hungry. PD. PU. Mouth, lips: dry, pruritic.
	Stomach: cancer with persistent vomiting of coffee-like material.
	Colic: tympanitic: improves by bending and eating.
	Diarrhoea: bloody, offensive, bloody.
CARDIOVASCULAR	Haemolytic anaemia in juveniles. Reduce side effects when undergoing chemotherapy without negating beneficial effects.
RESPIRATORY	Coughing: expectorant: bloody, mucopurulent.
LAMENESS	Lumbar: muscular pain and weakness.
SKIN	Lupus: eruptions: dry, lichenous, papules, vesicles.
MODALITIES	Agg: morning. Movement. Walking.
	Amel as eruptions appear. Bending. Bandaging. Cold therapy.
COMPARE	Other Cadmium salts. Ars Bry
CONSIDER	Important:
	• Anaemias that are haemolytic and profound.
	• Chemotherapeutic side effects.
	• Erythema of lupus.
	• Poisoning from heavy metals.
	The general weakness may improve as skin lesions appear.
POTENCY	12X. 30CH. 200CH.

Caj
CAJUPUTUM
Cajput oil Plant

Severe flatulence in hysterical individuals, averse to company.

GASTROINTESTINAL	Hiccoughs. Swollen tongue. Oesophagus: choking, constricted.
	Colic: tympanitic. Dysentery: spasmodic.
UROGENITAL	Urine smells of cats.
LAMENESS	Interesting, dignified walk.
MODALITIES	Agg: night. Five am.
COMPARE	Asaf Bapt Bov Ign Nux-m.
CONSIDER	• Choke of the oesophagus.
	• Tongue swelling of unknown origin.
POTENCY	6X – 12X.

Calc

CALCAREA CARBONICA *HAHNEMANNI*
Carbonate of calcium Mineral

Polycrest. Apprehensive: worse towards evening. Placid and shy, they become confused and easy to discourage as they have fears, of animals, dark, shadows, thunder, trifles. Mood swings from cheerful to anger with violence.

A major constitutional remedy featuring impaired nutrition. Mental or physical weakness from overwork. Chronic abscess, polyps, and exostoses. Pituitary and thyroid dysfunction. Stimulant to the periosteum. Juvenile obesity.

CNS	Epilepsy: backward, deprived juveniles.
HEAD	**Sub-maxillary** glands painfully swollen.
	Cataract. Corneal spots and ulcers. Photophobia. Pupils: chronically dilated.
	Lachrymation outdoors and early morning. Lachrymal ducts: blocked, fistulae.
	Otitis externa: mucopurulent. Polyps: bleed easily.
	Nose, nostrils: blocked, bloody, dry, purulent, ulcerated, yellow snot alternates with colic.
ABDOMEN	Hernia: umbilical: enlarged, hard.
	Liver: painfully swollen.
	Inguinal, mesenteric glands, painfully swollen.
GASTROINTESTINAL	**Appetite** good. Dentition delayed, difficult and gums bleed. Stomatitis: exudate: sour, thick, yellow. Tonsils swollen. Halitosis.
	Parotid fistula.
	Constipation: hard, large, whitish, watery, sour faeces. Prolapsed anus.
	Diarrhoea with good appetite: foetid, undigested food, sour, watery. Neonatal diarrhoea.
RESPIRATORY	Bronchitis, pharyngitis: recurrent. Cough: dry, irritating, nocturnal. **Chest** painful on palpation. Exudate: mucous, thick, yellow.
UROGENITAL	PU: bloody, brown, sour. Or foetid with white sediment. Enuresis.
	Mammae: engorged, hot. Uterine polyps.
	Male. Signs worse after mating. Irritable, weak.
LAMENESS	Neck, wither: painfully stiff.
	Periostitis: shins, splints: juvenile: soft and swollen.
	Arthritic nodes. Stifle bursitis. Distal muscles: painfully weak. Tendonitis. Soles: raw, tender.

COMPETITION	Accelerates healing process in periostitis.
JUVENILE	Young animals particularly 2-y-o racehorses are backward, cough, and produce typical thick yellow mucous exudate.
	Tend to eczema: pimply mange, neonates.
SKIN	Unhealthy: ulcerates easily.
MODALITIES	Agg: exertion: mental or physical. Cold in every form. Moist air. Wet weather. Full moon. Dark.
	Amel: dry climate and weather. Lying on affected side.
COMPARE	Anth Lyc Sil.
CONSIDER	A great anti psoric remedy with a role in the treatment of:
	• Coughing dry, nocturnal, and persistent.
	• Bone abnormalities: including juvenile periostitis.
	• Debility from impaired nutrition.
	• Diarrhoea of undigested food.
	• Eczema in neonates.
	• Otitis externa.
	Often overweight, eat well, lazy, and hate cold.
POTENCY	12X. 30CH. 200CH.

Calc-fl
CALCAREA FLUORICA NATURALIS
Fluoride of lime Mineral

Polycrest. Concentration is poor and when pressed leads to irritability and depression. A powerful tissue remedy where lymph glands are stone hard. Chronically enlarged and damaged veins. Malnutrition of bones. Hard knots in mammae. Cataracts.

HEAD	Scalp ulcers: calloused, hard edges.
	Teeth: hard swelling on mandible over gums.
	Cataract, keratitis, spots on cornea. Conjunctivitis. Palpebral cysts.
	Calcium deposits on tympanum. Sclerosis of middle ear bones, with deafness.
	Otitis media: chronic.
	Rhinitis: atrophic: crusts, dry. Coryza: copious, greenish to yellow, thick.
GASTROINTESTINAL	Tongue: cracked, hardened, indurate, with or without pain. Teeth loose. Vomiting: neonates.
	Pharyngitis: follicular: plugs of thick mucoid exudate.
	Proctitis: helminthiasis: *Oxyuris spp.* Flatulence.
	Perianal fissures: intensely painful.
CARDIOVASCULAR	Endocardium, valves: fibrous deposits.
	Vascular tumour: dilated blood-vessels.
RESPIRATORY	**Spasmodic cough.** Expectoration of tiny lumps of yellow mucous.
UROGENITAL	Mammae: hard knots.
	Testes: cryptorchid. Indurate, hydrocele.
LAMENESS	Lumbar pain. Bone tumour.

	Ligaments: annular and carpal: chronic, hard, irregular lumps. **Joint:** exostoses. Synovitis: chronic: digital: firm lumps in joint capsules.
JUVENILE	**Tendon** contractures or laxity in neonates. Jaw: bony swelling.
SKIN	**Adhesions** and scar tissue after surgery. Chapping and cracks. Fissures or hard skin in extremities. **Ulcers:** edges raised and hard. Surrounding skin: purple and swollen. Fistulous wounds: indolent, indurate. Exudate: thick, yellow, purulent. Fascia: subcutaneous lumps.
MODALITIES	Agg: rest. Changeable weather. Amel: after food. Heat and warm applications. Massage.
COMPARE	Bar-m Calc Calc-p Con Hekla Lap-a Rhus-t Thiosin.
CONSIDER	• Actinomycosis and Actinobacillosis. • Adhesions and scar tissue. • Bone malnutrition. • Cataract. • Chronic infection in juveniles. • Deafness. • Mouth ulceration. • Rhinitis: atrophic and chronic. • Skin fissures and ulceration. • Tendons that are weak or contracted in neonates.
POTENCY	12X. 30CH. 200CH.

Calc-p
CALCAREA PHOSPHORICA
Phosphate of lime Mineral

Polycrest. Natural anxiety becomes anger when aggravated by consolation during fears, dark, thunder. Irritable during teething with restless, wandering. Like Calc but with a greater influence on problems associated with dentition and juvenile bone disease. Juvenile anaemia.

HEAD	Cranial bones: neonate: soft, thin. Cornea: **diffuse opacity** after infection. Otitis: acrid exudate. **Dentition: tardy,** rapid decay.
ABDOMEN	Vomiting of unknown origin in juveniles. Constipation: bleed after hard stool. Diarrhoea at dentition. Perianal fissures.
GASTROINTESTINAL	Anaemia from malnutrition.
UROGENITAL	FLUTD. Balance Ca / P ratios. PU. Back pain. Milk: sour. Orchitis.
LAMENESS	Sacroiliac: **muscle pain and stiffness of** flexors worsens as weather changes.
JUVENILE	Important to establish healthy bone and blood in

95

	neglected juveniles. Neonates nurse poorly from vomiting sour milk. Rapid growth in adolescence. Chronic lymphadenitis.
MODALITIES	Agg: exposure to cold, damp weather. Melting snow. Amel: dry, warm summer.
COMPARE	Other Calciums. Bar-c Psor Sil Sulph.
CONSIDER	• Bone weakness and debility. • Dentition slow. Often tall, skinny, fast-growing juveniles.
POTENCY	6X – 12X. 30CH.

Calc-s
CALCAREA SULPHURICA
Plaster of paris Mineral

Sad, bossy individuals who are jealous, oversensitive, and restless. Fear of birds. Calcium remedy with the most marked effect on abscess, infected eczema, and glandular swellings with copious exudation. Pimples, pustules, and crusts. Thick, lumpy bloody and offensive. Herpes.

HEAD	Eczema: offensive eczema. Conjunctivitis. Deafness. Otitis media. Rhinitis.
GASTROINTESTINAL	Painful hepatitis. Tongue: flabby, clay-like, yellow base. Tonsillitis after abscess ruptures. Peri-anal: abscess, fissure. Diarrhoea: bloody, purulent, slimy.
RESPIRATORY	Fever: cough, purulent expectorant. Laryngitis, pleurisy, empyema.
LAMENESS	Soles are sensitive.
SKIN	Unhealthy, easily infected. Juvenile eczema: dry, lupus.
JUVENILE	Tummy pimples, puppies: adaptive mange.
MODALITIES	Agg: cold. Damp. Exercise. Amel: open air. Heat. Warmth, including hot water. Bandaging.
COMPARE	Bapt Hep Pyrog Sil.
CONSIDER	• Anal abscess and fissures. • Conjunctivitis. • Coughing. • Eczema. • Tonsillitis. Thick, lumpy, yellow, and offensive exudates.
POTENCY	12X. 30CH.

Calen
CALENDULA OFFICINALIS
Marigold Plant

Polycrest. Painful postsurgical neuroma and neuritis where reactions appearing excessive, make them irritable, restless, and fearful creatures.

Remarkable wound healing, including those resistant from chronic granulation and ulceration. Significant antibacterial agent.

Haemostasis after extraction. Must use, even in the absence of the mental picture

HEAD	Eye, lachrymal sac: injury, surgery: infection and pain.
	Deafness: develops slow, distant sounds still heard.
	Nasal exudate: greenish, unilateral.
GASTROINTESTINAL	Vomiting. Ranula.
UROGENITAL	Cervical Injury and warts.
	Metritis, uterine hypertrophy: chronic.
BREEDING	Postpartum injury, bacterial infection.
SKIN	Burns: deep, superficial. Cancer. Granulation, scarring.
	Unpleasant sequels to slow healing wounds.
COMPARE	Arn Ham Hyper Led Symph.
CONSIDER	• Wounds: Acute, chronic.
POTENCY	2X topically. 6X – 12X. 30CH. Topical.

Calth
CALTHA PALUSTRIS
Cowslip Plant

GASTROINTESTINAL	Gastritis and diarrhoea with restlessness.
UROGENITAL	Dysuria. Cervical cancer.
SKIN	Eczema around one eye.
	Pemphigus: bullae surrounded by a ring.
COMPARE	Ars.
CONSIDER	Pemphigus.
POTENCY	4X – 12X. 30CH.

Camph
CAMPHORA
Cinnamomum camphora Camphor Plant

Hahnemann's famous cholera treatment. Fixed, staring look with dilated pupils. Aggressive and destructive. Fear: being alone, night. Vocal.

CNS	Epilepsy with screaming rage. Vertigo.
HEAD	Dilated pupils: fixed, staring look.
	Persistent ozena.
GASTROINTESTINAL	Mouth, tongue: cold, hypersalivation.
	Jaw: clenched.
	Dysentery: disgusting, great weakness.
RESPIRATORY	Laryngitis: dyspnoea, hacking cough: exudate: copious, thick mucous.
UROGENITAL	Retention of urine.
LAMENESS	Back and large joints: muscles and ligaments are stiff and painful.
JUVENILE	**Lifesaver in parvovirus.** Combine with Cupr and Verat.
MODALITIES	Agg: chilly air. Covering. Movement. Night. Touch.
	Amel: warmth.
COMPARE	Ars Carb-v Cup Verat.
CONSIDER	• Food poisoning.
	• Neonatal Diarrhoea – parvovirus.
	• Salmonellosis.

	• Shock.
POTENCY	4X – 8X. 30CH.

Cann-i
CANNABIS INDICA
Hashish Marijuana Plant

Mental instability with excitement and an odd, stupid look with restlessness. In view of its popularity, worth stating C indica is more potent in pain control. May be more relaxing and calming than C sativa.

HEAD	Epilepsy. Involuntary shaking. Noise sensitive.
GASTROINTESTINAL	Tenacious mucous sticks to lips.
	Pyloric spasm. Tympany.
RESPIRATORY	Asthma: deep breathing, slow pulse.
UROGENITAL	Dribble slimy mucous.
	Back pain referred from sex organs.
	Penis: drips thick, white mucous.
LAMENESS	Ataxia: weak, painful back muscles. Sensitive soles.
MODALITIES	Agg: morning.
	Amel: chilly water. Fresh air. Rest.
COMPARE	Agar Anh Bell Cann-s Hyos Lach Stram.
CONSIDER	• Back weakness associated with deteriorating behaviour.
POTENCY	4X – 12X.

Cann-s
CANNABIS SATIVA
American hemp Plant

Deteriorating behaviour including mood swings ends in confusion and excitement. Hurried individuals swing from being cheerful, to dull. Fear the dark and noise. Slowly progressive. More popular for recreational use with a tendency to energise.

CNS	Epilepsy: tetanic spasms, unconsciousness.
HEAD	Opacity: cornea, lens.
GASTROINTESTINAL	Choke on swallowing.
CARDIOVASCULAR	Palpitation. Pericarditis.
RESPIRATORY	Pneumonia: coughing, rales, wheezing.
	Exudate: bloody, greenish, thick.
UROGENITAL	Cystitis, urethritis. Exudate: acrid, bloody, mucopurulent.
	FLUTD with blockage.
	Habitual foetal loss.
	Balanitis. Orchitis.
MODALITIES	Agg: climbing stairs. Lying down. Travel.
	Amel: slow exercise. Rest.
COMPARE	Apis Cann-i Canth Cop Kali-chls Thuj.
CONSIDER	• Balanitis and Orchitis.
	• Behavioural deterioration.
	• Corneal opacity.
	• Cystitis, urethritis.
POTENCY	4X – 8X. 30CH.

CANTHARIS VESICATORIA
Spanish fly Animal

Fear of approach, touch, and water. Violent inflammation of urinary tract when pain makes them deteriorate from irritability to vocal rage.

CNS	Epilepsy followed by unconsciousness.
HEAD	Ophthalmia: loss of vision.
	Eczema: painful, vesicles.
GASTROINTESTINAL	Peritonitis. Swallowing of liquids difficult.
	Tongue, mouth: deeply furred, vesicles have red edges.
	Dysentery: painful.
RESPIRATORY	Dyspnoea. Epistaxis and pleurisy.
	Cough: dry, frequent.
UROGENITAL	Painful cystitis, nephritis. Urinate drop by drop. FLUTD.
	Dysentery.
LAMENESS	Referred spinal pain. Tender soles.
SKIN	Insect bites.
	Burns. Sunburn.
	Genital eczema: pruritic, raw, vesicles.
MODALITIES	Agg: drinking chilly water. Touch. Urinating.
	Amel: cold bandaging, therapy. Grooming after initial resistance.
COMPARE	Apis Ars Merc-c.
CONSIDER	• Cystitis, urethritis.
	• Dysentery.
	Always intolerably painful.
POTENCY	4X – 12X. 30CH.

CAPSICUM ANNUUM
Cayenne pepper Plant

Lazy, irritable, and easily offended, these homesick, often obese animals need warmth. Suppuration of mucous membranes in awkward, confused, and fearful individuals.

HEAD	Otitis media: severe, purulent. Head shaking, whining.
GASTROINTESTINAL	Stomatitis: mucous, tenacious, offensive, ulcerated.
	PD: great, shudder when drinking. Diphtheria.
	Dysentery.
RESPIRATORY	Dyspnoea with bronchospasm.
	Cough: dry, explosive.
UROGENITAL	Cystitis, urethritis. FLUTD: bloody, painful.
	Male impotence: atrophy of testes.
LAMENESS	Generalised painful stiffness of large muscles as movement begins.
SKIN	Rodent ulcer.
MODALITIES	Agg: drafty open air.
	Amel: food. Gentle, continuous exercise. Heat.
COMPARE	Bell Lyc Puls.
CONSIDER	• Diphtheria.
	• Purulent otitis media.
	• Rodent ulcer.

POTENCY	6X – 12X. 30CH.

CARBO ANIMALIS

Animal charcoal Animal

Anxiety at night. Being averse to company, confusion exaggerates their fears: of crowds, dark. Homesick. Sad. Quiet. Vertigo Debilitated geriatrics. Painful, chronic, and destructive with offensive exudations.

HEAD	Vision reduced. Purulent otitis externa.
GASTROINTESTINAL	Gums: mucous, swollen, vesicles.
	Colic: tympanitic.
CARDIOVASCULAR	Lymphadenitis: axillary, parotid.
RESPIRATORY	Pleurisy. Exudate: fluent, greenish, mucous.
UROGENITAL	PU. Acrid genital pruritus.
	Mammary: cancer: indurate, nodular, painful.
	Uterine cancer.
LAMENESS	Painful stiffness of large muscles. Strain of carpus and hocks.
SKIN	Congested and discoloured. Dermatitis: excoriating, fissures: moist, painful.
	Warts and wartlike, soft tumours: face, genitals.
GERIATRIC	General debility reduces healing.
	Colic: tympanitic after eating.
MODALITIES	Agg: loss of body fluids.
	Amel: open air. Cold, dry weather. Eating.
COMPARE	Bad Carb-v Con Merc-i Sep Sulph Plb.
CONSIDER	• Cancer of the mammae.
	• Chronic colic.
	• Geriatric debility.
	• Skin ulcers.
POTENCY	6X – 12X. 30CH.

CARBO VEGETABILIS

Wood charcoal Plant

Anxious, apprehensive, and fearful of dark, of strangers and odd, unreasonable situations. Confusion with poor concentration makes them insecure and desire company and carried. Oversensitive, which leads to them being irritable, unreasonable, and easily offended.

Overweight, lazy creatures. Easily fatigue. Recovery slow.

Mental and physical collapse.

HEAD	Eyes agglutinated on awakening.
	Otitis externa: part of a systemic problem. Cerumen peels off in flakes.
	Nose: cracks, red, scabby, painful.
	Epistaxis with every exertion.
GASTROINTESTINAL	Mouth: ulcerated: gums bleed. Tongue: thickly coated brown to white or yellow with bloody, dark exudation.
	Liver pain.

	Colic: tympanitic of the most severe kind. **Will not lie down.** Extensive offensive flatus.
CARDIOVASCULAR	A weak, poorly oxygenated circulation.
RESPIRATORY	Cough: hoarse, spasmodic. Gag from thick expectorate.
	Asthma: noisy, mucous rales, epistaxis.
UROGENITAL	Metritis: exudate: acrid, greenish milky, thick, greenish. Genital pruritus.
LAMENESS	Hind quarters: flabby, weak muscles.
	Circulation: poor to extremities. Chronic laminitis.
SKIN	Weak circulation causes falling hair. Evening pruritus. Wounds heal slow.
	Moist, offensive exudate.
GERIATRIC	Asthma, COPD: overweight ponies prone to laminitis.
FEVER	Hectic, exhausting sweating.
COMPARE	Ars Carb-a Chin Kali-c Lyc.
CONSIDER	Important: • Debility. • Digestive upsets after food changes. • Laminitis. • Prevents sequels of overeating. • Toxaemia. Remember patients are often geriatric and chronically weak.
POTENCY	6X – 12X. 30CH.

Carbn-o
CARBONEUM OXYGENISATUM
Carbonous oxide Mineral

Skin and nervous problems in sleepy, easily excited individuals.

CNS	Cerebral oedema with circling, unconsciousness, and vertigo.
HEAD	Optic nerve: atrophy, neuritis. Ocular paralysis.
	Pupillary reaction weak. Retinal haemorrhage.
SKIN	Pemphigus where vesicles follow nerve paths.
COMPARE	*Carboneum hydrogenisatum* Carbn-h. Tetanic spasms. Eyeballs oscillate.
	Arn Nat-s.
CONSIDER	• Cerebral irritation from viral infection. • Pemphigus.
POTENCY	6X – 12X. 30CH.

Carbn-s
CARBONEUM SULPHURATUM
Bisulphide of carbon Plant

Anxious individuals that lacking in concentration may exhibit marked mood swings when, from dull and sad, they swing to being irritable, excitable, and angry.
Fear: dark and night. Tissue degeneration.

CNS	Cranial nerves insensitive. Paralysis. Unconscious.
HEAD	Optic disc: atrophy, cloudy, pale. Vessels: congested.

	Sight and hearing poor.
GASTROINTESTINAL	Lip ulcers. Noisy, painful flatus.
UROGENITAL	Male: Semen quality variable: good to poor.
	Libido fluctuates from good to nothing.
LAMENESS	Neuritis: ataxia and muscle cramping.
	Oedema: extremities.
SKIN	Cancer: develops slow. Eczema: chronic, pruritic. Skin lacks sensitivity. Wounds infect easily. Furuncles and ulcers.
MODALITIES	Agg: bathing, After breakfast. Damp warm weather.
	Amel: open air.
COMPARE	Acid-sal Caust Carb-s Carb-v Cinch Potassium salts. Rad Sulph.
CONSIDER	• Neuritis with loss of sensitivity.
POTENCY	8X. 30CH. 200CH.

Carc
CARCINOSINUM BURNETT
Carcinosin Nosode Animal

Miasm. Shy, hypersensitive creatures who enjoy work when well-treated, but easily offended. Fear: anticipation and thunder. Insomnia. Cancer prophylactic if family history.

GASTROINTESTINAL	Diabetes mellitus. Helminthiasis: anaemia.
	Colic: constipation, impaction, tympany.
RESPIRATORY	Asthma, bronchitis: tickling cough. Exudate: acrid, thick.
LAMENESS	Chronic, one sided DJD. Osteomyelitis.
SKIN	Lipoma: benign, small.
JUVENILE	Chronic debility after illness.
MODALITIES	Agg: chilly air. Washing.
	Amel: evening. Rest.
COMPARE	Maland Sulph Thuj Tub Vac Variol.
CONSIDER	• Asthma and bronchitis as sequel to virus.
POTENCY	30CH. 200CH.

Carp-b
CARPINUS BETULUS
Hornbeam (Ironwood) tree Plant

Often weak and exhausted from chronic low grade respiratory disease.

Immune modulation with a particular role in conditions associated with excessive mucous production in the respiratory tract.

RESPIRATORY	Cough: persistent from excessive mucous production in the upper tracts and sinuses.
COMPARE	Ant-t Dulc Lyc.
CONSIDER	• Persistent coughing.
POTENCY	2X – 4X.

Cart-a
CARTILAGO ARTICULUS
Cartilage Nosode Animal

Of value when used concurrently with selected arthritis remedies to support and enhance effectiveness.

LAMENESS	DJD. Dysplasias and physis. Polyarthritis. Ringbone.
COMPARE	Specifies specific nosodes.
	Cart-eq, etc. Lith-c Mang.
CONSIDER	• Arthritis.
	• DJD.
	• Dysplasias and physis.
POTENCY	2X – 4X in treatment. 30CH for prevention.
	Species specific where possible.

Cast-eq
CASTOR EQUI
Equine ergot Animal

UROGENITAL	Nipples cracked and painfully swollen. Female genital warts.
LAMENESS	Improved exercise after strengthening brittle hoof and nails.
SKIN	Inadequate quality. Thickened and distorted.
COMPARE	Acid-oxal Calc Graph Hipp.
CONSIDER	• Brittle feet in horses.
	• Nipple problems when suckling.
POTENCY	6X – 12X.

Caul
CAULOPHYLLUM THALICTROIDES
Blue cohosh Plant

Polycrest. Fearful during pregnancy with severe irritability and nocturnal restlessness. Main sphere is in pregnancy and parturition.

BREEDING	Spasmodic uterine activity during late pregnancy threatens premature labour. Contractions: strong before cervix dilates.
	Afterbirth: expulsion: delayed, painful.
LAMENESS	Pain and stiffness of digit joints.
SKIN	Aesthetic discoloration of hair after neutering.
COMPARE	Cimic Gels Puls Sep Viol-o.
CONSIDER	• Habitual abortion.
	• Modulate excessive contractions.
	• Premature labour.
	• Ringwomb where cervix does not dilate.
POTENCY	2X – 6X. 30CH.

Caust
CAUSTICUM HAHNEMANN
Tinctura acris sine kali Mineral

Polycrest. Interesting individuals who respond to good management. Amorous. Anxious. Excitable: open air but fear approach, crowds, noise, and unexpected, irrational events. Slow developing and chronic illness develops after sudden, severe emotional trauma. May develop into long-lasting grief leading to an oversensitive phase when easily offended.

Sleepy: can hardly keep awake yet are restless and suspicious at night.

Chronic arthritic, paralytic pains in muscular and fibrous tissues leads to joint deformity with progressive weakness. Local paralysis of vocal cords, muscles of swallowing, of tongue, eyelids, face, bladder, and extremities.

Neonates and juveniles with walking difficulties. Often on left.

HEAD	Cataract. Paralysis of ocular muscles.
	Eyelid: inflammation: ptosis, ulceration.
	Otitis media: chronic catarrh.
	Dental fistula. Facial, jaw bones: pain, paralysis: right.
	Warts. Nose: chronic nasal mucous. Pimples, scales, and ulcers.
GASTROINTESTINAL	Arthritis of mandible. Gums bleed. Difficult to open the mouth. Tongue paralysis.
	Colic: impaction: hard to soft, mucous, small, tough faeces. Tenesmus. Pruritus. Fistula. Partial paralysis.
RESPIRATORY	**Laryngitis** with chest pain. 'Roaring' worse during early morning exercise. Voice is weak, lost.
UROGENITAL	**Urination** involuntary: coughing, excited, sleeping, sneezing. Retention post-surgical.
	Metritis: worse at night.
	Uterine inertia: labour ceases or slows.
LAMENESS	Neck, withers, and sacroiliac: stiff, **left**.
	Joints: carpal, hock: deformed, enlarged, painfully weak. Muscles: front left leg are weak.
	Tendon: contracted, tight, weak.
JUVENILE	Foals and calves born with contracted tendons and weak joints. May walk on floppy fetlock joints.
GERIATRIC	Arthritis of digits with deformity and pain.
SKIN	Severe burns. Old scars reopen. Sores in folds.
	Warts and sarcoid: bleed, jagged, large. Often on extremities.
MODALITIES	Agg: music. Weather: cold dry air. Fine, cold winds.
	Amel: warmth. Damp, warm weather.
COMPARE	Am-p Ars Gels Nat-m Puls Rhus-t.
CONSIDER	An important remedy to consider in:
	• Arthritis with deformity.
	• Bladder incontinence.
	• Joints contracted or floppy in neonates.
	• Lameness of back and muscles.
	• Paralysis of isolated parts.
	Often juveniles and elderly are weak, wrinkled and worn out.
POTENCY	10X. 30CH. 200CH.

Cean

CEANOTHUS AMERICANUS
New Jersey tea Plant

GASTROINTESTINAL	Painfully enlarged liver and spleen in excitable individuals with anaemia.
	Diabetes mellitus. PU.

	Diarrhoea with tenesmus.
RESPIRATORY	Dyspnoea: chronic, mucous cough.
UROGENITAL	PU. Constant urge to urinate. Glycosuria: frothy, green urine.
MODALITIES	Agg: lying on left side. Movement.
	Amel: warm weather.
COMPARE	*Ceanothus thrysiflorus* Cean-r. Tonsillitis and pharyngitis.
	Agar Berb Cedr Myric.
CONSIDER	• Anaemia.
	• Splenic disease.
POTENCY	6X. 30CH.

Cedr
CEDRON
Simaruba ferroginea Rattlesnake bean Animal

Restless individuals resent confinement. Vocal, scream before and during fits. Parasitic blood disease and infected bite wounds.

HEAD	**Facial neuralgia: Severe,** left, pain.
	Iritis with profuse, acrid lachrymation.
CARDIOVASCULAR	Anaemia of parasitism including Babesiosis, Erhlichia.
LAMENESS	Spinal arthritis. Widespread synovitis.
SKIN	Bite induced abscess and cellulitis.
COMPARE	Ars Chin.
CONSIDER	• Babesiosis with nervous signs.
	• Cat-bite abscess and cellulitis.
POTENCY	4X. 30CH.

Cench
CENCHRIS CONTORTRIX
Copperhead snake Animal

Dyspnoea with great restlessness and mood swings in jealous, suspicious individuals. Dreamy.

HEAD	Facial paralysis: frontal eminence.
	Toothache: left, painful.
UROGENITAL	Nymphomania and satyrs.
LAMENESS	Spine: **right:** sitting / lying down difficult.
MODALITIES	Agg: afternoon. Night. Lying down. Pressure.
COMPARE	Ars Lach.
CONSIDER	• Dyspnoea.
	• Facial right sided paralysis with great local swelling.
POTENCY	30CH. 200CH.

Ip
CEPHAELIS ACUMINATA
Ipecacuanha Plant

HEAD	Facial muscle twitch. Lachrymation: acrid, painful.
GASTROINTESTINAL	Great salivation with constant vomiting.

105

	Severe dysentery.
RESPIRATORY	Kennel Cough with haemoptysis.
	Asthma: recurrent.
UROGENITAL	Uterine haemorrhage: arterial, flows freely.
LAMENESS	Spasmodic jerking of front leg.
	Hind limb held in extension.
MODALITIES	Agg: moist warm wind. Lying down. Periodically.
COMPARE	*Emetinum* Emet. The alkaloid.
	Ant-t Ars Cham Puls.
CONSIDER	• Persistent, severe vomiting.
POTENCY	12X. 30CH. 200CH.

Cere-b
CEREUS BONPLANDII
Night blooming cactus Plant

CARDIOVASCULAR	Endocarditis. Hypertrophy. Mitral valve insufficiency. Palpitation with severe pain.
RESPIRATORY	Dyspnoea. Haemoptysis.
UROGENITAL	Bladder muscle spasm, retention of bloody, clotted urine.
	Left sided back pain during oestrous.
LAMENESS	Back: pain may extend down legs to stifles.
	Painful digits with distal oedema.
FEVER	Persistent, low grade with haemorrhage and ice-cold sweats.
MODALITIES	Agg: lying on left side. Noon. Walking.
	Amel: open air.
COMPARE	Cact Conv Dig Spig Kalm Naja.
CONSIDER	• Cardiac disease with severe pain.
POTENCY	2X – 6X.

Chel
CHELIDONIUM MAJUS
Greater celandine Plant

Bossy, aggressive Individuals, reluctant to exercise who develop painful, debilitating liver disease.

GASTROINTESTINAL	Jaundice from enlarged painful liver. Vomiting.
	Tongue: flabby, swollen, teeth imprint.
	Colic: diarrhoea alternates with impaction. Faeces: hard, round, bright yellow to pasty balls. Proctitis.
RESPIRATORY	Dyspnoea with rales and an exhausting, harsh, sharp cough.
UROGENITAL	PU is dark, turbid, yellow, and foams.
LAMENESS	Stiff **right**: back muscle pain referred from liver. Paralytic rigidity of distal joints. Bones: metacarpal and others, painful.
SKIN	Dry and wilted looking. Pruritic, painful, yellow pustules. Old spreading painful ulcers.
MODALITIES	Agg: lying on right side. Early mornings. Motion. Touch. Changeable weather.

	Amel: food. Defecating. Firm pressure.
COMPARE	Ars Bry Lyc Nux-v Op Pod Sang Sulph.
CONSIDER	• Painful hepatitis.
POTENCY	4X – 8X. 30CH.

Chelo
CHELONE GLABRA
Snakehead Plant

GASTROINTESTINAL	Hepatitis. Jaundice. Gastritis. Helminthiasis.
COMPARE	Chel Lyc.
CONSIDER	• Liver disease secondary to helminthiasis.
POTENCY	2X – 6X.

Chim
CHIMAPHILA UMBELLATA
Ground ivy Pipsissewa Plant

HEAD	Painful left eye with epiphora.
GASTROINTESTINAL	PD. Toothache aggravated by eating and exercise.
CARDIOVASCULAR	Left sided cancer of lymph glands.
UROGENITAL	Cystitis, nephritis: offensive. PU: haematuria, mucous, tenesmus, turbid. Female genitalia: pruritic, painful, swollen.
	Mammae: atrophy. Milk: excessive.
	Cancer: Non-ulcerative, painful. Prostatitis.
MODALITIES	Agg: cold floor. Damp weather.
	Amel: walking.
COMPARE	Epig Led Uva.
CONSIDER	• Cystitis, nephritis
	• Mammary cancer.
POTENCY	6X – 12X. 30CH.

Chin-ar
CHININUM ARSENICOSUM
Arsenite of quinine Mineral

Chronic infection associated with great weakness from anaemia. Vertigo.

HEAD	Severe acrid lachrymation. Photophobia. Spasm of eyelids.
GASTROINTESTINAL	Anorexia. PD. Tongue: furred, slimy, yellow. Gastritis.
CARDIOVASCULAR	Myocardial insufficiency: post virus.
	Relapsing fever. Anaemia from parasitism such as Babesiosis and helminthiasis.
	Significant antibacterial agent.
RESPIRATORY	Dyspnoea with collapse.
COMPARE	Bapt Chin Chin-s.
CONSIDER	• Babesiosis.
POTENCY	4X – 12X. 30CH.

Chin-s
CHININUM SULPHURICUM
Sulphite of quinine Mineral

Anaemia with nervous signs including headaches. Vertigo caused by blood parasitism.

UROGENITAL	Albuminuria and haematuria. Urine: clay-like, greasy, turbid.
LAMENESS	Spinal pain: neck to thorax.
SKIN	Pruritic erythema with pustules. Shrivelled.
MODALITIES	Fever at 3pm.
COMPARE	Ars Chin-ar.
CONSIDER	• Babesiosis, particularly with fever and nervous signs.
POTENCY	4X – 8X. 30CH. 200CH.

Chion
CHIONANTHUS VIRGINICUM
Fringe tree Plant

GASTROINTESTINAL	Angry, irritable. Hepatitis and pancreatitis.
	Diabetes mellitus.
	Tongue: furred, thick. Jaundice.
	Constipation: clay coloured, pasty, soft, yellow.
UROGENITAL	PU: dark, high SG, glycosuria. Prostatomegaly.
SKIN	Pruritic and moist. Jaundice.
MODALITIES	Agg: jarring. Movement.
	Amel: Lying on abdomen.
COMPARE	Berb Calc Card-m Cean Chel Cinch Lept Podo.
CONSIDER	• Hepatitis.
POTENCY	4X – 12X.

Chlol
CHLORALUM HYDRATUM
Chloral hydrate Mineral

Urticaria. Sad and vocal at night. Fearful on awakening.
Hysteria during pregnancy and parturition.

CNS	Cerebral oedema from inflammation.
HEAD	Conjunctivitis: epiphora: watery.
RESPIRATORY	Asthma: dyspnoea, sleeplessness.
SKIN	Pruritic urticaria after a chill. Purpura.
MODALITIES	Agg: chilling. Eating. Night.
COMPARE	Apis Bell Op.
CONSIDER	• Urticaria.
POTENCY	12X. 30CH.

Chloram
CHLORAMPHENICOLUM
Chloramphenicol antibiotic Mineral

Confused, sad and restless individuals. A growing reputation in diarrhoea.

HEAD	Epistaxis. Otitis interna: right.
GASTROINTESTINAL	Anterior enteritis. Colitis: diarrhoea: chronic, neonatal. IBD.
LAMENESS	Gonitis: right, dry.
SKIN	Urticaria.

MODALITIES	Agg: after eating.
	Amel: gentle massage. Wrapping.
COMPARE	Ars Verat Rhus-t.
CONSIDER	• Arthritis with dry, sticky joint.
	• Neonatal and juvenile diarrhoea aggravated by drugs.
POTENCY	12X. 30CH.

Chlf
CHLOROFORMIUM
Chloroform anaesthetic Mineral

Anaesthetic overdose. Epilepsy with profound muscular relaxation.

HEAD	Facial chorea with rapid twitching.
	Eyelids: open, close rapid. Pupils: contracted.
RESPIRATORY	Dyspnoea with short shallow rhythm.
	Cough: dry, ticklish, nocturnal.
UROGENITAL	PD and PU.
COMPARE	Ether: postsurgical bronchitis.
CONSIDER	• Anaesthetic overdose.
POTENCY	4X – 12X. 30CH.
	Greater than 8X for competition animals.

Chlorpr
CHLORPROMAZINUM
Chlorpromazine Mineral

A growing reputation in the management of behavioural problems in dominant, irritable patients. May be sad, indifferent and concentrate poorly. Cerebral inflammatory conditions.

CNS	Ataxia. Cushing's disease. Diabetes insipidus. Encephalitis. Epilepsy. Facial paralysis.
HEAD	Blepharitis. Conjunctivitis. Keratitis.
GASTROINTESTINAL	Hepatitis: jaundice. Diabetes mellitus. Gastric ulcers. Stomatitis.
CARDIOVASCULAR	Arrhythmia. Agranulocytosis.
	Capillary fragility. Low platelet count.
RESPIRATORY	Asthma, COPD, emphysema, pneumothorax. Bloody cough. Soft palate disease.
UROGENITAL	PU. Hypergalactia. Prostatitis. Prostatomegaly. Impotence.
SKIN	Dark, progressive pigmentation. Urticaria. Photosensitization.
MODALITIES	Agg: evening.
COMPARE	Anh Cic Phos Sabal Syph Tub.
CONSIDER	• Encephalitis.
	• Gastric ulceration.
	• Prostate disorders.
POTENCY	12X. 30CH.

Chlor

109

CHLORUM
Chlorine gas in water Mineral

Great mood swings. Nymphomania. Severe choking respiratory disease.

HEAD	Rhinitis: acrid, excoriation, fluent, severe.
RESPIRATORY	Cyanosis. Severe spasm of the rima glottis. Asthma and bronchitis. Dyspnoea: choking, loud prolonged rales, sudden. Inspiration easier than expiration.
COMPARE	Brom.
CONSIDER	• Asthma. • Spasm of rima glottis including postsurgical.
POTENCY	6X. 30CH. 200CH.

Chol
CHOLESTERINUM
Cholesterol nosode Animal

COMPARE	Berb Chel Lyc.
CONSIDER	• Liver disease.
POTENCY	30CH. 200CH.

Chrysar
CHRYSAROBINUM
Goa powder Plant

HEAD	Blepharitis. Conjunctivitis. Keratitis. Photophobia. Otitis externa: crusts, thick, scabs. Ear may appear one huge single scab.
SKIN	Offensive pruritic eruptions with confluent, crusty, dry, thick scabs over pus.
COMPARE	Psor Seneg.
CONSIDER	• Eczema with crusty, disgusting scabs.
POTENCY	6X – 12X. 30CH.

Cic
CICUTA VIROSA
Water hemlock Plant

Severe neurological disturbances with marked mood swings. Change from being cheerful to become distrustful and violent, particularly before fits. May begin with them becoming sad and suspicious.

Fear of people is severe, averse to company. May appear insane. Extremely vocal.

CNS	Encephalitis and meningitis. Opisthotonos, torticollis: fall to the side. Fearful screaming sessions precede fits. Severest spasm of neck muscles. Drag head backwards. Jerk violently.
HEAD	Pupils alternate between contracted and dilated. Fixed staring look. Strabismus.
GASTROINTESTINAL	Pica: swallowing difficult. Grind teeth.
RESPIRATORY	Dyspnoeic owing to severe muscle spasms.
SKIN	Crusty eruptions: pustular, yellow. **No pruritus**.
MODALITIES	Agg: cold. Touch. Amel: warmth.

COMPARE	*Cicuta maculata* Cic-m. Similar, more powerful. Bell Con Oena.
CONSIDER	Important in behavioural disturbances: • CCN, encephalitis, meningitis, tetanus. • Canine distemper complications. • *Clostridial spp* infections.
POTENCY	12X. 30CH. 200CH.

Cimx
CIMEX LECTULARIUS
Acanthia lectularia Bedbug Animal

LAMENESS	Tight hamstrings in anxious, angry, destructive puppies and rehomed juveniles.
MODALITIES	Agg: chill. Exercise. Amel: rest.
COMPARE	Cham.
CONSIDER	• Destructive puppies.
POTENCY	12X. 30CH.

Cimic
CIMICIFUGA RACEMOSA
Actea racemosa Black cohosh Plant

Apprehensive. Easily excited when they show fear of touch and travel. Sad, indifferent, restless, suspicious, and easily startled. Chorea. Photophobia and oversensitive to noise. Severe neuralgic pains in females.

GASTROINTESTINAL	PU. Vomiting. Pharyngitis: left. Constipation alternates with Diarrhoea.
RESPIRATORY	Cough: dry, short, spasmodic.
UROGENITAL	PU. Habitual foetal loss. Ovaritis. Salpingitis. Delayed ovulation.
BREEDING	Improve ovulation. Maintain early pregnancy.
LAMENESS	Spine: severe muscle spasm from spinal nerve neuritis. Painful sacroiliac, hip, and hock. Ovarian pains, referred: erratic, cyclical.
SKIN	Excessive pigmentation in female neonates and juveniles.
COMPETITION	Erratic back pains in working mares with ovarian problems.
MODALITIES	Agg: chilly morning. During oestrous. Amel: eating. Walking quietly. Warmth.
COMPARE	Agar Arist Caul Lil-t Puls.
CONSIDER	Important: • Habitual abortion. • Lameness from neuralgia. • Ovaritis with infertility. • Pyometra with nervous signs. These patients are anxious, sad, and easily discouraged.
POTENCY	4X – 12X. 30CH. 200CH.

111

Chin

CINCHONA SUCCIRUBRA

Peruvian bark Plant

Anxious, indifferent, and easily provoked to dangerous anger when unable to cope with their fear of animals, dogs, examination, and noise. May suddenly be very vocal with great restlessness. Debility after fluid loss.

CNS	Vertigo on awakening.
HEAD	Photophobia. Nose bleeds on awakening.
GASTROINTESTINAL	Liver and spleen enlarged. Hungry, yet poor appetite. Jaundice. Hiccough. Vomit undigested food.
CARDIOVASCULAR	Anaemia.
	Arrhythmia: rapid, weak beats followed by strong beats.
RESPIRATORY	Dyspnoea of asthma: epistaxis. Cough: constant, suffocative. Painful left lung.
UROGENITAL	Chronic painful nephritis. Pyuria. Debilitated breeders.
LAMENESS	Generalised muscle pain over back, referred from kidney.
SKIN	Gentle palpation resented then improves on pressure. Eczema: local glands: indurate, swollen.
MODALITIES	Agg: alternate days. Bending. Drafts. After eating. Night. Vital fluid loss.
	Amel: bending double. Open air. Pressure. Warmth. Wrapping.
COMPARE	Ars Cedr Chin-ar Chin-s.
CONSIDER	• Debility from fluid loss.
	• Chronic, purulent nephritis.
	• Chronic purulent respiratory disease.
	• Pre- and post-surgery.
	The great exhaustion and fluid loss are important signs.
POTENCY	4X – 12X. 30CH.

Cinnm

CINNAMOMUM CEYLANICUM

Ceylon cinnamon Plant

Control of arterial haemorrhage. Pain of cancer.

HEAD	EIPH: arterial, profuse.
GASTROINTESTINAL	Rectum: arterial haemorrhage.
RESPIRATORY	EIPH. Arterial. Often diagnosed endoscopically in trachea after work.
UROGENITAL	Postpartum arterial haemorrhage.
COMPETITION	Can prevent loss of use in racehorses affected by EIPH of physiological origin. Combines well with Mill and Trill.
MODALITIES	Agg: exercise.
	Amel: rest.
COMPARE	Ip Sil Tril.
CONSIDER	• Arterial haemorrhage.
	• EIPH.

CAUTION	*Aconitum napellus* interferes with its action.
POTENCY	6X − 12X: preventative. 30CH treatment.

Cist
CISTUS CANADENSIS
Canadian rock rose Plant

Apprehensive, anxious, and restless at night. Anti-psoric with powerful action in chronic glandular problems.

HEAD	Disgusting, open cancer of the face.
	Lupus: right: crusty lupus over zygomatic arch.
	Otitis externa.
	Sinusitis. Exudates: crusty, offensive, purulent, watery.
	Cancer of neck glands.
GASTROINTESTINAL	Pyorrhoea. PD of lesser amounts. Glossitis and tonsillitis.
RESPIRATORY	Frequent recurrent respiratory infection. Epistaxis.
UROGENITAL	Mastitis: chronic, indurate.
LAMENESS	Carpitis.
SKIN	Eczema: chronic, small painful pimples. Lupus. Skin cracked, dry, hard. Sepsis after bites.
MODALITIES	Agg: chilly air. Excitement. Exertion. Movement. Touch. Amel: after eating. Expectoration.
COMPARE	Arg-n Calc Carb-a Con.
CONSIDER	• Lymphoid cancer.
POTENCY	6X − 12X. 30CH.

Coloc
CITRULLUS COLOCYNTHIS
Bitter cucumber Plant

Polycrest. Pain is often severe. Of particular importance when associated with angry, easily irritated individuals. Colic and spinal problems respond well. Angry and dangerous because they will bite and kick. During painful colic attacks they prove difficult to examine but respond fast to treatment.

GASTROINTESTINAL	Hunger. Colic: throw themselves around, difficult to manage, requiring lots of restraint.
	Faeces: jelly-like to dysentery.
LAMENESS	Painful. Lumbar to sacroiliac. Hip, stifle, and hamstring. Hind limb tendon strains.
MODALITIES	Agg: anger. **Resistance.** Restraint.
	Amel: curling up. Rolling. Warmth.
COMPARE	Anth Cocc Dios Mag-p Merc Plb.
CONSIDER	• **Colic.** Violent pain, roll, and curl up.
POTENCY	12X. 30CH. 200CH.

Clem
CLEMATIS ERECTA
Virgins bower Plant

Sad, dull irritable individuals that fear being alone and irrational fears. Easily become homesick. Significant role in the reproductive tract

113

HEAD	Neuralgia: facial, painful.
	Blepharitis, conjunctivitis, iritis: chronic pustular. Pain in Meibomian glands.
	Blisters on nostrils.
CARDIOVASCULAR	Lymphadenitis of sub maxillary and other glands.
UROGENITAL	Urethritis: recurrent: drops, painful.
	Cancer: mammary: indurated. mammary cancer.
	Cryptorchid. Orchitis: right, painful. Scrotum swollen.
SKIN	Severe pruritus with scabs, scales, and vesicles on face and feet.
JUVENILE	Cryptorchid in neonates.
MODALITIES	Agg: movement. Night. Touch.
	Amel: open air.
COMPARE	*Clematis vitalba* Clem-vit. Skin ulcers.
CONSIDER	• Cancer of mammae.
	• Eczema, particularly on face and feet.
	• Orchitis.
POTENCY	4X. 30CH.

Cob-n
COBALTUM NITRICUM
Cobalt nitrate Mineral

Great fatigue. Back pain better for exercise.

CNS	Encephalitis. Meningitis. Neuralgia. Hemiplegia.
HEAD	Conjunctivitis. Keratitis. Ophthalmia. Deaf.
	Rhinitis: epistaxis, pus.
GASTROINTESTINAL	Appetite poor. Morning vomit. Constipation or diarrhoea.
CARDIOVASCULAR	Pericarditis, pleurisy. Anaemia in juvenile females. Leukaemia.
UROGENITAL	Metritis, fibroids: bloody. Ovaritis.
	Orchitis.
LAMENESS	Juveniles with spinal developmental problems.
MODALITIES	Agg: awakening in morning.
	Amel: afternoon. Evening. Eructation.
COMPARE	Ferr Merc.
CONSIDER	• Brain disorders.
	• Spinal weakness in juveniles.
	Profound fatigue is always present.
POTENCY	12X. 30CH.

Cocain
COCAINUM HYDROCHLORICUM
Alkaloid of *coca* Plant

CNS	Ataxia. Chorea. Paralysis: local sensory.
HEAD	Pupils: dilated, insensitive to light.
GASTROINTESTINAL	Poor appetite. Swallowing difficult: constricted, dry, paralysed throat.
	Rectal haemorrhage.
COMPARE	Coca.

CONSIDER	• Ataxia.
	• Chorea.
	• Paralysis.
POTENCY	12X. 30CH. 200CH.

COCCULUS INDICUS
Indian cockle Animal

Anxious, dull, indifferent, and apprehensive creatures that startle easily, and tremble with excitement. When deteriorating their mental attitude worsens when they become irritable. Irrational fears make them restless and even degenerate into hysteria. Spasmodic, paretic problems affecting one half of the body.

Painful, tetanic contracture of limbs.

CNS	Brain involvement. Muscles weak and numb. Epilepsy. Seasickness: profound: fainting, vomiting.
GASTROINTESTINAL	Anorexia. Oesophageal spasm. Colic: tympanitic: inguinal ring.
RESPIRATORY	Dyspnoea from bronchospasm.
UROGENITAL	PU. Metritis with great weakness: exudate: clotted, dark, gushing, even purulent.
LAMENESS	Neuralgia: severe pains, anywhere along the back, shoulders, and stifles with spasm of large muscles. Trembling and twitching.
COMPETITION	Easily exhausted.
MODALITIES	Agg: afternoon. Open air. After eating. Emotional upsets. Flexion. Jarring.
	Amel: Lying on preferred side. Massage. Swimming.
COMPARE	Nux-v Petr Puls.
CONSIDER	• Lameness associated with great pain and weakness.
	• Profound travel sickness.
	Look out for the deteriorating behaviour signs.
POTENCY	6X – 12X. 30CH.

COCCUS CACTI
Cochineal Animal

Severe coughing and cystitis in sad, apprehensive individuals that enjoy gentle work.

RESPIRATORY	Kennel Cough laryngitis: mucous: abundant, thick, white, very viscid. Cough: harsh, suffocative.
UROGENITAL	Cystitis, nephritis. PU: bloody, calculi, tenesmus. Pruritus of female genitalia.
MODALITIES	Agg: after work. After sleep. Touch.
	Amel: gentle work.
COMPARE	Cact Canth Sars.
CONSIDER	• Coughing.
	• FLUTD.
	• Nephritis.
POTENCY	6X-12X.

Coff
COFFEA CRUDA
Coffea arabica

Initially cheerful and excitable but become irritable and angry with irrational fears. Oversensitive and restless. Stimulatory effect on the whole animal. Pains felt excessively and associated with vocalisation.

GASTROINTESTINAL	Excessive appetite. Impaired digestion. Intestinal stasis. Ruminal atony.
CARDIOVASCULAR	Arrhythmia. Pulse: tense, palpitation.
UROGENITAL	Nymphomania. Mood swings during parturition.
LAMENESS	Various erratic, transient joint pains.
JUVENILE	Restless hyperactivity of new puppies.
COMPETITION	Excellent in helping lean, intelligent juveniles to adjust to training. Make mistakes from being keen to please.
MODALITIES	Agg: open air. Cold. Emotional excitement. Night. Noise. Strange smells. Touch. Amel: lying down. Rest. Warmth.
COMPARE	*Coffea tosta* Coff-t. Nutritional deficiencies and neuralgia. *Caffeinum* Coffin. Heart stimulant with a diuretic effect. Acon Anth Nux-v Passi.
CONSIDER	Behavioural control: • Hyperactive puppies. • Cheerful, inattentive horses.
POTENCY	12X-30CH.

Colch
COLCHICUM AUTUMNALE
Meadow saffron Plant

Confused, sad and weak, they become irritable, restless, and oversensitive when mood can escalate into rage. Great debility from severe arthritis. Colic.

HEAD	Facial: muscles: painfully inflamed, oedematous. Lachrymation: excessive outdoors. Pupils: left contracted, unequal. Jaw: right: pain behind the angle.
ABDOMEN	Ascites: liver: enlarged, painful.
GASTROINTESTINAL	PU with a dry mouth, yet salivation profuse. Vomiting of food or mucous. Colic: tympanitic: colon, cecum, noisy, severe. Roll with outstretched legs. IBD: diarrhoea: jelly-like, scant, transparent, tenesmus.
UROGENITAL	Cystitis, nephritis. Urine: albumin, bloody, dark, glycosuria, scant. May contain offensive clots of decomposed blood. Female genitalia: pruritic.
LAMENESS	Lumbosacral: pain amel by rest, pressure. Left front leg may be painful. Right leg with absent plantar reflex. DJD: periostitis: hot, painful, gout-like.

SKIN	Extremities: poor circulation, oedema.
	Facial eczema: blotchy, papular rash. Urticaria.
MODALITIES	Agg: mental exertion. Smell of food in evening. Jarring and movement. Night.
	Amel: defecation. Rest.
COMPARE	Arn Ars Lil-t Verat.
CONSIDER	An important arthritis remedy:
	• DJD with severe periarticular involvement.
	• Nephritis.
POTENCY	12X. 30CH. 200CH.

Coll

COLLINSONIA CANADENSIS

Horse balm Stoneroot Plant

Rectal disease.

HEAD	Rhinitis: chronic, mucous.
GASTROINTESTINAL	Mouth, tongue: coated yellow.
	Constipation and diarrhoea alternate during pregnancy.
	Retained meconium. Dysentery.
	Rectal fissures painfully constricted.
CARDIOVASCULAR	Heart failure with oedema.
RESPIRATORY	Painful larynx: dry cough: excess vocalisation.
UROGENITAL	Female genitalia: swollen, painful during pregnancy.
MODALITIES	Agg: cold. Excitement.
	Amel: heat.
COMPARE	Aesc Aloe Ham Grat Lyc Nux-v Rat Sil Sulph.
CONSIDER	• Rectal fissures.
	• Retained meconium.
POTENCY	4X – 8X – 12X.

Colos-b

COLOSTRUM BOVIS

Bovine colostrum Animal

Cancer and immune mediated conditions.

HEAD	Keratitis from Feline Herpes Virus infection.
	Chronic sinusitis.
RESPIRATORY	Various Acute, chronic viral infections.
	Secondary infections.
BREEDING	In its natural form, when administered to pregnant queens, has proven value in reducing kitten mortality.
SKIN	Cancers: various, including melanoma.
JUVENILE	Neonatal support against infection.
COMPARE	Species specific colostrum.
	Echi Eleuth Gins.
CONSIDER	• Feline herpes virus.
	• Immune modulation.
	• Neonatal debility.
POTENCY	2X – 4X – 12X.

Con

117

CONIUM MACULATUM
Poison hemlock Plant

Confused and averse to company when reacting to their fears: approach, thunder, become irritable and easy to startle. Geriatric weakness and debility. Spinal problems.

CNS	Vertigo. Paralysis.
HEAD	Photophobia with intense lachrymation. Corneal ulcers, abrasions, and pustules.
	Otitis: chronic, acrid. Hearing defective.
	Epistaxis. Polyps.
ABDOMEN	Hepatitis: chronic, jaundice, painful.
GASTROINTESTINAL	Gastritis. Vomiting. Constipation. Tenesmus. Tremulous weakness after every stool.
RESPIRATORY	Laryngitis: cough: continuous, hacking.
UROGENITAL	Dysuria, difficulty voiding, interrupted.
	Dribbling in geriatric males. Cysts and tumours.
	Mammae: hard, shrunken, pain to touch.
	Ovaries indurate.
	Prostatomegaly: benign. Orchitis: chronic, hard.
LAMENESS	Pain: anywhere along the spine between shoulders. Spinal injuries. Weary, paralysed hindquarter movement of cauda equina disease, CDRM.
GERIATRIC	An important remedy in the control of premature aging, and in debility and weakness.
SKIN	Injury that leads to excessive scar tissue. Pigmentation.
MODALITIES	Agg: Exertion. Lying down.
	Amel: Dark. Fasting. Motion. Pressure.
COMPARE	Bar-c Carc Cur Hydr Hyos Iod Kali-p.
CONSIDER	• Debility.
	• Paralysis of degenerative myelitis.
	• Senility.
POTENCY	6X – 12X. 30CH.

Conv

CONVALLARIA MAJALIS
Lily of the Valley Plant

Dull, irritable individuals lack concentration and may be hysterical.
Heart failure with hypertrophy and widespread oedema. May be ascites and epistaxis.

CARDIOVASCULAR	Arrhythmia. Endocarditis. Failure. Hypertrophy. Palpitation from slight exercise. Pulse: fast.
RESPIRATORY	Dyspnoea: congestion, oedema. Exercise intolerant.
UROGENITAL	Scant, offensive urine. Uterine pain referred to back.
LAMENESS	Back muscles painfully stiff over lumbar and sacroiliacs.
MODALITIES	Agg: warm room.
	Amel: open air.
COMPARE	Adon Crat Dig Lil-t.
CONSIDER	• Heart disease.
POTENCY	2X – 4X – 12X. Combines well with Crat.

Cop
COPAIVA
Peruvian balsam Plant

Mucous inflammation in dull, oversensitive, and restless individuals. Exudates and urine are offensive, grey to green, profuse, and mucopurulent.

GASTROINTESTINAL	Colic: impacted, tympanitic.
	Colitis. IBS. IBD: mucous.
RESPIRATORY	Laryngitis, bronchitis; cough.
UROGENITAL	Cystitis: drop by drop. Pruritic female genitalia. Metritis.
SKIN	Mottled. Eczema: abdomen: circumscribed, red, swollen, ulcer-like. Chronic juvenile urticaria.
MODALITIES	Agg: morning. Starch.
	Amel: bending double. Walking.
COMPARE	Apis Cann-i Canth Cub Erig Sen Sep Vesp.
CONSIDER	• Cystitis, urethritis.
	• Eczema when associated with cystitis.
	• Pyometra.
POTENCY	4X – 12X.

Cor-r
CORALLIUM RUBRUM
Red coral Animal

HEAD	Photophobia. Rhinitis: blocked, bloody, dry, mucous, profuse, ulcerated.
GASTROINTESTINAL	Arthritis of mandible in whiny individuals.
RESPIRATORY	Laryngitis: Kennel Cough-like, suffocative.
UROGENITAL	Ulcers on male genitalia.
SKIN	Psoriasis on feet. Red spots. Flat red ulcers.
MODALITIES	Agg: open air. From warm to cold room.
COMPARE	Bell Caust Dros.
CONSIDER	• Coughing.
	• Penile ulcer.
POTENCY	8X. 30CH.

Corn
CORNUS CIRCINATA
Round-leaved dogwood Plant

Sad individuals who because they find concentrating difficult, are averse to work. Chronic complicated blood parasitism

GASTROINTESTINAL	Fungal and ulcerated stomatitis.
	Diarrhoea: flatulent after food.
CARDIOVASCULAR	Anaemia from Babesiosis and Erhlichia.
SKIN	Juvenile eczema with widespread debilitating vesicles on face and mouth when nursing.
COMPARE	*Cornus alternifolia* Corn-a. Swamp willow. Eczema with cracked skin. Restless and weak.
	Cornus florida Corn-f. Dogwood. Intermittent fever and debility from fluid loss. Bapt Chin Echi.
CONSIDER	• Anaemia from parasitism.
POTENCY	6X – 12X. 30CH.

Cortico
CORTICOTROPHINUM
ACTH Animal

Active in mornings. Irritable. Often coupled with Cortiso in the management of iatrogenically induced Diabetes insipidus and Cushings Disease.

HEAD	Conjunctivitis. Corneal ulceration.
	Rhinitis: purulent rhinitis.
GASTROINTESTINAL	PD. Stomatitis, pharyngitis.
	Ulcer: stomach, duodenum.
CARDIOVASCULAR	Thrombosis. High triglycerides.
	Arrhythmia. Extrasystoles.
RESPIRATORY	Bronchitis, COPD, emphysema: chronic.
UROGENITAL	PU. Cushings Disease. Glycosuria.
	Oestral irregularities: amenorrhea, silent heat.
	Balanitis. Impotence: loss of libido. Testicular atrophy.
LAMENESS	Spinal pain and stiffness from neck to sacroiliac.
	Arthritis of left hip and stifle joints: associated gluteal muscle stiffness.
SKIN	Hypertrichosis. Lupus of the extremities. Urticaria.
COMPETITION	To improve joint and muscle suppleness.
	Urticaria pre-race.
MODALITIES	Agg: coughing. Exercise.
	Amel: afternoons.
COMPARE	Cic Cortiso Dios.
CONSIDER	• Corticosteroid detoxification.
	• Cushings Disease.
	• Lameness of indeterminate nature.
	Often thirsty, lazy individuals.
POTENCY	30CH. 200CH.

Cortiso
CORTISONUM
Hydrocortisone Animal

Suggested as a new **Polycrest**. Impatient, irritable, and suspicious, they experience rapid mood swings from being excitable to being lazy. The therapeutic employment of this remedy focuses on iatrogenic conditions directly caused by the overuse of cortisone. Immune system modulation.

CNS	Cushings Disease. Diabetes insipidus.
HEAD	Conjunctivitis: inner canthus dry, agglutinated.
ABDOMEN	Ascites from weak liver. Detoxification.
	Diabetes mellitus.
GASTROINTESTINAL	Insatiable appetite with PD. IBD: colic: flatus.
CARDIOVASCULAR	Fast weak pulse.
RESPIRATORY	Laryngitis: dyspnoea: exudate: mucous, painful, tenacious. Worse for effort, excitement.
UROGENITAL	PU to oliguria. Glycosuria, nocturia and proteinuria.
LAMENESS	Sacroiliac and other joint disease with osteoarthritis and osteoporosis.

	Spavin. Windgall.
	Oedema of extremities.
SKIN	Cracked, dry unhealthy. Prone to eczema: allergic, hot, pruritic. Abdomen and feet. Lupus.
GERIATRIC	Rapid aging with joint and skin disease.
COMPETITION	Prolongs career in maturing athlete.
MODALITIES	Agg: heat. Morning. Rest.
	Amel: evening. Walking
COMPARE	Cortico Psor Puls.
CONSIDER	Increasingly important:

- Arthritis.
- Behavioural abnormalities.
- Cortisone toxicity.
- Cushings Disease.
- Eczema that is chronic with severe scratching.
- Immune system modulation.

POTENCY	12X. 30CH. 200CH.

Coryl-a
CORYLUS AVELLANA
Hazelnut Plant

ABDOMEN	Diarrhoea: acute, chronic.
	Liver: chronic insufficiency. hepatitis.
RESPIRATORY	COPD. Mucous thick. Fibrosis.
COMPARE	Am-c Ant-t Calc-fl Carb-v Lob Lyc.
CONSIDER	• COPD.
POTENCY	4X – 12X.

Yohim
CORYNANTHE YOHIMBE
Yohimbine Plant

UROGENITAL	Urethritis. Female impotence, hypergalactia.
	Balanitis: erection extreme. Impotence.
COMPARE	Canth.
CONSIDER	• Impotence: libido good but poor erection
	• Urethritis.
POTENCY	4X – 12X.

Crat
CRATAEGUS OXYACANTHA
Hawthorn Mayflower Plant

Polycrest. Best heart tonic.

CARDIOVASCULAR	Dilated: first sound weak. Palpitation: extreme on slight exertion, slight increase in pulse rate.
	Protection and recovery from surgery.
	Murmurs. Post-virus cough and weakness.
UROGENITAL	Adjunctive therapy in juvenile Diabetes mellitus.

COMPETITION	**Invaluable** for its ability to treat heart strain from virus infection.
MODALITIES	Agg: warm room.
	Amel: open air. Quiet. Rest.
COMPARE	Cact Dig Iber Naja Stroph-h.
CONSIDER	• Heart tonic in athletes.
POTENCY	2X – 4X – 12X. Important adjunctive remedy.

Kres
CRESOLUM
Kreosote BP88 Mineral

Chronic anaemia, anorexia, and debility. Indifferent to irritable. Vocal with great mood swings.

CNS	Ataxia. Epilepsy. Paralysis. Vertigo.
HEAD	Blepharitis. Keratitis. Otitis interna: females.
GASTROINTESTINAL	**Gastritis.**
CARDIOVASCULAR	Vascular disease: obstructive, thrombosis. Lymphadenitis.
RESPIRATORY	Asthma. COPD. Emphysema: oedema.
UROGENITAL	Nephritis: interstitial, glomerular.
	Male genitalia: oedema.
LAMENESS	Polyarthritis: deformed.
SKIN	Abnormal pigmentation. Genital sarcoid.
COMPARE	Arg-m Caust Con Plb.
CONSIDER	• Behavioural abnormalities.
	• Epilepsy.
	• Polyarthritis.
POTENCY	12X. 30CH.

Croc
CROCUS SATIVUS
Saffron Plant

Happy affectionate creatures who love everyone. Can also be timid, startle easily and during disease may show severe mood swings and become angry. Haemorrhage of dark, stringy blood.

HEAD	Glaucoma. Photophobia. Pupils dilated, react slow. Drooping eyelids. Epistaxis.
GASTROINTESTINAL	Proctitis: chronic constipation: juveniles with distended abdomen: helminthiasis.
RESPIRATORY	Respiration: frothy, wheezing, offensive. EIPH.
UROGENITAL	Uterine haemorrhage before foetal loss.
LAMENESS	Chorea. Weak hindquarters.
MODALITIES	Agg: hot weather. Hunger. Lying down. Morning. Warm room.
	Amel: music. Open air.
COMPARE	Chin Ip Plat Sab Tril
CONSIDER	• Chronic constipation in juveniles.
	• Threatened foetal loss.
	• Venous haemorrhage.
POTENCY	2X – 6X. 30CH.

Crot-h
CROTALUS HORRIDUS
Rattlesnake Animal

Polycrest. Confused when anxious, this makes them averse to company during fearful attacks: crowds, public places. Become impatient, irritable, sluggish, and timid. Will run away. Vocal Septic states with marked blood abnormalities, including haemorrhage and jaundice. Copious venous haemorrhage from anywhere. Significant antibacterial agent.

CNS	Cerebrospinal meningitis. Cerebrovascular incidents. Right sided weakness, paralysis.
HEAD	Intraocular haemorrhage.
	Pain; non-inflammatory.
ABDOMEN	Liver: painfully swollen.
GASTROINTESTINAL	Jaundice. PD.
	Cancer: tongue: dry, dark, haemorrhage, red, swollen. Tonsillitis. Oesophageal spasm.
	Stomach: **cancer:** vomiting: bile, blood, food, slimy mucous. Ulcer.
CARDIOVASCULAR	**Haemorrhage.** Copious bleeding from any orifice. Constant slow venous haemorrhage. Clots poorly. Palpitation. Tremulous pulse.
RESPIRATORY	Laryngitis.
UROGENITAL	Cystitis, nephritis: albuminuria, casts, dark, haematuria, PU.
	Uterine haemorrhage. Offensive metritis with parturient fever.
LAMENESS	Right sided ataxia.
COMPETITION	EIPH.
SKIN	**Discoloured,** swollen, tense.
	Purpura haemorrhagica.
MODALITIES	Agg: Annually. Damp. Evening and morning. Jarring. Open air. Sleep.
	Amel: spring: warming weather. Slow walking.
COMPARE	*Crotalus cascavella* Crot-c. Brazilian rattlesnake. Jealous. Love crowds. Separation anxiety.
	Both Elaps Naja Lach.
CONSIDER	• Haemorrhage is dark slow to clot.
	• Lymphangitis.
	• Sepsis.
	• Septicaemia.
POTENCY	8X. 30CH. 200CH.

Crot-t
CROTON TIGLIUM
Purging croton Plant

HEAD	Corneal pustules. Eyelids: granular, raw, red.
GASTROINTESTINAL	Diarrhoea: flatulent: copious, explosive. Tenesmus.
RESPIRATORY	Asthma: painful. Cough when lying down.

123

UROGENITAL	Diurnal urine: greasy, pale, turbid, white sediment. Nocturnal urine: foams, orange.
SKIN	Eczema: intensely painful: face and genitalia. Vesicles: confluent, ooze pus.
MODALITIES	Agg: least food or drink. Night and morning. Summer. Touch. Washing. Amel: gentle massage. After sleep.
COMPARE	Anac Anag Rhus-t Sep.
CONSIDER	• Severe flatulent Diarrhoea • Moist, severe eczema.
POTENCY	6X – 12X. 30CH.

Cub
CUBEBA OFFICINALIS
Piper cubeba Plant

RESPIRATORY	Angry and impatient. Throat full of offensive mucous.
UROGENITAL	Cystitis, urethritis: females: bloody, mucous. Prostatitis: exudate: thick, yellow.
COMPARE	Cuc-p Cop.
CONSIDER	• Cystitis, urethritis.
POTENCY	4X – 8X.

Cuc-p
CUCURBITA PEPO
Pumpkin seed Plant

GASTROINTESTINAL	Vomiting during pregnancy, seasickness, and tapeworm.
COMPARE	*Cucurbita citrullis* Cuc-c. Watermelon. Urethritis. Fil.
CONSIDER	• Vomiting of seasickness.
POTENCY	2X – 6X.

Cund
CUNDURANGO
Condor Plant

CNS	Ataxia with digestive problems.
GASTROINTESTINAL	Mouth: painful cracks: corners. Oesophagus: choke, stricture. Stomach, rectum: epithelial cancer. Fissures, ulcers: mucocutaneous junctions.
COMPARE	Ars Aster Con Hydr.
CONSIDER	• Cancer of mouth and rectum. • Perianal fissures.
POTENCY	6X – 12X. 30CH.

Cupr-ars
CUPRUM ARSENICOSUM
Arsenite of copper mineral

Kidney and intestinal disease in confused, restless individuals that can degenerate into hysterical screaming from uremic convulsions and epilepsy.

GASTROINTESTINAL	PD. Tongue: coated: dirty brown, dry.
	Gastroenteritis, dysentery: violent. Faeces: dark liquid.
CARDIOVASCULAR	Bacterial endocarditis.
RESPIRATORY	Asthma. COPD. Emphysema.
UROGENITAL	Diabetes mellitus.
	Nephritis with acetones, high SG.
	Painful prostatomegaly.
LAMENESS	Muscle cramps.
SKIN	Pustular eczema. Ulcers at extremities.
MODALITIES	Agg: damp. During Diarrhoea. Movement. Touch.
	Amel: bandaging and wrapping.
COMPARE	Other Cuprums. Bell Camph Con Dulc Hep Lach.
CONSIDER	• Neonatal Diarrhoea including parvovirus.
	• Dysentery.
	• Nephritis.
POTENCY	6X. 30CH.

Cupr

CUPRUM METALLICUM
Copper Mineral

Anxious and excitable with fears: of approach, dark and of strangers. Show odd gestures and will bite and kick but usually give clear warning.
Tonic or clonic spasms of epilepsy.

HEAD	Muscles of face and jaw tightly clamped during epileptic fits.
	Eyes crossed, fixed, glassy, stare, roll.
ABDOMEN	May be hot, tense, and tender.
GASTROINTESTINAL	Mouth: foam. Tongue: paralysed or constantly moves in and out. Vomit. Constant borborygmi when asleep.
	Colic: intermittent, tympanic, violent. Intussusception.
	Tapeworm. Diarrhoea: black, bloody, tenesmus.
RESPIRATORY	Asthmatic coughing attacks are suffocative and worse at 3am. Alternate with vomiting.
BREEDING	Parturient anxiety.
MODALITIES	Agg: hot weather. Stress. Vomiting.
	Amel: drinking. Sweating.
COMPARE	*Cuprum aceticum* Cupr-acet. A similar action, but more effective for allergic rhinitis with an acrid exudate. Coughing with tenacious mucous. Chronic eczema with slight itch.
	Cuprum oxydatum nigrum Cupr-o. Parasitic larval migrans and lungworm infestation.
	Bell Camph Con Dulc Hep Lach.
CONSIDER	Important in:
	• Ataxia of unknown origin.
	• Colic.
	• Coughing with cyanosis.
	• Diarrhoea.
	• **Epilepsy**.

POTENCY	12X. 30CH. 200CH.

Cur
CURARE
Chondrodendron tomentosum Arrow poison Plant

Reduced reflexes in sad, angry, destructive individuals. Hydrophobia.

CNS	Motor paralysis.
HEAD	Right sided ptosis.
GASTROINTESTINAL	Cirrhosis. Diabetes mellitus.
	Buccal and facial paralysis. Tongue drawn from right to left. Vomit when coughing.
RESPIRATORY	Slow respiration when asleep. Cough: dry, short.
UROGENITAL	Azoturia / myositis. Urine: offensive, thick, purulent. Pruritus.
SKIN	Pruritic, bloody boils.
MODALITIES	Agg: damp. Cold and cold winds.
COMPARE	Caust Con Crot-h Nux-v.
CONSIDER	• Paralysis of extremities and single parts.
POTENCY	12X. 30CH. 200CH.

Curc
CURCUMA LONGA
Turmeric Plant

Anxiety and the fatigue of EMS. Obesity from overeating. Various painful inflammatory conditions. Significant antibacterial agent.

GASTROINTESTINAL	Diarrhoea. PD and PU.
RESPIRATORY	Fast, weak respiration.
UROGENITAL	Cystitis. Mastitis: chronic, fibrosis.
LAMENESS	Severe back and bone pain.
	Osteoporosis. Sequestrum.
SKIN	Encouraging evidence suggests a role in management of inflammatory skin diseases.
COMPARE	Caust Con Crot-h Nux-v.
CONSIDER	• EMS
	• Obesity.
POTENCY	6X – 12X.

Ang
CUSPARIA FEBRIFUGA
Angustura vera Plant

Severe lameness in oversensitive, easily frightened individuals with poor concentration.

CNS	Epilepsy: tetanic spasms induced by noise or touch. Tetanus.
HEAD	Eye fixed, prominent. Eyelids: agglutinated, red.
GASTROINTESTINAL	PD. Tongue white in dry mucous mouth.
	Chronic bacterial Diarrhoea. Tenesmus.
UROGENITAL	Scant, orange urine.
LAMENESS	Severe back and bone pain. Osteoporosis. Sequestrum.
SKIN	Deep, painful infiltrative ulcers.

MODALITIES	Agg: exercise. Jarring. Noise.
COMPARE	Merc Ruta Nux-v.
CONSIDER	• Bone spurs and spavin.
	• Chronic bacterial Diarrhoea.
	• Geriatric osteoarthritis.
POTENCY	4X – 12X.

Cycl
CYCLAMEN EUROPAEUM
Sow bread Plant

Agoraphobia. Apprehensive during fears: of lightning when they become indifferent, irritable, and easily offended. Sad and averse to work. Anaemia and breeding problems.

HEAD	Diplopia and vertigo.
GASTROINTESTINAL	Diurnal thirstless.
CARDIOVASCULAR	Anaemia.
UROGENITAL	Cyclic abnormalities. Painful postpartum haemorrhage.
LAMENESS	Periosteal pain.
SKIN	Pruritus of female genitalia at puberty.
MODALITIES	Agg: cold application. Evening. Sitting. Standing.
	Amel: after oestrous. Massage. Warm room.
COMPARE	Ambr Chin Cinch Ferr-cit Puls.
CONSIDER	• Painful oestral abnormalities with irritability.
	• Postpartum haemorrhage.
POTENCY	4X – 12X.

Cyt-l
CYTISUS LABURNUM
Laburnum Plant

Depressed, indifferent, and debilitated after viral infection. Fear travel.

CNS	Convulsions. Meningitis. Travel sickness. Vertigo.
HEAD	Facial muscles twitch. Pupils: unequal.
GASTROINTESTINAL	PD. Vomit. Painful, debilitating, and flatulent Diarrhoea.
RESPIRATORY	Constricted larynx with Kennel Cough-like cough.
UROGENITAL	Urethritis: urine: green, pain.
MODALITIES	Agg: afternoon and evening. Cold.
	Amel: after Faeces. Flatus.
COMPARE	Acid-phos Agar Gels Nux-v Tab Verat.
CONSIDER	• Chronic Diarrhoea.
	• Meningitis.
POTENCY	6X – 12X. 30CH.

Daph
DAPHNE INDICA
Spurge laurel Plant

GASTROINTESTINAL	Tongue coated on one side. Halitosis.
LAMENESS	Painful, fluctuating pains in distal muscles in sad, confused, and excitable individuals.
	Lameness: odd, difficult to diagnose.
UROGENITAL	Urine: offensive, thick, turbid, yellow.
COMPARE	Acid-fl Aur Mez Stram.

CONSIDER	• Odd hind limb lameness.
POTENCY	6X – 12X.

Mez

DAPHNE MEZEREUM

Spurge olive Plant

Confused, dull, sad, and unable to concentrate, may experience severe restlessness from separation anxiety. Chronic, painful teeth and bones with profuse salivation. Significant antibacterial agent.

HEAD	Face: eczema: crusty, disgusting, leathery, red, purulent, thick.
	Eye and ear pain after surgery.
	Nose: exudate: acrid, chronic, mucous, pruritic.
GASTROINTESTINAL	Gastritis: chronic, disgusting.
	Vomit is chocolate-like.
	Rodent and gastric ulcers.
	Colic: tympany: debilitated puppies.
	Rectum: constriction and rectal prolapse. Constipation after parturition.
	Green diarrhoea with small, flaky white particles.
UROGENITAL	Urethritis: bloody, flakes, hot.
	Metritis: acrid, albumen-like.
	Orchitis: painfully swollen. Violent sexual desire.
LAMENESS	Widespread pain from neck to stifle with neuralgia of long bones.
SKIN	Intolerably pruritic eruptions with thick purulent scabs.
	Fiery red areola of ulcers surrounded by vesicles.
MODALITIES	Agg: chilly air. Evening until midnight. Warm food. Movement. Touch including riding.
	Amel: eating. Open air.
COMPARE	Merc Phyt Rhus-t Syph.
CONSIDER	• Disgusting eczema.
	• Neuralgic bone pain.
	The eruptions ulcerate and form thick scabs over pus.

Stram

DATURA STRAMONIUM

Thorn apple Plant

Polycrest. CNS abnormalities in cheerful individuals who desire company. But when ill, become destructive, will bite, kick, and run away. Fears: alone, approach, dark, irrational, moving water. Rapid mood changes from happy to violent, dangerous, vocal rage.

Can develop into severe mental illness when they do odd things including 'fly-catching' at imaginary objects. Significant antibacterial agent.

Odd rhythmical movements, including head shaking, nodding, pacing, and weaving.

CNS	Chorea after injury. **Epilepsy.** Staggers with tendency to fall forward and to the left. Trembling. Meningitis. Unconscious with eyes fixed. Induced by contact and movement.
HEAD	Eyes: prominent, staring wide open. Pupils: dilated.

	Strabismus. Vision: lost.
GASTROINTESTINAL	Odd chewing motion. Thirst: violent. Swallowing: difficult from throat spasms.
RESPIRATORY	Bronchitis: emotional trauma. Expectorant: greenish to yellow phlegm.
UROGENITAL	Eclampsia. Uterine haemorrhage.
LAMENESS	Chorea: particularly if induced by injury or vaccination. Incoordination.
FEVER	High, with profuse sweating.
MODALITIES	Agg: being alone. Dark room. Bright or shiny objects. After sleep.
	Amel: company. Good light. Swallowing. Warmth.
COMPARE	Bell Bry Hyos.
CONSIDER	• Ataxia.
	• Brain injury: Acute, chronic.
	• Chorea.
	• Encephalosis and meningitis.
	• Mineral deficiencies with CNS signs.
	• Movements that are odd: gyratory, OCD.
POTENCY	12X. 30CH. 200CH.

Staph

DELPHINIUM STAPHYSAGRIA
Housewort Stavesacre Plant

Polycrest. Anger with violence. Nervous conditions range from apathy to great sensitivity, with marked irritability. Become averse to company and will bite and kick. Complete loss of control with impetuous, violent outbursts. Extremely sensitive animals with great mood swings. Disease of the urogenital tract and skin. Significant antibacterial agent.

CNS	Brain trauma: emotional and physical.
HEAD	Eczema: orbital: pruritic, scabby.
	Corneal laceration, surgery. Hordeolum: recurrent.
	Otitis externa: thick, pruritic scabs.
	Lymphadenitis: sub maxillary glands.
GASTROINTESTINAL	Always hungry, even when stomach full. Gums: pyorrhoea: bleed, salivation, spongy. Teeth: black, decay, osteomalacia. Vomiting.
	Colic: impaction postsurgical, tympanitic: after anger.
CARDIOVASCULAR	Arrythmia after anger.
UROGENITAL	Cystitis with dyspnoea. Incontinence after surgery or catheterisation. Bladder: empty, tenesmus.
	Female genitalia: injury, after mating or rape.
	Metritis. Prolapse.
BREEDING	**Pain** after mating in irritable, younger females. May give confidence to virgin bitches before mating.
LAMENESS	Painfully stiff muscles of back, sacroiliac, hip, right shoulder, and calf are worse in morning before rising. Arthritic nodes.
COMPETITION	Helps working mares focus. Impossible when anxious.

129

SKIN	Eczema on body, ears, face, and head. Scabs are dry. Pruritus. Warts and sarcoid are fig-like, pedunculated.
MODALITIES	Agg: anger. After grief. Least touch on affected parts. Music.
	Amel: after breakfast. Night. Rest. Warmth.
COMPARE	Acid-phos Calad Caust Coloc Ign.
CONSIDER	• Alveolar osteomalacia and periostitis.
	• Behavioural abnormalities; violent mood swings.
	• Eczema.
	• Surgical pain.
POTENCY	12X. 30CH. 200CH.

Dna
DEOXYRIBONUCLEIC ACID
DNA Animal

Immune system modulation. Mental and physical backwardness. Company desire for. Poor concentration. Courageous. Hypersensitive to light and noise. Actual Dna carries the genetic instructions for growth and repair, indicating its sphere of usefulness.

CNS	Epilepsy. Neuralgia post virus.
HEAD	Conjunctivitis. Frontal sinusitis.
GASTROINTESTINAL	Painful, enlarged liver. Pancreatitis. Anorexia. Gingivitis. Proctitis.
UROGENITAL	Female genitalia: pruritus.
	Prostatomegaly. Poor libido.
JUVENILE	Improve growth rate in backward juveniles.
LAMENESS	Spondylitis. Fractures with non-union. Osteomyelitis. Arthritis of large joints.
	Tendon contractures and strains.
SKIN	Alopecia. Burns. Psoriasis. Seborrhoea.
MODALITIES	Agg: movement.
	Amel: dark. Rest.

Dig
DIGITALIS PURPUREA
Common foxglove Plant

Anxiety: in evenings, movement, and during vomiting. Apprehensive, disobedient, excitable, and irritable. Fear: movement. Startle: easily. Suspicious. Cardiac disease where pulse is weak, irregular, intermittent, slow.

HEAD	Eyes agglutinated in mornings. Eyelids: red, swollen margins. Diplopia, irregular. Retina detached.
GASTROINTESTINAL	Cyanosis. Halitosis. Salivation. Vomiting. Diarrhoea with jaundice. Faeces: ashy, chalk-like and pasty.
CARDIOVASCULAR	Terribly slow pulse. Movement triggers palpitation. Atrial fibrillation. Failure after fever. Dilatation.
	Mitral valve incompetence. Oedema.
	Pericarditis with serous exudate.
RESPIRATORY	Bronchitis: chronic: cough: raw. Breathing: congestion, deep sighing, difficult, irregular. Dyspnoea with

	constant desire to breathe deeply. Senile pneumonia.
UROGENITAL	Cystitis, urethritis. Brick red sediment. Tenesmus.
GERIATRIC	General senile degeneration of heart and lungs.
MODALITIES	Agg: after meals. Exercise. Heat. Music. Sitting erect. Amel: empty stomach. Open air.
COMPARE	*Digitoxinum* Digox. Extract of Dig. Severe vomiting. Adon Con Crat Kalm Liat Ner Spig.
CONSIDER	• Heart disease with irregular, slow pulse.
POTENCY	2X – 6X.

Dios
DIOSCOREA VILLOSA
Wild yam Plant

GASTROINTESTINAL	Offensive, profuse eructation. Colic: great restlessness, fear of people. Exhausting morning diarrhoea.
UROGENITAL	Uterine pain.
LAMENESS	Severe, right sided, back, and joint pain with cramp. Brittle hooves.
MODALITIES	Agg: doubling up. Evening, night. Lying down. Amel: open air. Movement. Pressure. Standing. Stretching.
COMPARE	Anth Bry Coloc Nux-v.
CONSIDER	• Painful colic. • Severe lameness.
POTENCY	12X.

Diosm
DIOSMA LINCARIS
Buku Plant

CNS	Epilepsy in dull, stupid individuals with pruritic, weepy eyes.
GASTROINTESTINAL	Liver atrophy, cirrhosis, hepatitis. Gastroenteritis. Splenitis. Diarrhoea: frequent, nocturnal, yellow.
UROGENITAL	Painful nephritis with bloody urine. Ovaritis.
LAMENESS	Weak, restless legs.
CONSIDER	• Gastroenteritis. • Epilepsy. • Liver disease. • Nephritis.
POTENCY	6X – 12X. 30CH.

Dros
DROSERA ROTUNDIFOLIA
Round-leaved sundew Plant
Apprehensive and sad, they become restless, suspicious, and easily startled when ill.

RESPIRATORY	Cough is irritating, **Kennel Cough-like** and worse after midnight. Bronchitis, laryngitis, pneumonia.

	Asthma and chronic pleurisy after viral infections.
MODALITIES	Agg: drinking. After midnight. Lying down.
CONSIDER	• Any severe cough.
POTENCY	6X – 12X. 30CH.

Dub
DUBOISINUM
Corkwood elm Plant

CNS	Ataxia. Fall backwards. Excitable and restless.
HEAD	Acute, chronic conjunctivitis. Dilated pupils. Distended tortuous retinal vessels.
GASTROINTESTINAL	Pharyngitis coated with black, stringy mucous.
RESPIRATORY	Laryngitis with a dry, hoarse cough. Dyspnoea.
COMPARE	*Duboisia myoporoides* (sulphate) Dubo-m. Hysterical epilepsy.
CONSIDER	• Ataxia.
POTENCY	6X – 12X.

Echi
ECHINACEA ANGUSTIFOLIA
Narrow-leaved Purple coneflower Plant

Polycrest. Apprehensive, confused, and depressed when ill. Control and prevention of infection. Powerful immune modulator. Can improve quality of life in terminal cancer. An influence in snake, insect, and other animal bites. Significant antibacterial agent.

CNS	Brain: meningitis, vertigo.
HEAD	Nose: mucous exudate: offensive.
	Nostril: right: bloody, raw.
GASTROINTESTINAL	Mouth: cancer: gums recede, bleed easily.
	Corners: cracked. Saliva: profuse.
	Tongue: dry, swollen.
	Tonsil: black or purple: mucous: grey, ulcer.
CARDIOVASCULAR	Blood: septicaemia. Lymphadenitis.
UROGENITAL	Urine: albuminuria, frequent, involuntary, scant.
	Female: postpartum metritis: excoriating, offensive.
BREEDING	Parturition: infection control.
LAMENESS	Joint: infection: omphalophlebitis. Pain.
SKIN	Abscess: recurrent.
	Bites / infection / stings / reactions: insect, plant.
JUVENILE	Profound importance in the prevention and treatment of infection associated with the umbilicus.
	Septic fever.
MODALITIES	Agg: cold.
	Amel: effort. Recumbent. Rest. Warmth.
COMPARE	*Echinacea purpurea*: Echi-p. Remarkably similar, but less effective.
CONSIDER	Any situation compromised by bacterial infection including.
	• Animal and insect bites and their sequel.
	• Arthritis that is septic.
	• Granuloma including acral.

- Immune system modulation.
- Pre- and post-surgery: particularly of joints.

POTENCY	2X–12X when immune system underactive. 30CH or 200CH when immune system overactive.)

Elaps
ELAPS CORALLINUS
Coral snake Animal

Disgusting exudates. Angry, dangerous individuals with Irrational fears. Hate being alone.

HEAD	Periorbital oedema: intolerably pruritic. Otitis externa. Rhinitis. Exudates: black, green, hard, offensive. Eruptions around nostrils.
GASTROINTESTINAL	Pharyngitis and oesophageal spasms: exudate: crusty, dry, green to yellow. Swallow: difficult.
CARDIOVASCULAR	Distal capillaries: blocked, constricted. Lymphadenitis.
RESPIRATORY	Cough: right sided pneumonia with bloody epistaxis.
UROGENITAL	Female genitalia: pruritic. Metritis with black exudate.
LAMENESS	Laminitis. Lymphangitis. Phleg-leg. Navicular disease.
SKIN	Severe, peeling eczema in axilla. Vesicles on extremities.
COMPARE	Alumn Ars Carb-v Crot-h Sec Lach.
CONSIDER	• Laminitis. • Lymphadenitis including snake bite. • Navicular disease. • Sepsis.
POTENCY	6X – 12X. 30CH.

Elat
ELATERIUM OFFICINARUM
Squirting cucumber Animal

Violent gastroenteritis in sad, homesick individuals with a tendency to startle.

GASTROINTESTINAL	Painfully debilitating vomiting. Painful diarrhoea is copious, squirted out with force, frothy, olive green and watery.
CARDIOVASCULAR	Anaemia: chronic parasitism.
LAMENESS	Swollen joints from hips downwards.
SKIN	Severe, pruritic angioneurotic eruptions with oedema.
MODALITIES	Agg: damp bedding.
COMPARE	Bry Crot-t.
CONSIDER	• Babesiosis. • Gastroenteritis.
POTENCY	4X – 8X. 30CH.

Eleuth
ELEUTHEROCOCCUS SENTICOSUS
Siberian ginseng Plant

Chronic disease control, and in immune system modulation. Profound fatigue. Significant antibacterial agent.

HEAD	**Conjunctivitis** with profuse lachrymation and pruritus.
ABDOMEN	Hepatitis. Splenitis.
GASTROINTESTINAL	Chronic gastritis with vomiting. **Chronic Diarrhoea**.
UROGENITAL	Nephritis with bloody urine. Ovaritis.
LAMENESS	Legs are weak.
COMPARE	Acid-phos. Echi (combines well). Gins.
CONSIDER	Chronic conditions:
	• Gastritis.
	• Hepatitis.
	• Immune system modulation.
	• Nephritis.
	• Splenitis.
POTENCY	2X. 8X. 30CH.

Epih
EPIHYSTERINUM
Uterine fibroid nosode Animal

UROGENITAL	Uterine haemorrhage from tumour.
COMPARE	Ergot Foll Thlas.
CONSIDER	• Chronic bloody exudate from uterus.
POTENCY	12X.

Equis
EQUISETUM HIEMALE
Rough horsetail Plant

GASTROINTESTINAL	Faecal incontinence in geriatric females. Debility, irritability, and restlessness.
UROGENITAL	Cystitis, nephritis. Urine: mucous, drop by drop. Tenesmus. Dysuria: retention during pregnancy.
MODALITIES	Agg: movement. Pressure. Sitting. Touch. Getting wet. Amel: afternoon. Lying down.
COMPARE	Apis Canth Chim Ferr-p Hydrang.
CONSIDER	• Cystitis, nephritis.
	• Urinary problems during pregnancy.
POTENCY	4X – 8X. 30CH.

Ergot
ERGOTINUM
Alkaloid of ergot Plant

HEAD	Intermittent deafness.
UROGENITAL	Enuresis and genital pruritus in females. Anxious, sad and mood swings during oestrous.
SKIN	Alopecia post neuter.
COMPARE	Foll Ign Lil-t Sec Thyr.
CONSIDER	• Mood swings during oestrous.
	• Genital pruritus.
POTENCY	12X.

Erig
ERIGERON CANADENSIS
Leptilon canadense Fleabane Plant

GASTROINTESTINAL	Flatulent dysentery.
UROGENITAL	Bloody cystitis.
	Postpartum haemorrhage. Prolapse of uterus.
COMPARE	Ter.
CONSIDER	• Postpartum haemorrhage.
POTENCY	2X – 6X.

Coca
ERYTHROXYLUM COCA
Divine plant of the Inca Plant

Anxious, apprehensive and insomnia. Swing from bright to exhausted and timid, with a desire for solitude. Irritability, even hysteria when ill. Palpitation and dyspnoea.

GASTROINTESTINAL	Dental decay. Tympanitic colic.
CARDIOVASCULAR	Heart weakness with palpitation.
RESPIRATORY	Laryngitis from overuse: cough: harsh. Exudate with small, transparent pieces of mucous. Air hunger of asthma.
UROGENITAL	Diabetes mellitus in impotent males.
COMPETITION	Tonic in asthma, COPD, and lower airway disease. Adjust to altitude living and training.
MODALITIES	Agg: exercise.
	Amel: lower altitudes.
COMPARE	Acid-phos Anth Cypr.
CONSIDER	• Exercise intolerance.
POTENCY	2X – 6X.

Eucal
EUCALYPTUS GLOBULUS
Tasmanian blue gum tree Plant

HEAD	Rhinitis, sinusitis: chronic (ethmoid and frontal).
	Exudates: offensive, thin, watery.
	Significant antibacterial agent.
GASTROINTESTINAL	PD. Painfully contracted spleen. Salivation excessive. Tonsillitis with severe ulceration and bloody vomiting. Stomach cancer with copious mucous. Diarrhoea and dysentery. Salmonellosis.
CARDIOVASCULAR	Anaemia: blood parasitism.
RESPIRATORY	Asthma, bronchitis, bronchiectasis, COPD: exudates are copious and mucopurulent.
UROGENITAL	Cystitis, pyelonephritis. PU. Haematuria, pus.
	Metritis: acrid, purulent, ulcers at meatus.
LAMENESS	Swollen, nodular joints of carpus, hock, and digits.
SKIN	Herpetic-like ulcers heal slow.
COMPETITION	Exercise tonic during low grade allergic, lower airway disease. Individuals try hard but limited by excess mucous.

MODALITIES	Agg: food. Morning. Movement. Touch.
	Amel: lying down.
COMPARE	*Eucalyptus tereticoris* Eucal-t. Exhausting cough.
	Eucalyptus rostra Eucal-r.
	Anac Hydr Kali-s.
CONSIDER	• Allergic lower airway disease.
	• Babesiosis.
	• Bronchitis.
	• Nephritis.
POTENCY	2X in nebulizer. 6X. 30CH.

Eug
EUGENIA JAMBOSA
Rose-apple Plant

Interesting range of mental signs from depression to excitement. Mood swing from cheerful to being sad and averse to company.

HEAD	Epiphora: warm tears. Brachycephalic cat breeds.
SKIN	Cracks. Purulent fissures that recede from digits.
COMPARE	*Eugenia cheken* Myrt-ch. Chronic bronchitis.
CONSIDER	• Chronic Feline epiphora.
	• Pododermatitis in terrier breeds.
POTENCY	2X – 8X.

Euon
EUONYMUS EUROPAEA
Wahoo spindle tree Plant

Anxious and confused. Easily exhausted.

HEAD	Pain in malar bones.
GASTROINTESTINAL	Acute, chronic hepatitis.
	Mouth: dry, painful tongue, thirstless.
	Colic: tympanitic.
	Constipation alternates with diarrhoea.
UROGENITAL	Chronic nephritis. Urine, albumen, casts, discoloured, tenesmus.
LAMENESS	Back pain referred from kidney.
MODALITIES	Agg: evening.
	Amel: pressure of bandaging and wrapping.
COMPARE	*Euonymus atropurpurea* Euon-a. Similar, but less intense.
	Chel Podo.
CONSIDER	• Chronic nephritis with gastroenteritis.
POTENCY	2X – 6X – 12X.

Eup-per
EUPATORIUM PERFOLIATUM
Boneset Thoroughwort Plant

Bone pain, fever, and bronchial mucous in anxious, restless, and vocal individuals.

CNS	Vertigo. Fall to left.
HEAD	Occipital bone painful. Mucopurulent rhinitis.

GASTROINTESTINAL	PD. PU. Yellow tongue. Chronic vomiting of bile. Greenish diarrhoea alternates with clay coloured constipation.
CARDIOVASCULAR	Anaemia from chronic parasitic and viral infection.
RESPIRATORY	Viral bronchitis: cough, mucopurulent.
LAMENESS	Severe polysynovitis. Pain in various bones.
MODALITIES	Amel: stimulation.
COMPARE	*Eupatorium aromaticum* Eup-a. Chorea, hysteria. Sore nipple.
	Other Eupatoriums.
	Bry Chel Hyos Lap-a Nat-m Passi Sep.
CONSIDER	• Babesiosis.
	• Bronchitis.
	• Fever in viral infections.
	• Polysynovitis.
POTENCY	2X in nebulizer. 8X. 30CH.

Eup-pur

EUPATORIUM PURPUREUM

Queen of the meadow Plant

CNS	Diabetes insipidus. Homesick, lethargic and whine constantly.
UROGENITAL	PD. PU. Cystitis: acute, chronic: albuminuria, dysuria, haematuria, pain.
	Threatened foetal loss. Agalactia. Painful left ovary. Prostatomegaly. Impotence.
COMPARE	Other Eupatoriums.
	Acid-phos Aven Cann-i Epig Helon Senec Trit.
CONSIDER	• Diabetes insipidus.
	• Cystitis FLUTD.
	• Prostatomegaly.
	Always associated with great lethargy and bone pain.
POTENCY	4X – 8X. 30CH.

Euph-l

EUPHORBIA LATHYRIS

Gopher plant

CNS	Great weakness associated with gastroenteritis.
HEAD	Pruritic erythema begins on face and spreads in 3-4 days. Oedema: glossy or rough.
GASTROINTESTINAL	PD. PU. Musty halitosis. Tongue coated and slimy. Vomiting. Diarrhoea: bloody, copious, clear, mucous: gelatinous, watery.
	Constipation follows diarrhoea.
CARDIOVASCULAR	Arrhythmia with a fast, hard pulse.
RESPIRATORY	Associated with Kennel Cough-like signs.
MODALITIES	Agg: chilly air. Touch.
	Amel: closed room. Topical oil massage.
COMPARE	*Euphorbia prostata* Euph-pr. Insect and snake bite.
	Euphorbia polycarpa Euph-po. Snake bite.

137

	Gymnema sylvestre Gymne. Snake bite.
	Plumeria cellinus Plume. Snake bite.
	Rhus-v Verat.
CONSIDER	• Eczema.
POTENCY	4X − 12X

Euph-r
EUPHORBIA RESINIFERA
Wood spurge Plant

HEAD	Erysipelas with yellow blisters.
	Conjunctivitis: morning: agglutinated.
	Rhinitis, pharyngitis: mucous, violently pruritic.
GASTROINTESTINAL	PD. Hungry. Colic: spasmodic, tympanitic.
	Faeces: clay coloured, fermented, profuse.
RESPIRATORY	Asthma with a constant dry cough.
LAMENESS	Intense pain in lower back and hip.
SKIN	Pruritic vesicular erysipelas. Chronic, painful, and indolent ulcers. Gangrene. Ulcerated carcinoma and epithelioma.
COMPARE	*Euphorbia amygdaloides* Euph-a. Nose pain. Painful Diarrhoea.
	Euphorbia corrolata Euph-c. Severe vomiting.
	Euphorbia marginata Euph-m. Severe eczema.
	Euphorbia pilulifera Euph-pi. Rhinitis, urethritis, metritis.
	Colch Crot-t Jal.
CONSIDER	• Pain of cancer.
	• Severe eczema.
POTENCY	4X − 8X. 30CH.

Euph
EUPHRASIA OFFICINALIS
Eyebright Plant

Apprehensive, lazy, and mild mannered with restlessness during illness. Mucous membranes of eyes and nose. Profuse acrid lachrymation and bland exudate: worse, evening. Significant antibacterial agent.

HEAD	Conjunctivitis: acrid, blisters, epiphora: constant, mucous, sticky, thick. Corneal blisters. Iritis. Opacities. Photophobia.
	Swollen eyelids blink constantly. Ptosis.
	Nasal exudate: bland, fluent, profuse.
GASTROINTESTINAL	Frequent vomiting from excessive coughing.
RESPIRATORY	**Cough:** Kennel Cough-like, diurnal.
UROGENITAL	Male cystitis: dribbling, nocturnal pain. Prostatitis.
COMPARE	All-c Ars Cine (combines well) Gels Kali-i Sabad.
CONSIDER	• **Eye** disease associated with an acrid watery exudate.
	• Bland rhinitis with severe diurnal coughing.
POTENCY	2X topically. 8X − 12X.

Ferr-ars
FERRUM ARSENICOSUM
Iron arsenate Mineral

Like Ferr, but more severe anaemia and nephritis. Sad, anxious, restless individuals. Significant antibacterial agent.

GASTROINTESTINAL	Liver, spleen: painfully enlarged.
	Thirstless. Constipation to diarrhoea: mucous, undigested food.
CARDIOVASCULAR	Anaemia: parasitism: destructive, life threatening.
UROGENITAL	Anaemia: Acute, chronic: nephritis.
SKIN	Dry and debilitated. Psoriasis.
COMPARE	Other Ferrums. Ars Chin Ham Rumx.
CONSIDER	• Anaemia. • Babesiosis. • Ehrlichiosis. • Nephritis.
POTENCY	6X – 12X. 30CH.

Ferr
FERRUM METALLICUM
Iron Mineral

Polycrest. Anxieties, including fever, at night, and irrational ones, develop into irritability, then anger when aggravated by consolation. Cheerful, excitable when well, but dull when finding the pressure of company, confrontational. Mood swings when oversensitive, and hysteria is possible.

Special role in the treatment of juveniles with flabby, relaxed muscles, and exercise intolerance. Anaemic, cold, and weak.

HEAD	Photophobia. Eyes: red, watery.
	Nasal mucous membranes: pale, relaxed.
GASTROINTESTINAL	Halitosis. Appetite varies from anorexia to voracious.
	PD. Vomit: up to 2 hours after eating, after midnight.
	Intolerant of eggs. Constipation, hard.
	Neonates with prolapse and pruritus.
CARDIOVASCULAR	Anaemia: Acute, chronic. Pulse: full, but soft.
	Palpitation: aggravated by movement.
RESPIRATORY	Dyspnoeic cough: bloody, dry, spasmodic.
UROGENITAL	PU. Diurnal incontinence.
	Habitual foetal loss. Metritis: mucous plugs. Painful vaginal prolapse.
	Male: impotency.
LAMENESS	Back and lumbar pain.
	Arthritis: right, shoulder and hind joints.
COMPETITION	Useful for improving general condition of anaemic, debilitated and overworked individuals.
JUVENILE	Weak and backward.
	Urinary incontinence from excitement.
FEVER	Extremities cold. Mid night. Profuse, debilitating sweat.
MODALITIES	Agg: night. First movement. Overheating. Rest. Sitting still. Sweating. Chilly water.
	Amel: rising. Slow walking.

COMPARE	*Ferrum aceticum* Ferr-a. Thin, weak juveniles grow too fast. Allergic respiratory problems such as asthma, throat infections and sinusitis. *Ferrum cyanatum* Ferr-cy. Irritable, hypersensitive, chorea, epilepsy. *Ferrum iodatum* Ferr-i. Sad. Nephritis. Glands enlarged, tumour. *Ferrum muriaticum* Ferr-m. Polyuria. Interstitial nephritis at puberty. Other Ferrums. Rumx Chin Alum Ham.
CONSIDER	• Juveniles with anaemia and debility.
POTENCY	6X – 12X. 30CH. 200CH.

Ferr-p

FERRUM PHOSPHORICUM
Iron phosphate Mineral

Polycrest. Like Ferr, but milder in the mental sphere when apprehension, excitement, and fear of crowd triggers of depression. Effective in the initial stages of inflammatory conditions before exudation. Particularly associated with mucous affections of the respiratory tract. A feature of this remedy is low fever and localised congestions. Significant antibacterial agent.

CNS	Encephalitis. Meningitis. Vertigo.
HEAD	Conjunctivitis. Optic disc; retina: hyperaemia. Eustachian tubes inflamed. Otitis media: acute, prevents suppuration. **Nasal** exudates: frequent, recurrent, slowly develop. Epistaxis: arterial.
GASTROINTESTINAL	**Appetite: poor.** Eructation is sour. Halitosis. PD. Tonsillitis: red and swollen. Vomiting: blood, undigested food. Dysentery.
CARDIOVASCULAR	Pulse: rapid, regular, soft. Acute post virus. Palpitation.
RESPIRATORY	**Cough:** dry, hard, painful, short, tickling. Lung: congestion, pneumonia: haemoptysis: arterial.
UROGENITAL	**Acute, irritating cystitis,** urethritis where urine spurts with every cough. Diurnal incontinence. PU.
LAMENESS	Neck stiff. Arthritis.
FEVER	Respiratory conditions, before exudate becomes purulent.
MODALITIES	Agg: jarring. Early morning. Motion. Night. Touch. Amel: cold application. Gentle exercise.
COMPARE	Other Ferrums. Acon Ars Chin Graph Petr.
CONSIDER	• **Acute** infections in animals that are anaemic, weak fevered and haemorrhage.
POTENCY	8X. 30CH. 200CH.

Ferr-pic

FERRUM PICRICUM
Iron picricum Mineral

HEAD	Slow developing deafness.
GASTROINTESTINAL	Dental neuralgia. PD. Furred tongue.
UROGENITAL	Nocturnal PU. Cystitis, urethritis. Prostatomegaly.
SKIN	Epithelial cancer. Wart-like.
COMPARE	Other Ferrums.
CONSIDER	• Benign, warty skin cancers.
	• Prostatomegaly associated with cystitis.
POTENCY	12X. 30CH.

Fic
FICUS RELIGIOSA
Pakur Plant

GASTROINTESTINAL	Arterial haemoptysis. Painful gastritis.
CARDIOVASCULAR	Anaemia with fast, thread pulse. Sad and restless.
RESPIRATORY	Exercise intolerance. EIPH: arterial.
UROGENITAL	Haematuria. Postpartum haemorrhage.
COMPARE	Acal Fic-v Ip Mill Thlas.
CONSIDER	• Arterial haemorrhage.
POTENCY	4X – 12X.

Flav
FLAVUS
Bacterial nosode of *Neisseria flava* Animal

HEAD	Frontal and maxillary sinusitis with dry cough.
LAMENESS	Painful arthritis of upper spine and left hip.
COMPARE	Kali-bi Zinc.
CONSIDER	• Adjunctive therapy in arthritis and sinusitis.
POTENCY	6X – 12X.

Flor-p
FLOR DE PIEDRA
Stone blossom *Lopophytum leandri* Plant

THYROID	Thyroid dysfunction. Active, but easily discouraged.
GASTROINTESTINAL	Hepatitis and pancreatitis: acute.
SKIN	Severe pruritus.
COMPARE	Iod Thyr. Combines well with these.
CONSIDER	• Pancreatitis.
	• Thyroid dysfunction.
POTENCY	12X. 30CH.

Foll
FOLLICULINUM
Ripe ovarian follicle Nosode Animal

UROGENITAL	Behaviour modification. Severe oestral mood swings.
	Ovary: infertility: inactive.
SKIN	Hormonal alopecia and eczema.
MODALITIES	Agg: noise. Ovulation. Rest.
	Amel: anoestrous. Gentle work.
COMPARE	Lach Lyc Murx Ov Puls Sep.

141

CONSIDER	• Alopecia. • Behavioural problems in females. • Eczema. • HRT. • Infertility.
POTENCY	2X – 6X to improve ovulation. 30CH for behaviour control.

Form-ac
FORMICICUM ACIDUM
Formic acid Mineral

HEAD	Chronic intermittent rhinitis.
GASTROINTESTINAL	Flatus with tenesmus in mornings.
RESPIRATORY	Dry, hoarse, and painful throat.
UROGENITAL	Cystitis: albuminuria, haematuria, tenesmus.
LAMENESS	Ataxia with restlessness and great weakness. Right sided. Arthritis: digits, hip: periarticular stiffness.
SKIN	Pruritic, painful periarticular urticaria.
COMPETITION	Useful training tonic in non-specific lameness.
MODALITIES	Agg: cold and cold washing. Damp. Before snowstorm. Amel: grooming. Massage. Warm bandaging and soaking.
COMPARE	Dulc Juni-c Rhus-t Rhus-v Urt-u.
CONSIDER	• Acute, periarticular polysynovitis.
POTENCY	6X – 12X.

Frag
FRAGARIA VESCA
Wood strawberry Plant

GASTROINTESTINAL	Prevents and removes **dental tartar**. Tongue swollen and strawberry-like.
UROGENITAL	Agalactia.
SKIN	Erysipeloid urticaria with petechial swellings. Localised or widespread.
GERIATRIC	Important in dental management as adjunctive therapy.
CONSIDER	• Dental disease.
POTENCY	6X – 12X.

Fuc
FUCUS VESICULOSUS
Sea kelp Plant

THYROID	Obesity from hypothyroidism in dull, slow individuals.
GASTROINTESTINAL	Obstinate constipation with flatulence.
COMPARE	Bad Flor-p Iod Phyt Thyr. Combines well with these.
CONSIDER	• Hypothyroidism.
POTENCY	2X – 6X.

Fuli
FULIGO LIGNI
Soot Plant

GASTROINTESTINAL	Epithelial carcinoma. Chronic, ulcerative stomatitis.
UROGENITAL	Pruritic female genitalia.
	Uterine cancer with haemorrhage.
	Scrotal cancer.
SKIN	Chronic, pruritic eczema. Obstinate ulcers.
COMPARE	Kres.
CONSIDER	• Cancer of genitalia.
	• Precancerous, ulcerative stomatitis.
POTENCY	12X.

Gali
GALIUM APARINE
Goose grass Plant

GASTROINTESTINAL	Cancerous nodules and ulcers on the tongue.
UROGENITAL	Urethritis and nephritis. Calculi. Dysuria.
SKIN	Excessive granulation tissue. Ulcers.
CONSIDER	• Cancer of the tongue.
	• Promote healing where granulation is exuberant.
POTENCY	2X topically. 30CH.

Galph
GALPHIMIA GLAUCA
Thyrallis glauca Plant

HEAD	Allergic pruritus of conjunctiva, eyelids, and rhinitis.
SKIN	Allergic dermatitis and urticaria.
CONSIDER	• Allergies.
POTENCY	12X. 30CH.

Gaul
GAULTHERIA PROCUMBENS
Wintergreen Plant

CNS	Vertigo in sad individuals.
HEAD	Conjunctivitis: better for rubbing.
	Dirty brown pigmented spots.
GASTROINTESTINAL	Anorexia. Halitosis. PD. Tongue: dirty, furry, yellow at base. Vomiting.
	Constipation: tenesmus after faeces passed.
	Painful diarrhoea: bright green to yellow, liquid, mucous, offensive.
RESPIRATORY	Congested right lung.
UROGENITAL	Lithiasis with haematuria. Calcium oxalates. Turbid with a muddy colour. High SG.
	Metritis: white, mucous.
LAMENESS	Arthritis of right sided digits.
MODALITIES	Agg: eating. Movement. Warm room.

	Amel: frequent small feeds.
COMPARE	Chel Chin Lac-c Lyc.
CONSIDER	• Hepatitis.
	• Lithiasis.
POTENCY	12X. 30CH.

Gels

GELSEMIUM SEMPERVIRENS
Yellow jasmine Plant

Polycrest. Illness follows excitement, fright, or grief. Anxiety: anticipation, downward motion. Desires: alone, light, quiet. Dull, listless and will bite / kick when rudely disturbed.

Fears: crowds, during diarrhoea, performing in public, public places, thunder. Oversensitive, sad, and timid during parturition, and may become dangerous when hysterical.

Vocal. Influence on the nervous system in the control of motor paralysis and emotional trauma. Paralysis of various groups of muscles: eyes, throat, chest, larynx, sphincters, and extremities.

Muscular incoordination and weakness, with complete relaxation and prostration possible. Sluggish circulation. Significant antibacterial agent.

CNS	Mental trauma. Paralysis of various muscles. Vertigo.
HEAD	Jaw: muscles contracted, quiver when hanging. Descemitis. Eyelids heavy: can hardly open them. Ptosis. Glaucoma.
	One pupil dilated, the other contracted. Retina detached. Coryza: acute, dry, excoriating, watery. Turbinates swollen.
GASTROINTESTINAL	Halitosis. PD. Tongue: coated, paralysed, thick, trembles, yellow. Tonsillitis. Emotional Diarrhoea: fear, excitement.
	Faeces: involuntary, painless. Rectal paralysis.
CARDIOVASCULAR	Pulse: slow, soft, weak. Palpitation.
RESPIRATORY	Acute bronchitis: dry cough. Diaphragmatic contractions of *thumps*. Spasm of glottis. Vocal cord paralysis: LSLH.
UROGENITAL	PU. Dysuria. Clear, watery. Partial bladder paralysis with flow intermittent. Retention from excitement.
	Cervix: rigid os at parturition. False labour efforts.
BREEDING	An aid in parturition, particularly ring womb in sheep. Hysteria during pregnancy and parturition.
LAMENESS	Ataxia: painfully stiff muscles of neck, lumbar, sacroiliac, hip, and extremities. Trembling and weakness.
	Cramp of forearms.
COMPETITION	Preparation of nervous animals for competition. Irrational fears: with diarrhoea, appearing in public.
	Early cases of inspiratory noises such as 'roaring and whistling' have responded.
JUVENILE	Behavioural problems.
GERIATRIC	Ataxia: progressive. Pulse: slow, weak.

FEVER	Heat and sweats are long, exhausting.
SKIN	Pruritic: eruptions: dry, hot. Erysipelas.
MODALITIES	Agg: emotion. Excitement. Damp, foggy weather. 10.00 am. Before thunderstorm.
	Amel: open air. Bending forward. Continuous movement. PU.
COMPARE	Acon Bapt Bell Cimic Con Ign Mag-p.
CONSIDER	Of significant importance in:
	• Behaviour problems.
	• Incoordination and paralysis.
	Important indicators are the apprehension, generalised sleepiness, weakness, and stiffness.
POTENCY	6X – 12X. 30CH. 200CH.

Ger
GERANIUM MACULATUM
Wild cranesbill Plant

GASTROINTESTINAL	Tongue has a hot, dry tip. Pharyngitis. Gastritis with mucous and hematemesis. Ulcer.
	Chronic constipation; mucous, offensive.
	Diarrhoea: mucous.
RESPIRATORY	Pulmonary haemorrhage.
UROGENITAL	Postpartum haemorrhage. Painful nipples.
COMPARE	*Erodium cicutarium* Erod.
	Geranium Gerin.
CONSIDER	• Haemorrhaging gastric ulcer.
POTENCY	4X – 12X.

Gink-b
GINGKO BILOBA
Maidenhair tree Plant

GASTROINTESTINAL	PD. Colic: tympanitic, then diarrhoea.
RESPIRATORY	Dyspnoea. Laryngitis. Cough: virus.
UROGENITAL	Nephritis: acute: dysuria, milky. Metritis.
COMPETITION	May improve memory in working dogs.
MODALITIES	Agg: cold. Walking.
	Amel: heat. Rest.
COMPARE	Canth Rhus-t.
CONSIDER	• Nephritis
	• Viral infection. Prophylactic for in-contact animals.
POTENCY	4X – 12X for treatment. 30CH for prevention.

Glon
GLONOINUM
nitro-glycerine mineral
Circulatory problems including cerebral congestion of sun, heatstroke, and meningitis. Dull, sad, delirious and cannot concentrate. May desire to run away.

GASTROINTESTINAL	Variable appetite and pica. Gastritis. Vomiting. Constipation, diarrhoea: dark, copious, lumpy.
CARDIOVASCULAR	Extreme palpitation. Fainting from slight exertion. Anaemia.
RESPIRATORY	Dyspnoea and generalised stiffness.
SKIN	Pruritus of extremities.
MODALITIES	Agg: fire. Heat. Mornings. Sun.
COMPARE	Bell Op Stram Verat.
CONSIDER	• Overheating during transport • Sunstroke.
POTENCY	6X. 30CH.

Grat
GRANATUM
Pomegranate Plant

CNS	Persistent vertigo. Irritable.
HEAD	Dilated pupils.
GASTROINTESTINAL	Constant hunger. Nocturnal vomiting. Poor digestion. Tapeworm and anal pruritus.
RESPIRATORY	Suffocative laryngeal spasm.
LAMENESS	Withers, shoulders: pain.
SKIN	Pruritus of extremities.
COMPARE	*Pelletierinum* Pelin. Anthelmintic of tapeworm. Cina Fil Kou.
CONSIDER	• Spasm of glottis. • Adjunctive tapeworm therapy.
POTENCY	2X – 6X.

Graph
GRAPHITES
Black lead Mineral

Anxious, apprehensive and startle easily. Fears crowds, people, and thunder. Anticipates danger when revisiting places that were earlier difficult. Healing of scars. Often obese. Significant antibacterial agent.

HEAD	Eczema: face: eruptions: humid, offensive, purulent. Blepharitis. Eyelids: dry, red, scabbed, swollen. Otitis externa. Nostrils: eruptions, fissures.
GASTROINTESTINAL	Halitosis. Tongue blisters with excessive salivation. Pyloric cancer: vomit after every meal. Colic: tympanitic, offensive flatus. Gastric and duodenal ulcer. Anal fissures with pruritus. Prolapse. Constipation: large, knotty stools united by threads of mucous. Diarrhoea: less common: chronic, undigested food. Offensive, brown liquid.
CARDIOVASCULAR	Lymphadenitis: indurate.
RESPIRATORY	Vocal cord paralysis. LSLH with roaring and whistling.
LAMENESS	Spine: muscular pain and stiffness. Excoriations between thighs.

	Shoulders: weak, stiff, painful.
	Hooves and nails: blackened, rough, thick, and crumble on shoeing.
	Oedema of the extremities.
SKIN	Inferior quality with cracks and eruptions around the anus, mouth, nipples, toes. Raw behind ears, on limb bends, neck, and groin. Every injury suppurates: exudate: honey-like, sticky. Sweet itch and veld mange. Early fibroma. Ulcers: exudation: glutinous, fluid, thin, sticky liquid.
GERIATRIC	Nail and hoof problems in the overweight.
COMPETITION	Excellent for improving hoof quality. LSLH if early.
MODALITIES	Agg: cold. Night. Music. Warmth.
	Amel: bandaging and wrapping. Dark. Walking.
COMPARE	Acid-nit Arg-n Ars Petr Sep Sulph.
CONSIDER	Important:
	• Cancer of the stomach.
	• Duodenal and gastric ulcer.
	• Eczema that is offensive with a sticky honey-like exudate.
	• Gastroenteritis is chronic.
	• Hooves that are weak, deformed and crumble.
	• LSLH in obese juveniles with bad feet.
POTENCY	6X – 12X. 30CH.

Grat

GRATIOLA OFFICINALIS
Hedge hyssop Plant

Chronic mucous gastrointestinal and urogenital conditions. Ulcers. Is this the female Nux-v?

CNS	Vertigo before and after food.
	Angry: easily confused. Fears: approach, touch, work.
	Irritable and obstinate.
HEAD	Dry, painful conjunctivitis.
GASTROINTESTINAL	Colic: tympanitic and impaction: after evening meal and night.
	Diarrhoea: green, frothy water, painlessly forced out.
UROGENITAL	Metritis and nymphomania.
	Oversexed males.
LAMENESS	Lower back pain.
MODALITIES	Agg: PD.
COMPARE	Anth Dig Euph Nux-v Tab.
CONSIDER	• Behaviour modification in strong willed mares with a tendency to colic.
POTENCY	6X – 12X. 30CH. 200CH.

Gua

GUACO
Climbing hemp weed Plant

Spinal irritation. Antidote to scorpion and snake bite. Bulbar paralysis.

GASTROINTESTINAL	PD. Tongue: heavy, slow, swallowing difficult. Dysentery.
RESPIRATORY	Constricted larynx.
UROGENITAL	PU. Cystitis: cloudy, phosphaturia.
LAMENESS	Ataxia. Painful back, hindquarters, hock.
MODALITIES	Agg: movement.
COMPARE	Acid-oxal Caust Lath.
CONSIDER	• Ataxia of medullary origin. • Cancer.
POTENCY	6X − 12X. 30CH.

Guai
GUAIACUM OFFICINALE
Resin of *lignum vitae* Plant

HEAD	Periorbital pimples. Dilated pupils in dull, sluggish individuals.
GASTROINTESTINAL	Averse to milk. Furred tongue. Weak throat muscles. Acute tonsillitis. Tympanitic colic. Severe juvenile Diarrhoea.
RESPIRATORY	Lungs, pleura. Cough: dry, offensive, tight.
UROGENITAL	Urethritis with tenesmus. Ovaritis. Epididymitis.
LAMENESS	Arthritis: spine, shoulder, hock. Growing pains.
MODALITIES	Agg: heat. Motion. Night. Cold, wet weather. Amel: firm bandaging and wrapping.
COMPARE	Caust Mez Merc Rhod Rhus-t.
CONSIDER	• Arthritis.
POTENCY	6X − 12X.

Gunp
GUNPOWDER
Black gunpowder Mineral

GASTROINTESTINAL	Rectal fissures. Penetrating wounds anywhere.
COMPARE	Arn Calen Pyr.
CONSIDER	• Septic conditions.
POTENCY	4X − 12X.

Halo
HALOPERIDOL
Butyrophenol Mineral

Anxious, depressed and fear being alone. Restless in evenings. Poor concentration leads to mood swings. Allergic and behavioural problems.

HEAD	Allergic conjunctivitis. Early cataract. Photophobia. Painful left ear.
GASTROINTESTINAL	Poor easily satisfied appetite. Eructation. Hypersalivation. Daytime vomiting. Salt desire. Chronic constipation. Incontinence with pruritus.

CARDIOVASCULAR	Asthma. Heart: fainting attacks. Rapid and weak. BP low. Poor peripheral circulation.
UROGENITAL	Incontinence and urinary retention. Male libido reduced.
LAMENESS	Spasm of neck muscles.
SKIN	Eczema: blotchy, pruritic, yellow. Excessive sweating.
MODALITIES	Amel: company. Walking.
COMPARE	Agar Anh Chlor.
CONSIDER	• Allergy. • Behaviour modification.
POTENCY	30CH. 200CH.

Ham

HAMAMELIS VIRGINIANA
Virginian witch hazel Plant

Polycrest. Calm, even during a significant, painful bleed. Dull. Solitary. Work: averse to. Venous congestion. Painful, passive haemorrhages. Open, painful wounds with major blood loss. Postoperative control of passive, profuse haemorrhage. Significant antibacterial agent.

HEAD	**Eyes** bloodshot, vessels injected. Intra-ocular haemorrhage. Hematoma. Epistaxis. Blood clots poorly.
GASTROINTESTINAL	Hematemesis: black. Halitosis. Thirst. Tongue blistered on sides. Pharyngitis, tonsillitis: congested, veins prominent. Dysentery.
CARDIOVASCULAR	Passive venous haemorrhage: clots slow. Hematoma.
RESPIRATORY	Cough: bloody, tickling.
UROGENITAL	**Cystitis** with haematuria. Female: genitalia: pruritic. Varicosities. Nipple: sore when suckling. Ovaritis. Male genitalia: painfully swollen. Epididymitis. Orchitis.
BREEDING	Useful postpartum to involute uterus. Pain control. Varicosities in mature mare. May preserve stud with acute orchitis.
LAMENESS	Painful stiffness of cervical and lumbar vertebrae and joints. **Extremities** swollen after snare entrapment. Snake bites. Lymphadenitis. 'Phleg leg.'
SKIN	Haemorrhage or increased venous vascularity: bruising, burns, ecchymosis, phlebitis, purpura haemorrhagica, trauma, venous. Pain is severe.
MODALITIES	Agg: moist air. Pressure at damaged site. Warmth. Amel: fresh air.
COMPARE	Acid-sul Arn Bell-p Calen Puls Symph Tril.
CONSIDER	• **Venous haemorrhage with poor** clotting. Pain is severe, yet animal does not panic.
POTENCY	4X – 8X. 30CH.

149

Harp
HARPAGOPHYTUM PROCUMBENS
Devil's claw Plant

LAMENESS	Painful joints, tendons, and muscles.
	DJD and OA of hip and carpus.
COMPARE	Caust Mang Ruta Sil.
CONSIDER	• Painful DJD and OA.
POTENCY	6X – 12X.

Hedeo
HEDEOMA PULEGOIDES
Penny royal Plant

GASTROINTESTINAL	Tongue coated white.
	Gastritis: painful, vomiting.
UROGENITAL	Cystitis, nephritis. Red, sediment and tenesmus.
	Metritis: painful, pruritic. Ovaritis.
LAMENESS	Painful muscle twitching.
MODALITIES	Amel: lying down. After urination.
COMPARE	Hed Lil-t Oci Sep.
CONSIDER	• Painful pruritic metritis.
POTENCY	6X – 12X.

Hed
HEDERA HELIX
European ivy Plant

CNS	Insomnia. Ability to work decreases as anxiety increases.
HEAD	Acute, chronic allergic rhinitis. Thyroiditis.
GASTROINTESTINAL	Toothache. Gastric and duodenal ulcers.
CARDIOVASCULAR	Arrhythmia and extrasystoles. Myocarditis. Tachycardia.
MODALITIES	Agg: 3am.
	Amel: fresh air. Cold therapy. Massage. Wrapping.
COMPARE	Calc-fl Iod Nat-m Thyr.
CONSIDER	• Cardiac disease with thyroiditis.
POTENCY	4X. 30CH.

Hekla
HEKLA LAVA
Lava scoriae Mineral

Necrosis of the jaw bones. Mild mannered but can erupt.

HEAD	Abscess and epulis on gums.
	Toothache with a swollen jaw. Actinomycosis. Maxillary and nasal bones enlarged: cancer: osteomyelitis, osteoporosis, periostitis.
	Neuralgic pain: diseased teeth, extraction.
	Lymphadenitis: cervical.
MODALITIES	Agg: damp air. Touch.
COMPARE	Merc Phos Sil.

CONSIDER	• Jaw and other head bone disease.
POTENCY	8X. 30CH.

Hell
HELLEBORUS NIGER
Christmas rose Plant

Trauma and CNS infections. Great anxiety with fears: irrational, and of being alone, yet averse to company. Mood swings lead to depression and OCD. Marked weakness: senses suppressed. Oedema and effusions.

Automatic rhythmical movements: weaving, stretching.

CNS	Head / brain injuries. Head shaking, weaving. Meningitis with unconsciousness. Odd automatic gestures.
HEAD	Dilated pupils. Left facial neuralgia. Dirty, dry nostrils.
GASTROINTESTINAL	Lips dried and cracked. Chewing difficult. Teeth: grinding, loose. Hypersalivation. Tongue: red, dry. Colic; tympanitic. Faeces: involuntary, mucous.
CARDIOVASCULAR	Cardiac incompetence. Bradycardia. Hydrothorax.
UROGENITAL	Distended juvenile bladder with difficulty urinating. Scant, red urine with sediment.
LAMENESS	Ataxia: obvious at a slow walk. Distal oedema.
SKIN	Weak, falling hair. Hooves: brittle, crumble. Vesicular eruptions between digits.
MODALITIES	Agg: chilly air. Covering. Dark. Exertion. Evening until morning. Amel: bandaging. Rest. Warmth. Wrapping.
COMPARE	*Helleboris foetidus* Hell-f. Bears foot. Similar but also spleen and sciatic neuralgia. *Helleboris orientalis* Hell-f. Apis Cic Cinch Iod Tub Zinc.
CONSIDER	Traumatic and infectious CNS problems including: • Brain injury. • Meningitis. • Sudden onset paralysis.
POTENCY	6X – 12X. 30CH. 200CH.

Helo
HELODERMA SUSPECTUM
Gila monster Animal

GASTROINTESTINAL	Tongue: cold, dry, tender. Swallowing difficult.
CARDIOVASCULAR	Great palpitation.
LAMENESS	Ataxia with numbness, trembling, and staggering. Odd goose-step walking. Stretching. Upper spine stiff.
COMPARE	*Lacerta agilis* Lacer. Green lizard. Mouth constantly full of saliva with vesicles under tongue. Dermal eruptions.
CONSIDER	• Ataxia.

151

POTENCY	30CH.

Helon
HELONIAS DIOICA
False unicorn root Plant

UROGENITAL	PD / PU. Diabetes mellitus.
	Nephritis with albuminuria, glycosuria and phosphaturia.
	Metritis after foetal loss.
LAMENESS	Back pain referred from kidney.
MODALITIES	Agg: motion. Touch.
	Amel: effort.
COMPARE	Alet Puls Senec Stann.
CONSIDER	• Diabetes mellitus.
	• Metritis.
POTENCY	4X – 12X.

Hep
HEPAR SULPHURIS CALCAREUM HAHNEMANN
Calcium sulphide Mineral

Polycrest. Anger with violence: bite, kick. Anxieties: evening, when exercising, separation. Apprehensive and discontented, always on guard. Company: appear to enjoy but need space, avoid touch. Fears: crowds, dark, exercise, open air, thunder, touch. Impetuous. Pain threshold is low. Sad with great sensitivity. Lesions show marked suppuration. Form small papules around old lesion. Offensive with an old cheesy smell. Often bloody and sensitive. Patients have a dirty, unkempt appearance. Significant antibacterial agent.

CNS	Vertigo on shaking the head.
HEAD	Facial eczema: pruritic, scab, smelly.
	Facial bones: pain on palpation.
	Conjunctivitis. Chemosis. Photophobia. Exudates: profuse, purulent. Eyeball: painful.
	Otitis externa, media: painful, purulent. Sinusitis.
	Pustules. Nostrils blocked outdoors, excoriated, ulcerated.
ABDOMEN	Chronic liver abscess. Hepatitis and peritonitis.
GASTROINTESTINAL	Eructation without taste or smell. Mouth, stomach: ulcers: bleed.
	Faeces: clay-coloured, offensive, soft, undigested.
CARDIOVASCULAR	Palpitation. Lymph gland abscess.
	Strangles: chronic.
RESPIRATORY	**Asthma: suffocating,** dry cough with mucous.
	Voice lost in dry, chilly wind.
UROGENITAL	Metritis: bloody, offensive.
LAMENESS	Fistulous wither. Digital joints sensitive.
	Nails, hooves: brittle, weak. Laminitis.
FEVER	Chilly outdoors or from slightest draught.
	Sweat: offensive, profuse, sticky, sour.
SKIN	Unhealthy: every small injury suppurates.

	Abscess with papules; extend, bleed easily and suppurate.
	Digits: deep cracks. Ulcers: offensive.
	Urticaria: chronic, recurrent.
MODALITIES	Agg: cool air. Drafts. Dry wind. Touch.
	Amel: eating. Warmth. Damp weather.
COMPARE	Acon Bry Calc-s Gunp Merc Myris Sanic Sil Spon Staph.
CONSIDER	Immense importance in bacterial infections:
	• The presence of pain and pus.
	• Strangles and other lymphadenitis scenarios.
	• Ulceration is offensive.
	Remember:
	• Great pain.
	• Hypersensitivity.
	• Cheesy offensive yellow pus.
POTENCY	4X to encourage pus formation.
	12X. 30CH. 200CH prophylaxis after injury.

Hipp
HIPPOMANES
Equine allantois Animal

Prostate and ligament problems in dull sad individuals that dislike company and fear dark

UROGENITAL	Prostatomegaly. Poor male libido.
LAMENESS	Constriction of annular and carpal ligaments.
	Radial paralysis.
COMPARE	Caust Ruta.
CONSIDER	• Tired breeding males with weak libido.
	• Constricted ligaments.
POTENCY	12X. 30CH.

Hippo
HIPPOZAENINUM
Glanders disease Animal

HEAD	Rhinitis, sinusitis: chronic, mucous, ulceration of nasal cartilage. Nocturnal delirium. Significant antibacterial agent.
CARDIOVASCULAR	Mucous asthma and bronchitis. Strangles. Lymphadenitis.
SKIN	Swollen with abscess and pustules. Periarticular.
COMPARE	Aur Bac Kali-by Psor.
CONSIDER	• Chronic mucous respiratory problems.
POTENCY	30CH. 200CH.

Hir
HIRUDO MEDICINALIS
Sanguisuga officinalis Leech Animal

HEAD	Bloody conjunctivitis in dull, sad individuals. Hematomata.
GASTROINTESTINAL	Haemoptysis. Tonsillitis. Stomach ulcers: bleed.
CARDIOVASCULAR	Anaemia. Thrombocytopenia. Lymphadenitis.
SKIN	Bruise easily. Hematoma.
MODALITIES	Agg: after Faeces.
	Amel: coughing.
COMPARE	Crot-h Lach Lat-m Lach Naja.
CONSIDER	• Any bruising and haemorrhage.
POTENCY	12X. 30CH.

Hist
HISTAMINUM MURIATICUM
Histamine Animal

Dull and adverse to company with restlessness. Abusive. and restless. Allergies with great weakness and dry mucous membranes.

HEAD	Blepharitis. Rhinitis. Conjunctivitis.
	Exudate: zero or thick, yellow.
GASTROINTESTINAL	Salivation either absent or profuse. IBD. Gastric, duodenal ulcers: painful. Diarrhoea: bloody, offensive.
CARDIOVASCULAR	Arrhythmia. Extrasystoles.
RESPIRATORY	Asthma, bronchitis, lower airway disease.
	Cough: chronic, dry, hacking, painful.
UROGENITAL	Dysuria. Metritis.
LAMENESS	Acute, painful muscle spasms.
SKIN	Alopecia. Dry. Hot spots.
	Urticaria may resolve fast enough to allow competition.
MODALITIES	Agg: heat. Movement.
	Amel: pressure.
COMPARE	Apis Ars Sec Urt.
CONSIDER	• Allergic conditions.
POTENCY	12X. 30CH.

Hoit
HOITZIA COCCINEA
Colibri flower Plant

CNS	Viral encephalosis, meningitis. Irrationally fearful, excitable.
HEAD	Blepharitis. Conjunctivitis. Epiphora. Photophobia; fixed gaze.
	Otitis media. Epistaxis: mild, recurrent.
	Sinusitis: frontal, maxillary. Nostrils: painful scabs, vesicles.
GASTROINTESTINAL	Gingivitis: dry, sticky, thick. Thirsty but vomit after.
	Tongue swollen. Painful gastritis.
	Constipation: dry, hard, balls.
CARDIOVASCULAR	Myocarditis. Pericarditis. Insufficiency.
	Pulse: full, fast.
RESPIRATORY	Laryngitis. Bronchitis. Pneumonia.

UROGENITAL	Cystitis. Frothy, haematuria, tenesmus.
	Uterine cancer.
	Prostate: adenoma.
LAMENESS	Periarticular muscle pain.
SKIN	Anthrax-like lesions. Alopecia. seborrhoea.
MODALITIES	Agg: movement.
	Amel: curling up.
COMPARE	Ars Bell Euph Rhus-t Thuj Vac.
CONSIDER	• Post viral problems.
POTENCY	6X – 12X.
	Thuj and Vac 30CH before vaccination.

Hydrang
HYDRANGEA ARBORESCENS
Seven barks Plant

UROGENITAL	PD / PU. Urethritis. Cystitis. Nephritis. Haematuria, calculi, mucous. Tenesmus. Prostatomegaly.
LAMENESS	Pain in left lumbar region referred from kidney.
COMPARE	**Berb** Chim Ferr-pic Lyc Pareir Sabal Uva.
CONSIDER	• Urinary calculi.
POTENCY	4X – 12X.

Hydr
HYDRASTIS CANADENSIS
Golden seal Plant

Individuals are often thin, exhausted, and chronically ill. Depressed, dull, and irritable after food. **Exudation** of mucous is thick, yellowish, and ropy.

HEAD	Conjunctivitis: chronic, mucopurulent.
	Deafness from blocked eustachian tube.
	Sinusitis: acrid, chronic, secondary, tenacious, thick, ulcerated, watery.
GASTROINTESTINAL	Tongue: flabby, teeth imprint. Slimy, swollen, ulcerated, white.
	Stomach: cancer, ulcer.
	Perirectal fissure, prolapse.
RESPIRATORY	Cough: dry, harsh: bronchitis, laryngitis, pharyngitis.
	Follicular pharyngitis: juvenile horses: chronic, copious, yellow, tenacious mucous.
UROGENITAL	Urine: smelly and sticky. Genital pruritus. Cervical erosion. Metritis: excoriating. Mammary cancer.
	Retracted nipple.
	Right sided Orchitis.
LAMENESS	Mares with referred pain: ovary, uterus.
SKIN	Cancer: benign, malignant. Unhealthy. Lupus.
COMPETITION	2-Y-O in training with follicular pharyngitis.
GERIATRIC	The thin and weak with a tendency to chronic bronchitis.
COMPARE	Ars-i Aster Con Kali-by Phyt Puls.
CONSIDER	Respiratory disease in thin individuals:
	• Bronchitis.

- Pharyngitis.
- Sinusitis.

Guiding signs are debility, tenacious, thick mucoid exudates.

POTENCY	6X – 12X. 30CH.

Hydrc
HYDROCOTYLE ASIATICA
Indian pennywort Plant

UROGENITAL	Cystitis at neck. Female genital pruritus.
	Metritis: granulating ulcers: uterus, cervix.
SKIN	Acne-like conditions with pruritus. Exudate: circular spots, dry, pustular, scales. Profuse sweating. Psoriasis of digits.
COMPARE	*Elaeis guineensis* Elae. South American Palm. Elephantiasis. Pruritic skin is hard and thick.
	Hura brasiliensis Hura. Assacu. Eczema. Snake bite. Ulcers.
	Ars Aur Hydr Sep.
CONSIDER	• Chronic eczema with marked thickening.
	• Lupus.
POTENCY	6X – 12X. 30CH.

Hydroph
HYDROPHIS CYANOCINCTUS
Sea snake Animal

CNS	Viral conditions. Dull, lack concentration. Fatigue.
HEAD	Left sided blepharitis, conjunctivitis, pruritic.
	Painful deafness. Acrid nasal exudate.
GASTROINTESTINAL	PD. Pharyngitis, tonsillitis: mouth dry.
	Colic: left colon. Constipation: painful after faeces.
CARDIOVASCULAR	Arrhythmia. Valvular incompetence.
RESPIRATORY	Laryngitis, bronchitis: cough tickling. Dyspnoea.
UROGENITAL	Cervicitis. Ovaritis. Vaginitis.
LAMENESS	Muscle: lameness: severely painful, even paretic.
COMPARE	Lach Lath.
MODALITIES	Agg: heat. Mornings.
	Amel: Lying flat or on one side.
CONSIDER	• Heart disease.
	• Painful left-sided paralysis.
POTENCY	12X. 30CH.

Hyos
HYOSCYAMUS NIGER
Black henbane Plant

disturbances. Illness from fear, grief, and jealousy.
Dangerous animals startle easily and become angry, violent, and will kick and bite.
Desire company but may be dull, sad, and easy to excite.
Fears: being alone, dogs, men, and water.

Foolish, demented behaviour with odd gestures. OCD. Nymphomania. Very vocal. Most severe mood swings in toy dog breeds who flash from cheerful to downright nasty. Offensive behavioural

CNS	Encephalosis with unconsciousness. Epilepsy during fever. Vocal then sleepy.
	Neuralgia: marked muscle twitching.
HEAD	Pupils: dilated, fixed. Strabismus.
GASTROINTESTINAL	Anorexia. Great foaming salivation with a slack, dropped jaw. Tongue: dry, immovable, red, stiff. Hiccough.
	Gastric dilatation: torsion, rupture.
	Vomit blood during fits.
	Colic: tympanitic, extreme pain.
	Diarrhoea is involuntary.
RESPIRATORY	Constricted throat causes a dry, nocturnal, and spasmodic cough with a bloody expectorant.
UROGENITAL	Bladder: incontinent: paralysis with retention and overflow.
	Nymphomania. Dangerous periparturient behaviour.
LAMENESS	Severe muscle spasms.
MODALITIES	Agg: after food. Oestrous. Lying down. Night. Postpartum. Touch.
	Amel: movement. Walking. Sitting up.
COMPARE	Agar Bell Gels Stram.
CONSIDER	Important:
	• Behavioural abnormalities.
	• Colic with tympany and great pain.
	These are acute conditions associated with seriously disturbing behaviour in dangerous animals.
POTENCY	30CH. 200CH.

Hyper
HYPERICUM PERFORATUM
St John's wort Plant

Polycrest. The remedy for injury to nerves, especially of toes and nails, from bites, and crushing. Bacterial infection. Anxiety. Claustrophobia. Confused. Depressed. Fear heights and are oversensitive to pain. **Excessive painfulness** is a guiding symptom to its use. Prevention and treatment of tetanus. Relieves pain and spasms after injury, operation. Significant antibacterial agent.

CNS	Brain and nerve injury. Shock. Neuritis.
	Pain: injury, surgery, excruciating. Tetanus.
HEAD	Painful right sided neuralgia. Hair loss.
GASTROINTESTINAL	Thirst. Tongue: coated white at base only.
	Ulcers: chronic, painful. Vomiting. Tenesmus.
RESPIRATORY	Asthma is worse during foggy weather.
LAMENESS	Pain: nape of neck, sacrum, coccyx. May radiate down legs from back. Spinal concussion: jerking, twitching.
	Cramp in calves. Pain: shoulders, ulnar nerve.
	Pain: hooves, nails, toes.
	Sole: control pain, prevent infection from puncture

157

	wounds.
COMPETITION	Prophylactic against infection and lameness after hoof prick. May relax anxious, spooky animals, particularly if they tend to sensitive feet.
SKIN	Hair loss: post injury. Photosensitisation.
	Eczema: pruritic: face and feet.
	Lacerated, surgical wounds: blood loss, prostration.
MODALITIES	Agg: Closed room. Touch. Weather: cold, damp, fog.
	Amel: Bending head backward. Lying down quietly.
COMPARE	Arn. Calen. Coff. Led. Ruta. Staph.
CONSIDER	Important remedy to consider in:
	• Behavioural abnormalities: anxiety and depression.
	• Injury including haemorrhage and nerve trauma.
	• Spinal nerve injury.
	• Surgery: prepare for and afterwards.
	• Tetanus treatment and prevention.
POTENCY	6X – 12X. 30CH. 200CH.

Pitu

HYPOPHYSIS POSTERIOR

Pituitary gland Animal

GASTROINTESTINAL	Hypersalivation. Vomit after food. Colic with tenesmus.
RESPIRATORY	Dyspnoea of asthma: with colic, great anxiety.
UROGENITAL	Incontinent: evenings: drop by drop. Albuminuria. Anuria.
SKIN	Pigmentation in females.
MODALITIES	Agg: evening. Heat.
	Amel: fresh air.
POTENCY	30CH.

Iber

IBERIS AMARA

Bitter candytuft Plant

GASTROINTESTINAL	Hepatomegaly. Clay-coloured Faeces.
CARDIOVASCULAR	Arrhythmia. Hypertrophy. Failure. Palpitation. Vertigo. Mucous. Heart conditions from viral infections. Distal oedema.
MODALITIES	Agg: after food. Morning. Warm, open air.
	Amel, when eating. Positional changes.
COMPARE	Cimic Kali-p Nat-m Sep Zinc.
CONSIDER	• Heart disease following viral infection.
POTENCY	4X – 12X.

Ign

IGNATIA AMARA

St Ignatia's bean Plant

Erratic signs match its changeable behaviour pattern. Anger, brooding, company, averse to. Fears: approach, vets. Hide. Sad.

Oversensitivity leads to destructive, behavioural changes. Great, chronic reactions to emotional trauma, including severe depression.

CNS	Epilepsy following mental trauma, shock, unconscious.
HEAD	Muscle twitch.
GASTROINTESTINAL	Colic: salivation, tympany.
	Pica results in foreign body.
	Tonsillitis with small ulcers.
	Range: from painful constipation to diarrhoea brought on by fear. Prolapse.
RESPIRATORY	Laryngeal constriction with spasmodic cough.
UROGENITAL	Female genital pruritus.
LAMENESS	Achilles tendonitis. Tender soles.
COMPETITION	Helps sensitive fillies to work better after poor training experience.
SKIN	Urticaria.
MODALITIES	Agg: after food. Morning. Open and warm air.
	Amel, when eating. Positional changes.
COMPARE	Cimic Kali-p Nat-m Sep Zinc.
CONSIDER	• Invaluable in epilepsy.
	• Acute, chronic mental trauma.
	Use even when correct mental picture absent.
POTENCY	12X. 30CH. 200CH.

Indg
INDIGO TINCTORIA
Dye from *Indigofera spp* Plant

Epilepsy. Sad, excitable, hysterical individuals that desire activity. Proceeded by vertigo.

GASTROINTESTINAL	Anorexia. Bloody sneezing. Helminthiasis.
	Colic: tympanitic: eructation, rectal pruritus.
UROGENITAL	Mucous, turbid urine with tenesmus.
LAMENESS	• Pain in sacroiliacs and thighs.
MODALITIES	Agg: after food. Rest. Sitting.
	Amel: grooming. Walking.

Infl
INFLUENZINUM
Human flu virus Animal

RESPIRATORY	Laryngitis, bronchitis, pneumonitis: acute, mucous.
MODALITIES	Agg: movement.
	Amel: rest.
CONSIDER	Respiratory virus infection:
	• Prophylaxis of.
	• Treatment of.
POTENCY	12X – 30CH.

Ins

159

INSULINUM
Insulin Animal

Fluctuating blood glucose levels. Juvenile obesity.

HEAD	Chronic otitis: exudate: thin.
UROGENITAL	Diabetes mellitus when insulin is difficult to balance.
SKIN	Unhealthy. Wounds easily infected.
COMPARE	Ars Chin.
CONSIDER	• Diabetes mellitus. • Otitis media.
POTENCY	12X in otitis. 200CH in diabetes mellitus.

Iod
IODUM PURUM
Iodine Mineral

Initially have fluent, hot exudates and are often right sided. Night fever. Anxious and depressed. Impulsive and always busy. Fear people.

HEAD	Oedema of eyelids. Dacryocystitis. Dilated pupils. Rhinitis with ulcers.
ABDOMEN	Hepatitis. Pancreatitis. Splenitis.
GASTROINTESTINAL	PD. Ravenous appetite with weight loss. Eructation. Gums: bleed, swollen. Hypersalivation. Offensive halitosis. Tongue thickly coated. Loose teeth. Ulcers. Constipation, diarrhoea alternate. Tenesmus. Diarrhoea: bloody, fatty, frothy, whitish.
CARDIOVASCULAR	Myocarditis: palpitation, fast pulse. Chronic vertigo. Hyperthyroidism. Thyroiditis.
RESPIRATORY	Bronchitis: acute, chronic, pleurisy, pneumonia. Cough: Kennel Cough-like. Fever.
UROGENITAL	PU: acrid, copious, dark, yellow to green, thick. Mammary atrophy. Painful ovarian dysfunction. Metritis: acrid, bloody, slimy, thick.
LAMENESS	Chronic bursitis and osteoarthritis. Ringbone.
SKIN	Dry, hot, withered, and yellow.
MODALITIES	Agg: rest. Warm room. Amel: open air. Walking.
COMPARE	Abrot Brom Hep Merc Nat-m Phos Sanic Tub.
CONSIDER	A powerful remedy in: • Arthritis with chronic deformity: ringbone. • Any chronic, relapsing conditions. • Emaciation. • Immune system modulation. • Chronic pneumonia. • Thyroid disease.
POTENCY	2X – 12X.

Iris
IRIS VERSICOLOR
Blue flag Plant

ABDOMEN	Hepatitis, pancreatitis, pancreatic insufficiency: acute, chronic.
GASTROINTESTINAL	Appetite is poor. Hypersalivation is ropy. Vomit: bilious, sour.
	Tympanitic colic.
	Constipation with pruritus.
	Gastroenteritis: acrid, green, nocturnal, watery.
CARDIOVASCULAR	**Modulator of thyroid function.**
LAMENESS	Vague, but severe, shifting back pains. Left hip.
SKIN	Pruritic, nocturnal, pustular eruptions. Psoriasis.
MODALITIES	Agg: evening. Night. Rest.
	Amel: walking.
COMPARE	Other Iris spp. Ars Ant-c Ip Podo Sang, Pancr Tryp.
CONSIDER	Adjunctive therapy in:
	• Gastroenteritis.
	• Liver tonic.
	• Pancreatic insufficiency.
	• Thyroid balancing.
POTENCY	6X – 12X.

Jac-c
JACARANDA CAROBA
Brazilian carob tree Plant

HEAD	Conjunctivitis, sinusitis: exudate: watery.
RESPIRATORY	Laryngitis, pharyngitis: constricted, dry, vesicles.
UROGENITAL	Urethritis. Sarcoid.
	Male genitalia: enlarged, pruritic.
LAMENESS	Weakness of lower back and right stifle.
COMPARE	*Jacaranda gualandai* Jac. Similar.
	Cor-r Thuj.
CONSIDER	• Enlarged, pruritic male genitalia.
POTENCY	2X – 8X.

Jal
JALAPA
Exogonium purga Plant

GASTROINTESTINAL	Painful, dry, gazed tongue. Vomit. Painful thin, muddy coloured diarrhoea: pruritus, tympany. IBD: juvenile.
LAMENESS	Synovitis of digits with stiff muscles.
COMPARE	Camph Coloc.
CONSIDER	• IBD in juveniles.
POTENCY	4X – 12X.

Jug-r
JUGLANS REGIA
British walnut Plant

CARDIOVASCULAR	Poor distal circulation: laminitis, phleg leg.
	Axillary lymphadenitis.
SKIN	*Crustea lactea.* Small red pimples on ears.

	Nocturnal pruritis.
COMPARE	**Juglans cinerea** Jug-c. Liver disease with eczema. Bry Chel Iris.
CONSIDER	• Eczema of ears.
POTENCY	4X – 12X.

Juni-c
JUNIPERUS COMMUNIS
Juniper berry Plant

UROGENITAL	Cystitis, nephritis, prostatitis, pyelonephritis: chronic, geriatric. Urine: bloody, scant, smells of violets.
COMPARE	*Juniperus virgimana* Juni. Red cedar. Severe tenesmus. Sabal Tereb.
CONSIDER	• Chronic, geriatric nephritis.
POTENCY	4X – 12X.

Kali-ars
KALIUM ARSENICOSUM
Fowler's solution Mineral

Morning anxieties make them indifferent, irrational, and suspicious. Fear of crowds. Anaemia, cancer, and chronic skin disease. Significant antibacterial agent.

UROGENITAL	Cervix: cancer: cauliflower-like, offensive, painful.
SKIN	Cancer: malignant: acute, often dramatically so with dry nodules under the skin. Sarcoid: scales, wilted. Eczema: fissures on bends of joints. Intolerably pruritic. Psoriasis. Lichenified patched. Pustules. Ulcers. *Veld mange.*
COMPARE	Other Kaliums. Ars Bov Mez Rad.
CONSIDER	• Cancer of the skin. • Eczema of the most severe kinds. • Insect bite sensitivities.
POTENCY	12X. 30CH. 200CH.

Kali-bi
KALIUM BICHROMICUM
Potassium bichromate Mineral

Polycrest. Fears: crowds, dark, men. Makes them impatient, irritable, and averse to work. Do not cope with pressure, and this leads to violence when they will bite and kick. Affinity for mucous membranes of the gastrointestinal and respiratory systems.
Important effects on bone, fibrous tissue, kidneys, heart, and liver. Significant antibacterial agent. Ulceration is common with distinctive small, punctate, round lesions. Exudates have diagnostic thick, yellow, ropy, stringy appearance. Left sided.

HEAD	Neuralgia: facial: right, supra-orbital. Conjunctivitis. Descemitis. Punctate deposits on inner cornea. Ulcers with little pain. Exudate: granular, ropy, yellow. Iritis. Eyelid oedema. Pannus. Otitis media, externa: pus, stringy, thick, and yellow. Rhinitis, sinusitis: acute, blocked, chronic, frontal,

ABDOMEN
GASTROINTESTINAL

mouth breathing, profuse, watery.
Septal ulcer. Sneezing: violent.
Liver enlarged, fatty.
Mouth: PD: dry, rough, viscid saliva.
Tongue: dry, indented, mapped, red, shiny, smooth, thickly coated.
Throat: dilated. Diphtheria: profound, prostration. Tonsils, soft palate: pseudo-membranous deposit.
Gastritis: ulcers: punctate, round, small. Vomiting: bright yellow, watery. Colic: after food.
Constipation: periodic.
Diarrhoea: gelatinous, jelly-like, worse in mornings. Dysentery: brown, frothy.

CARDIOVASCULAR
RESPIRATORY

Anaemia. Lymphadenitis: parotid.
Cough: hacking. Exudate: glutinous, membranous, profuse, sticky, stringy, yellow.

UROGENITAL

Cystitis, nephritis, and pyelonephritis. Albuminuria, casts, epithelial cells, haematuria, mucous, PU, pus.
Female genitalia: pruritis. Metritis: tenacious, yellow. Uterine prolapse.
Balanitis: painful, pruritic, pustular, ulcerated.

LAMENESS

Painful, left sided lumbar and sacroiliacs. Polybursitis, pain.
Achilles tendonitis.
Periostitis. Feet bruised and sensitive.

SKIN

Pruritic eruptions. Pustules, vesicles, ulcers with punched out edges. Exudation: sticky, tenacious.

MODALITIES

Agg: heat.
Amel: morning. Hot weather.

COMPARE

Kalium cyanatum Kali-cy. Similar, but has a profound influence on cancer of the tongue, and painful facial neuralgias. 30CH - 200CH.
Kalium muriaticum Kali-mur. Tissue salt 4. Chronic catarrhal inflammation including mouth, throat, and chest.
Kalium nitricum Kali-n. Similar, but has a profound influence on asthma, and purulent nephritis. 6X – 12X. 30CH – 200CH.
Kalium permanganicum Kali-perm. Like the other Kaliums, but has a profound influence on diphtheria, and sepsis with severe tissue destruction. 2X – 8X.
Other Kaliums. Ant-c Ant-t Brom Calc Hep Ind.

CONSIDER

An especially important remedy for its influence in:
- Gastro-enteritis.
- Nephritis.
- Pigeons with membranous crop.
- Rhinitis and sinusitis.
- Ulceration anywhere.

Signalment required for correct prescribing:
- Exudates must be yellow, stringy, and profuse.

	• Ulceration is usually round, punctate with raised edges.
POTENCY	6X – 12X. 30CH. 200CH.

Kali-br
KALIUM BROMATUM
Bromide of potash Mineral

Dull, depressed, sad, need company. Excitable, fidget and may be manic.
Anxiety at night.

CNS	Epilepsy with excitement and great restlessness. Agg: during oestrous.
GASTROINTESTINAL	PD. Persistent hiccough.
	Diabetes mellitus: albuminuria.
	Vomit after food: bloody.
	Diarrhoea is watery green.
RESPIRATORY	Larynx and pharynx: numb. Heart weak.
	Dry, spasmodic, tiring cough during pregnancy.
LAMENESS	Distal muscles: jerking, twitching, weak. Tonic.
SKIN	Offensive psoriasis. *Sweet itch:* chest, shoulders, hindquarters.
MODALITIES	Amel: regular slow work.
COMPARE	Other Kaliums. Ambr, Hyos Stram.
CONSIDER	• Diabetes mellitus.
	• Diarrhoea of neonates.
	• Mental degeneration from overwork.
	• Psoriasis.
POTENCY	6X – 12X. 30CH.

Kali-c
KALIUM CARBONICUM
Potassium carbonate Mineral

Juveniles are anxious when tired or hungry and lacking confidence, fear being alone when they desire   carried. Fears: irrational and of touch. Impatient and irritable. Timid and startle easily. Vocal. Pain and weakness are severe.
Exudates have crusts with thick, tacky, and greenish pus.
Significant antibacterial agent.

HEAD	Dry hair falls easily. Upper eyelids agglutinated. Parotitis. Tonsillitis. Rhinitis and postnasal drip.
GASTROINTESTINAL	Hepatitis: chronic, painful. PD. Dry mouth. Pyorrhoea. Swallow difficult. Hypersalivation.
	Sour vomiting.
	Hyperthyroidism.
	Constipation: bloody, large faeces.
	Rectum: pimples, prolapse, pruritic, ulcers.
CARDIOVASCULAR	Arrhythmia. Palpitation. Weak pulse.
RESPIRATORY	Asthma, bronchitis, hydrothorax, TB. Hard, dry cough.
UROGENITAL	PU. Incontinent. Urates.
	Constant postpartum haemorrhage.
	Weakness after foetal loss. Inexpert, tiring covering efforts.

LAMENESS	Lumbar and hind leg weakness. Soles sensitive.
MODALITIES	Agg: lying on left or painful side. After mating. 3am. Wintry weather. Amel: daytime effort. Moist, warm weather.
COMPARE	Other Kaliums. Bry Carb-v Lyc Natrums Phos Sep Stann.
CONSIDER	• Arthritis of hip and stifle. • Debility. • Hypothyroidism. • Postpartum problems.
POTENCY	12X. 30CH. 200CH.

Kali-chls
KALIUM CHLOROSUM
Potassium chlorate

GASTROINTESTINAL	Hepatitis. Anorexia. Mucosae: aphthous, gangrenous, jaundice, red, swollen, ulcerated. PD. Swollen tongue. Diarrhoea, vomit: black to greenish, flatus, profuse.
UROGENITAL	Anaemia: acute, chronic. Cystitis, nephritis. PU to scant. Albuminuria, bile, haematuria, phosphaturia.
SKIN	Miliary eruptions are pruritic and pigmented.
COMPARE	Other Kaliums.
CONSIDER	• Severe nephritis. • Disgusting stomatitis.
POTENCY	6X – 12X. 30CH.

Kali-i
KALIUM IODATUM
Potassium iodide Mineral

Meningitis in angry, irritable, and sad individuals. Exudates are acrid, greenish, profuse, and mucous or watery. Conditions are often chronic and destructive.

HEAD	Conjunctivitis, chemosis, pustular keratitis. Epiphora. Swollen nose with perforated septum. Sinusitis: bony enlargement, fissures.
GASTROINTESTINAL	Hypersalivation. Gastritis. Rectal fissures.
CARDIOVASCULAR	Heart weakness secondary to oedema of pneumonia.
RESPIRATORY	Asthma, hydrothorax, pneumonia: nocturnal cough.
UROGENITAL	Chronic nephritis. Uterine cancer and metritis.
LAMENESS	Periosteum: thick, sensitive. Lumbar and sacroiliac pain. Hip, stifle, digital: contractions, pain, thickening.
MODALITIES	Agg: bandaging. Night. Warmth. Damp weather. Amel: open air. Movement.
COMPARE	Other Kaliums Iod Merc Mez Sulph.
CONSIDER	• Meningitis. • Periostitis. • Rhinitis. • Sinusitis.

165

POTENCY	6X – 12X. 30CH.

Kali-p
KALIUM PHOSPHORICUM
Potassium phosphate Mineral

Shy, timid, and averse to work, easily frightened, they become irritable. Vertigo. Effect on nerve disease, cancer, and severe exhausting Diarrhoea. Significant antibacterial agent. Exudates may be bloody, brown to yellowish, and are offensive.

HEAD	Eyelids droopy. Rhinitis.
GASTROINTESTINAL	Dry mouth in mornings. PD. Gums: bleed, recede, spongy.
	Tongue gangrenous. Vomiting: incomplete.
	Bloody diarrhoea: blood.
RESPIRATORY	Asthma, laryngitis, vocal cord paralysis.
UROGENITAL	Cystitis, nephritis. PU to anuria, haematuria, incontinent.
	Incomplete labour effort. Metritis.
	Males find covering exhausting.
LAMENESS	Profound weakness of back muscles.
SKIN	Unhealthy, and wounds heal poorly. Gangrene.
MODALITIES	Agg: cold food. Excitement. Exertion. Morning.
	Amel: eating. Rest. Warmth.
COMPARE	Other Kaliums. Cimic Gels Lach Zinc.
CONSIDER	• Cancer: postsurgical healing.
	• Debility.
	• Diarrhoea.
POTENCY	12X. 30CH.

Kali-s
KALIUM SULPHURICUM
Potassium sulphate Mineral

Inherently timid, fear dark, and startle easily which leads to irritability, restless, and angry. Inflammatory conditions advance into profuse desquamation. Exudates intermittent, but profuse. They are usually mucopurulent slimy and offensive. Fevers. Significant antibacterial agent.

HEAD	Eustachian tube deafness. Acute rhinitis.
GASTROINTESTINAL	Tongue is slimy and yellow.
	Colic: tympanitic. Constipation. Diarrhoea.
RESPIRATORY	Asthma. Bronchospasm. Rales.
UROGENITAL	Nephritis with urate crystals.
LAMENESS	Generalised, shifting muscular pains.
SKIN	Bald spots, dandruff, papules, ringworm, scaly.
	Psoriasis. seborrhoea.
	Urticaria.
	Epithelioma. Polyps.
MODALITIES	Agg: evening. Heated room.
	Amel: open air. Cool.
COMPARE	Other Kaliums. Nat-m. Puls.
CONSIDER	• Eczema that is pruritic and offensive.
	• Nephritis with urate crystals.

- Ringworm associated with debility.

POTENCY	4X – 12X. 30CH.

Kalm
KALMIA LATIFOLIA
Mountain laurel Plant

CNS	Painful ataxia and vertigo. Early morning insomnia.
HEAD	Right sided, facial neuralgia.
CARDIOVASCULAR	Painful, sudden tachycardia.
UROGENITAL	PD / PU. Nephritis with albuminuria and vomiting.
LAMENESS	Sudden, sharp pains anywhere. Periarticular. Ulnar nerve. Feet hot and swollen. Soles: sensitive.
MODALITIES	Agg: bending forwards. Movement.
COMPARE	Spig Puls.
CONSIDER	Any sudden, sharp pains:

- Ataxia.
- Heart conditions.
- Periarticular arthritis
- Neuralgia.

POTENCY	2X – 8X.

Karw-h
KARWINSKIA HUMBOLDTIANA
Wild capuli Plant

Ataxia and various paralytic conditions of lip, pharynx, and throat. Bradycardia. Begins on left.

RESPIRATORY	Asphyxia from gradual, infection induced, paralysis of throat.
LAMENESS	Progressive, painful degeneration of muscle motor function.
COMPARE	Acid-hydr Lath Plb.
CONSIDER	• Encephalitis.
POTENCY	30CH. 200CH.

Kig
KIGELIA AFRICANA
Sausage tree Plant

SKIN	Developing remedy in the management of a variety of skin cancers from warts to melanoma and sarcoid.
POTENCY	2X topically. 12X.

Kou
KOUSSO
***Brayera anthelmintica* Plant**

GASTROINTESTINAL	Helminthiasis: tapeworms.
CARDIOVASCULAR	Arrhythmia: collapse, vertigo, vomiting.
COMPARE	*Kamala* Kam. Tapeworm. Fil Spig Teucr.
POTENCY	2X.

167

Lac-c
LAC CANINUM
Canine milk Animal

Apathy and sadness, easily startled into excitement, and become unpleasant. Throat conditions associated with great weakness. Exudates are bloody, purulent.

HEAD	Nostrils blocked alternately. Nasal bones: pain.
GASTROINTESTINAL	Cracked lips and nostrils. Tongue with bright edges. Diphtheria. Tonsillitis. Hypersalivation.
UROGENITAL	Painful mastitis.
LAMENESS	Instability of sacroiliac, hip, and stifle joints. Sensitive feet.
COMPETITION	2-y-o in training with pharyngitis and poor hind movement.
MODALITIES	Agg: morning one day, evening the next. Amel: cold, drinking chilly water.
COMPARE	*Lactis vaccinum defloratum* Lac-d. Skimmed milk. *Lac equinum* lac-e. Mare milk. Behavioural problems with severe aggression. Lac felis Lac-f. Cat milk. Separation anxiety. Con.
CONSIDER	• Throat infections with hind limb weakness. • Separation anxiety.
POTENCY	30CH.

Lach
LACHESIS MUTA
Bushmaster snake Nosode Animal

Polycrest. Anxious, cheerful, confused, dull and excitable, can progress into hysteria. Jealous, sad, suspicious. Sneaky hunter types.

Work: averse to. Control of infection, particularly when associated with venous haemorrhage. Severe depression. Left sided, painful conditions.

CNS	Epilepsy: cerebral excitement initially, followed by depression. Faint.
HEAD	Facial neuralgia: left jaw. Otitis: severe, waxy. Bloody nostrils.
ABDOMEN	Painfully swollen liver. Colic: tympanitic.
GASTROINTESTINAL	Gums: bloody, spongy, swallowing difficult. Tongue: cracked tip, dry, teeth marks, red. Diphtheria. Parotitis. Tonsillitis.
CARDIOVASCULAR	Arrhythmia. Cyanosis. Palpitation. Bruise easily, clots poorly.
RESPIRATORY	Laryngitis: spasmodic cough.
UROGENITAL	Ovaritis. Mastitis with blue milk. Nymphomania. HRT.
LAMENESS	Large hind joints with contracted tendons.
COMPETITION	Tendency to chronic swollen back legs and lymphadenitis. Mares: cyclical mood swings, referred lumbar pain.
SKIN	Cellulitis: discoloured, severe. Ulcer: discoloured.
MODALITIES	Agg: after sleep. Sun. Touch.

	Amel: after exudate. Warm water.
COMPARE	Acid-nit Crot-h Naja Nat-m.
CONSIDER	An important remedy with profound influence on:
	• Cellulitis: lymphangitis (phleg leg) in horses.
	• Mood swings.
	• Ovarian dysfunction.
	• Throat infections.
	Left side of throat is often sensitive on palpation.
POTENCY	12X. 30CH. 200CH.

Lap-a
LAPIS ALBUS
Silico-fluoride of calcium Mineral

HEAD	Appetite ravenous. Abscess anywhere.
	Purulent otitis media.
CARDIOVASCULAR	Lymphadenitis of cervical and mammary glands. Indurate.
UROGENITAL	Mammae: swollen, persistent, painful. Carcinoma and fibroma.
CANCER	Carcinoma, fibroma, sarcoma. Often in fat juveniles. Often associated with secondary fibrous: elastic-like swellings.
CONSIDER	• Otitis media.
POTENCY	12X. 30CH. 200CH.

Lappa
LAPPA ARCTIUM
Burdock Plant

LAMENESS	Painfully swollen synovitis of distal joints.
SKIN	Pruritus of extremities, eyelids, face, and neck. Pimples and pustules. *Sweet itch*-like.
MODALITIES	Agg: jarring. Standing. Walking.
CONSIDER	• Eczema.
POTENCY	12X.

Lath
LATHYRUS SATIVUS aut cicera
Chickpea Plant

Spinal cord problems with reflexes increased and non-painful. Ataxia and paralysis of extremities. Depressed and sleepy.

RESPIRATORY	Paralysis of larynx: LSLH.
UROGENITAL	PU. Retention with overflow.
LAMENESS	Ataxia, atrophy: myelitis.
	Weakness of small joints.
COMPARE	Sec.
CONSIDER	• Ataxia. Non-painful in juveniles
	• Roaring in horses if detected early.
POTENCY	4X – 12X.

Lat-m

LATRODECTUS MACTANS

Black widow spider Animal

CNS	Chorea-like twitch. Fatigue. Oversensitive.
CARDIOVASCULAR	Severe heart pain causing cramping in front legs.
RESPIRATORY	Dyspnoea: bronchospasm: acute, reversible.
COMPARE	*Latrodectus hasselti* Lat-h. New South Wales spider. Chronic septicaemia, pyaemia. Paralysis Wound oedema.
	Latrodectus katipo Lat-k. New Zealand spider. Lymphangitis and chorea-like twitch.
	Mygale lasiodora Mygale. Black Cuban spider. Great fear and chorea-like twitch.
	Theridion curassavicum Ther. Orange spider. Nervous, oversensitive to noise. Aran.
CONSIDER	• Chorea and other nervous twitching.
	• Heart pain.
POTENCY	6X – 12X. 30CH.

Led

LEDUM PALUSTRE

Marsh tea Plant

Anxious and restless, their fear of men may lead to violent anger.

Inflammatory conditions with tetanic spasms. Tetanus.

PD / PU. Significant antibacterial agent.

HEAD	Conjunctivitis. Corneal injury. Haemorrhage and keratitis. Epistaxis.
RESPIRATORY	Painful bronchitis, COPD, emphysema, and laryngitis with a bloody, soft cough.
LAMENESS	Hock, digits: painful bursitis.
	Prevention and treatment of infection after penetrating sole wounds.
SKIN	Painful eczema: bleed, infection: from puncture wound. Wounds: cold, blue.
COMPETITION	Keeps COPD horses working.
	If dressed immediately prevents unpleasant sequel of nail prick.
MODALITIES	Agg: water. Cold.
	Amel: heat. Night.
COMPARE	Arn Bell-p Cal Ham Hyper (combines well) Lob Ruta.
CONSIDER	• Combine with Cal 2X for the topical treatment of wounds.
	• Combines well with Lob against bronchospasm. Both in 4X for nebulisation.
POTENCY	2X – 4X. 8X. 30CH.

Lem-m

LEMNA MINOR

Duckweed Plant

HEAD	Mucopurulent rhinitis.

GASTROINTESTINAL	Dry mouth.
	Diarrhoea mucous and flatulent.
MODALITIES	Agg: heavy rain.
COMPARE	Calc Calen Dulc Nat-s Teucr.
CONSIDER	• Diarrhoea.
	• Rhinitis.
POTENCY	6X – 12X.

Lept
LEPTANDRA VIRGINICA
Culver's root Plant

GASTROINTESTINAL	Tongue furry and yellow.
	Liver tonic. Hepatitis.
	Diarrhoea: bloody, profuse, tarry.
COMPARE	Bry Iris Merc Myris Nux-v Podo.
CONSIDER	• Hepatitis.
	• Infectious Diarrhoea: Salmonellosis.
POTENCY	4X – 8X – 12X.

Levo
LEVOMEPROMAZINE
***Nozenan* drug Mineral**

Severe behavioural problems. Aggressive with extreme anxiety and panic attacks. Agoraphobia. Immune stimulant.

HEAD	Loss of sense of smell in working dogs.
GASTROINTESTINAL	Cirrhosis of liver.
CARDIOVASCULAR	Asthma and tachycardia of panic attacks.
LAMENESS	Periarticular arthritis of shoulder.
MODALITIES	Agg: crowds. Light.
	Amel: warmth. Wrapping.
COMPARE	Chlorp Sep Tub.
CONSIDER	• Aggression.
	• Agoraphobia.
	• Performance anxiety.
	• Loss of sense of smell.
POTENCY	12X. 30CH.

Liat
LIATRIS SPICATA
***Liatris serrulata* Colic root Plant**

GASTROINTESTINAL	Liver, spleen: chronic, weak.
	Diarrhoea with back pain.
CARDIOVASCULAR	Insufficiency with oedema: chronic anaemia.
UROGENITAL	Chronic nephritis with dysuria.
SKIN	Wounds heal slow. Ulcers.
COMPARE	Apis Aur-m Card-m Cean Chin Colch Lach.
CONSIDER	• Oedema of the extremities.
	• Tonic for general debility.
POTENCY	4X – 8X.

Lil-t
LILIUM TIGRINUM
Lilium lancifolium Tiger lily Plant

Behavioural problems related to female hormonal abnormalities. Difficult creatures with an indifferent, hurried, and impatient attitude that leads to anger. Easily offended and worse for consolation. Irrational fears. Left. Significant antibacterial agent.

GASTROINTESTINAL	Distended abdomen. PD: gastric tympany, vomiting. Constant urge to defecate in early mornings.
CARDIOVASCULAR	Painful heart conditions. Arrhythmia, palpitation, tachycardia.
UROGENITAL	Cystitis. Constant tenesmus before and after urination. Urine: hot, milky, scant. Metritis: acrid, pruritic. Ovaritis. Nymphomania.
BREEDING	Foetal loss and its complications. Behaviour deteriorates during and after parturition.
LAMENESS	Back pain with trembling muscles, referred from ovary. Hock pain.
MODALITIES	Agg: consolation. Heat. Standing. Warm room. Amel: effort outdoors. Company at a distance. Lying on left side.
COMPARE	Cact Helon Murx Sep Plat Pall.
CONSIDER	• Deteriorating behaviour in older females. • Behavioural problems around parturition.
POTENCY	12X. 30CH. 200CH.

Lith
LITHIUM CARBONICUM
Carbonate of lithium Mineral

HEAD	KCS.
CARDIOVASCULAR	Arrhythmia. Bradycardia. Cyanosis. Cough when recumbent.
UROGENITAL	Cystitis, nephritis, urethritis: chronic. Urine: acrid, dark, sandy, turbid, urates.
LAMENESS	Pain anywhere. Referred from kidney. Bursitis: carpus, hock, right, small joints.
SKIN	Widespread eruptions, particularly head. Dry, flaky, rash, raw, red, rough, scabs, tough.
MODALITIES	Agg: night. Amel: moving. Rising. Urinating.
COMPARE	Acid-benz Calc Lyc.
CONSIDER	• Arthritis. • Eczema. • FLUTD.
POTENCY	4X – 12X.

Lob
LOBELIA INFLATA
Indian tobacco Plant

Acts on muscles of gastrointestinal and respiratory tracts. Anxiety.

GASTROINTESTINAL	Good appetite. Saliva: acrid, profuse, tenacious. Tongue: coated, white. Tympany: exhausting vomiting.
RESPIRATORY	Asthma, COPD, emphysema: acute, reversible bronchospasm with great dyspnoea, worse after food.
LAMENESS	Severe muscular back pain.
GERIAT	Respiratory disease deteriorates with age.
COMPETITION	Lifesaver in allergic bronchospasm with late evening coughing and generalised muscle stiffness. Avoid
MODALITIES	Agg: chilly night. Cold washing and gentle exercise. Early morning work. Amel: afternoon. Exercise. Warmth.
COMPARE	Ars Led Tab Verat.
CONSIDER	Important: <ul><li>Asthma.</li><li>Back pains referred from lungs.</li><li>COPD.</li><li>Vomiting.</li></ul> Combine with Led 4X for nebulization in acute bronchospasm.
POTENCY	2X. 4X. 8X – 12X.

Lob-p
LOBELIA PURPURASCENS
Purple lobelia Plant

CNS	Ataxia post virus. Like Lob, exhaustion severe.
HEAD	Spasmodic closure of eyelids.
RESPIRATORY	Dyspnoea with shallow, slow respiration.
COMPARE	*Lobelia cardinalis* Lob-c. Red lobelia. Pain lungs and pleura. Bapt Lob.
CONSIDER	• Dyspnoea from infection.
POTENCY	2X in nebulizer. 4X – 12X.

Lol
LOLIUM TEMULENTUM
Darnel Plant

Painful ataxia. Restless and easily excited into rage. Oversensitive to noise.

GASTROINTESTINAL	Severe gastroenteritis.
LAMENESS	Ataxia with distal muscles trembling.
COMPARE	Astra-e Lath Oxyt Sec.
CONSIDER	• Ataxia. • Painful neuralgia.
POTENCY	6X – 12X.

Luf-op
LUFFA OPERCULATA
Esponjilla **Plant**

HEAD	Sad, irritable. Acute, chronic, purulent rhinitis and sinusitis.
RESPIRATORY	Asthma and bronchospasm.
COMPARE	Hep Merc-b-i.
CONSIDER	• Rhinitis. • Sinusitis.
POTENCY	6X – 12X.

Lyc

LYCOPODIUM CLAVATUM

Club moss Stags horn moss Plant

Polycrest. Anxieties, often when outdoors, affects the unconfident creatures. Because of their poor concentration poor, appear dull, even cowardly. Fears: alone, approach. Irritable. Mood swings from dull to real aggression.

Digestive and / or urinary disturbances. Significant antibacterial agent.

Right sided remedy with early morning and evening aggravation.

Deep seated chronic conditions with debility, flatulence, and weight loss.

Patients have a tired, worn-out look. Painful.

HEAD	Hordeolum: inner canthi, red, ulcer. Otitis: exudate: offensive, thick, yellow. Nostrils: blocked, fan-like movement, flaring. Food and drink regurgitated. Ulcer. Sinusitis.
ABDOMEN	Liver abscess, hepatitis. Ascites.
GASTROINTESTINAL	Mouth: including tongue and mucosa: black, blistered, cracked, dry. Halitosis. Hunger: pica. Thirstless. Pharyngitis, tonsillitis, and vocal cords diphtheritic and ulcerated. Tympanitic colic after small meal. Digestion: poor. Constipation; small, hard faeces. Tenesmus.
CARDIOVASCULAR	Palpitation. Cannot lie on left side.
RESPIRATORY	Dyspnoea. Asthma. COPD. Pneumonia. Rales with chronic, deep cough.
UROGENITAL	**Cystitis, nephritis:** PU: nocturnal, sediment, red and thick. Ovaritis: right. Metritis is acrid.
COMPETITION	Benefits working animals by improving them constitutionally. GSD breed.
LAMENESS	Painful stiffness from wither to sacroiliac. Osteitis, osteomyelitis. Severe pain in shoulder and elbow. Digits contracted: gout-like, immune mediated.
JUVENILE	Immature dogs. GSD males weak, inappetent, with poor digestion. Skin problems from weaning.
GERIATRIC	Support multiple organs.
SKIN	Abscesses under skin. Dermatitis: chronic, fissured, fleabite, indurate, offensive, pruritic. Lesions may be thick, ulcerated. Often secondary to chronic, yet undiagnosed, disease of other organs: kidney.
MODALITIES	Agg: evening: four to eight p.m. Heat. Early morning. Warmth: bandaging, poulticing, room, weather.

	Amel: cold: becoming. After midnight. Motion. Removing blankets.
COMPARE	Sulph Rhus-t Urt-u Merc Hep Alumn.
CONSIDER	In holistic medicine this remedy is a giant for its ability to save lives and improve comfort levels in a wide variety of conditions:

- Acetonemia.
- Arthritis.
- Colic.
- Conjunctivitis.
- Cystitis, nephritis.
- Debility.
- Dermatitis.
- Hepatitis.
- Respiratory: acute pneumonia.
- Respiratory: chronic COPD and pneumonia.

Remember:

- Debility.
- Digestive and urinary signalment together.
- Right sided.
- Time of aggravation.
- Worn, old looking.

| POTENCY | 12X. 30CH. 200CH. |

Lycps
LYCOPUS VIRGINICUS
Bugle weed Plant

HEAD	Protruded eyeballs. Excitable, irritable, and suspicious.
CARDIOVASCULAR	Valvular incompetence with arrhythmia and cyanosis. Hypertrophy: rapid, weak pulse.
RESPIRATORY	COPD: chronic cough and rhonchi.
UROGENITAL	PD / PU. Diabetes mellitus.
COMPARE	Crat Fuc.
CONSIDER	• Valvular incompetence.
POTENCY	2X – 6X.

Lyss
LYSSINUM
Hydrophobinum Animal

Oversensitive with vocal delirium and mood swings. Fear of animals, of water, will run away. Epilepsy Triggered by bright lights and with hypersalivation. Swallowing difficult.

COMPETITION	Can help water causes problems.
MODALITIES	Agg: dazzling lights. Water: sight or sound.
COMPARE	Bell Lach Nat-m Stram.
CONSIDER	• Behaviour problems with severe mood swings.
	• Competition horse with fear of water.
	• Detox rabies vaccination.
POTENCY	30CH for two days before and after rabies vaccination will reduce side effects and enhance immunity.

175

200CH for behaviour support.

Mag-c
MAGNESIA CARBONICA
Carbonate of magnesium Mineral

Angry. Bite. Anxious, often confused, and fearful; evening, night before sleep, irrational, thunder, touch. Mood swings from being pleasant to sudden, vocal violence.
Nervous exhaustion. Box walking.

HEAD	Intermittent and sudden deafness.
GASTROINTESTINAL	Dental abscess through malar bone.
	Bloody salivation and foul eructation. Green, offensive vomiting. Painful constipation brought on by fright.
	Diarrhoea: bloody, frothy, green, pain, watery.
RESPIRATORY	Dyspnoea: bloody cough.
LAMENESS	Shoulder: acute, chronic, right, severe, painful stiffness.
SKIN	Weak, thin with pruritic vesicles.
MODALITIES	Agg: periodically every two weeks. Moved to warmer housing.
	Amel: warm air, Defecating. Slow walking.
COMPARE	Other Magnesiums. Aloe Ant-c Kres.
CONSIDER	• Neonatal debility.
	• Neuralgia.
	Debility and fears are important pointers.
POTENCY	6X – 12X. 30CH.

Mag-f
MAGNESIA FLUORATA
Magnesium fluoride Mineral

HEAD	Chronic, purulent rhinitis with irritability.
GASTROINTESTINAL	Hepatitis, pancreatitis, pharyngitis, and tonsillitis.
CARDIOVASCULAR	Endocarditis, lymphadenitis, lymphangitis, oedema.
MODALITIES	Agg: 3am to morning. Napping.
	Amel: fresh air. Mild exercise.
COMPARE	Bar Kres Hep Stront Sulph.
CONSIDER	• Any problem where circulation and lymphatics need detoxification.
	• Any problem where healing is slow, unresponsive.
POTENCY	6X – 12X.

Mag-m
MAGNESIA MURIATICA
Magnesium chloride Mineral

Dull, anxious, and apprehensive. Restless when housed with box walking and weaving.
Vocal. Stasis of the gut. Liver weakness.
Often females.
Exudates are fluent, mucous, and offensive.

HEAD	Nose: blocked, mouth breath. Smell lost.

ABDOMEN	Hepatitis: pain, swollen, with constipation.
GASTROINTESTINAL	Poor appetite. Gums, lips, tongue: bloody, blistered, swollen. Maldigestion of milk.
RESPIRATORY	Painful dry, spasmodic heart cough.
UROGENITAL	Retention with tenesmus. Metritis: dark, clotted.
LAMENESS	Painful stiffness of back and hips.
NEONATES	Constipation from milk intolerance.
MODALITIES	Agg: after eating. Oestrous. Lying on right side. Night. Noise.
	Amel: open air. Movement. Wrapping.
COMPARE	Other Magnesiums. Am-m Calc Gels Nat-m Puls Sep Sil.
CONSIDER	• Hepatitis and liver tonic.
	• Neonatal milk intolerance.
	Note: chronic debility from weak liver in mature females.
POTENCY	6X – 12X. 30CH.

Mag-p

MAGNESIA PHOSPHORICA

Magnesium phosphate Mineral

Polycrest. Chronic debility from muscle cramping in tired, worn-out, irritable, even difficult individuals with poor concentration. Significant antibacterial agent.

CNS	**Chorea.** Vertigo: fall forward, ptosis, twitching.
HEAD	Lachrymation: increased. Nystagmus. Strabismus. Neuralgia, pain, right ear.
GASTROINTESTINAL	Toothache. Painful teething. Swollen tongue. IBD. Colic: spasmodic.
CARDIOVASCULAR	Lymphangitis: neck, throat glands.
RESPIRATORY	Asthma: cannot lie down. Laryngitis: cough: dry harsh, raw, spasmodic cough. Kennel Cough.
UROGENITAL	Ovaritis.
LAMENESS	Muscles: lumbar, sacroiliac: painfully stiff. Tetanic spasm.
	Neuralgia: chorea.
COMPETITION	Adjunctive therapy in azoturia / myositis and cramping.
JUVENILE	**Teething.**
GERIATRIC	**Neuralgic** pain: debility, muscle cramping.
MODALITIES	Agg: cold. Night. Touch.
	Amel: bending double. Warmth. Wrapping and bandaging after initial resistance.
COMPARE	*Nepeta cataria* Nepet. Catmint. Similar in painful, irritable, juvenile colic.
	Other Magnesiums. Coloc Dios Kali-p Zinc.
CONSIDER	Useful in:
	• Cramping weakness of muscles.
	• Hypomagnesemia.
	• Neuralgic pains.
	• Teething problems.
POTENCY	12X. 30CH.

Mag-s
MAGNESIA SULPHURICA
Epsom salts Mineral

Restless, anxious animals, with irrational fears, easily angered. Startle during sleep
Urinary and skin conditions with great debility.

GASTROINTESTINAL	Eructation: copious, offensive. PD.
UROGENITAL	Diabetes mellitus and urethritis.
	Urine: initially acrid, dribbles, easily interrupted, later glycosuria: PU that goes from yellow to red, turbid sediment.
LAMENESS	Painfully debilitating pain from withers to the lumbar area that improves with massage.
SKIN	Widespread juvenile pruritus that improves with grooming.
MODALITIES	Agg: cold.
	Amel: grooming. Massage.
COMPARE	Other Magnesias. Acid-lact Acid-phos Ars-br Sulph.
CONSIDER	Eczema with urethritis.
POTENCY	12X. 30CH.

Magn-gr
MAGNOLIA GRANDIFLORA
Southern magnolia Plant

CARDIOVASCULAR	Dyspnoea.
	Endocarditis, pericarditis with pain and fainting.
LAMENESS	Distal pain with pruritus.
MODALITIES	Agg: damp air. Lying on left side. Mornings.
	Amel: movement. Dry weather.
COMPARE	Aur-m Dulc Rhus-t.
CONSIDER	• Endocarditis.
POTENCY	2X – 4X.

Maland
MALANDRINUM
Equine 'grease' Nosode Animal

UROGENITAL	Acute, severe mastitis in dry cows.
SKIN	Severely pruritic, dry, scabby dermatitis of face and extremities.
	Agg: wintry weather and washing.
COMPARE	Thuj Sil.
CONSIDER	• Dry cow mastitis
	• Veld mange
	• Prophylaxis of pox viruses.
POTENCY	12X. 30CH.

Manc
MANCINELLA
Manganeel apple Plant

GASTROINTESTINAL	Hypersalivation is offensive.
	Vomit is black.
	Oesophagus: constricted, swallow difficult.
	Faeces are copious.
SKIN	Exudative dermatitis with erythema and blisters that ooze brownish and become crusty.
	Pemphigus-like in oversexed juvenile males.
COMPARE	Anac Canth Crot-t.
CONSIDER	• Severe dermatitis.
POTENCY	6X – 12X.

Mand
MANDRAGORA OFFICINARUM
Mandrake plant

Allergies and chronic inflammation. Epilepsy. Concentration poor. Irritable. Noise sensitive.

HEAD	Allergies. Blepharitis. Conjunctivitis. Iritis. Keratitis.
GASTROINTESTINAL	Hepatitis and pancreatitis.
	IBD: ulcers. Travel sickness.
RESPIRATORY	Laryngitis: allergic, chronic.
UROGENITAL	Lithiasis. Sterile females.
	Prostatomegaly.
LAMENESS	Arthritis: hip and digits. Severe spondylitis.
SKIN	Allergic dermatitis. Staphylococci infection.
	Lupus erythematosus.
MODALITIES	Agg: after initial movement. Weather changes.
	Amel: heat. Continuous movement.
COMPARE	Bell Dios Sulph.
CONSIDER	• Allergies.
	• Arthritis.
POTENCY	12X.

Mang
MANGANUM ACETICUM aut carbonicum
Manganese acetate Mineral

Severe anaemia and arthritis. Exudates are bloody to mucous.

GASTROINTESTINAL	Furry tongue. Chronic hepatitis.
CARDIOVASCULAR	Anaemia: chronic, destructive, severe.
RESPIRATORY	Laryngitis. Expectorate is tenacious. Hoarse.
UROGENITAL	Albuminuria and haemoglobinuria.
LAMENESS	Painfully stiff muscles and joints.
	Arthritis. Bursitis. Growing pains. Osteitis. Periostitis.
SKIN	Pruritic cellulitis is periarticular and purulent.
MODALITIES	Agg: weather changes to cold and wet.
	Amel: lying down.
COMPARE	Arg-m Rhus-t Sulph.
CONSIDER	• Anaemia of kidney, liver disease.
	• Arthritis.
	• Bone disease.
POTENCY	6X – 12X. 30CH.

179

Med
MEDORRHINUM
Gonorrhea nosode Animal

Polycrest. Miasm. Restless and hurried, with poor concentration, they fear dark. Chronic, often dormant infections that need stimulation to heal. Severe pain. Profuse acrid, serous to mucous, non-purulent exudates. Immune system modulation. Better at night. Often right sided. Significant antibacterial agent.

HEAD	Conjunctivitis. Tenacious mucous.
	Otitis externa and media.
ABDOMEN	Liver, spleen: pain, swollen.
GASTROINTESTINAL	PD. Pharyngitis. Proctitis.
RESPIRATORY	Dyspnoea of asthma. Laryngitis.
UROGENITAL	Cystitis, nephritis. PU. Slow stream of urine.
	Mastitis. Metritis. Ovaritis: left.
	Prostatitis, impotence.
LAMENESS	Arthritis of digits with exostoses such as ringbone. Peripheral oedema.
	Soles: sensitive, bruise easily.
SKIN	Sarcoid tumours and warts. Pruritic dermatitis.
MIASM	Med is psychosis. One of the five main miasms with a particular sphere in:
	• Cancer with small, slowly developing tumours.
	• Over function of tissues with mucous.
	• Secretory phases with oedema.
	Conditions need immune system modulation.
MODALITIES	Agg: cold. Day. Rest.
	Amel: lying on abdomen. Seaside.
COMPARE	Caust Sulph Syph Zinc.
CONSIDER	Conditions that need stimulation:
	• Arthritis.
	• Eczema.
	• Vaccinosis.
	• Nephritis.
POTENCY	12X. 30CH. 200CH.

Medus
MEDUSA
Jelly-fish Animal

UROGENITAL	Agalactia.
SKIN	Widespread urticaria.
COMPARE	*Homarus* Hom. Lobster. Urticaria. Conjunctivitis. Pharyngitis.
CONSIDER	• Widespread urticaria.
POTENCY	12X. 30CH.

Meli
MELILOTUS OFFICINALIS
Sweet clover Plant

Improves blood clotting. Insecure, hide.

CNS	Epilepsy: head injury.
HEAD	Nose: blocked, epistaxis.
RESPIRATORY	EIPH: arterial and causes air-hunger.
LAMENESS	Stifle muscles are painfully stiff or numb.
COMPETITION	EIPH: arterial.
MODALITIES	Agg: afternoon. Changeable weather.
COMPARE	Bell Glon Mill (combines well here).
CONSIDER	• Arterial haemorrhage.
POTENCY	4X in nebulizer. 12X. 30CH.

Merc-c
MERCURIUS CORROSIVUS
Mercuric chloride Mineral

Polycrest. From dull to excitable, they are irritable, easily startled into a dangerous, violent phase. Fears: dark, strangers, thunder. Tenesmus. Nephritis.

Ulceration appears and heals fast. Haemorrhage. Significant antibacterial agent.

Exudates are acrid, profuse, initially bloody, watery before degenerating into a chronic, purulent state with tissue swelling.

CNS	In advanced disease may become delirious then slip into stupor.
HEAD	Iritis with excoriated eyelids, photophobia and free of pus. Rhinitis and otitis externa.
GASTROINTESTINAL	Copious salivation. Painful throat and tongue. Vomit bile. Colitis and dysentery with shreds of slimy mucosa.
RESPIRATORY	Laryngitis with a bloody painful cough.
UROGENITAL	Cystitis, nephritis: chronic. Albuminuria. Metritis has a yellow to green exudate. Balanitis and Orchitis.
MODALITIES	Agg: defecating. Evening and night. Open air. Amel: rest.
COMPARE	*Mercurius biniodatus* Merc-i-r. Diphtheria, left, ulcer. *Mercurius cyanatus* Merc-cy. Acute left nephritis and pneumonia. *Mercurius iodatus flavus* Merc-i-f. Throat: glands enlarged, right, tongue: coated. Other Mercuries. Ars Lac.
MERCURY SALTS	The substantial number of mercury salts easily lead to confusion. In clinical practice bear in mind: **Merc-c** with acute, local, and severe pathology. Found with destruction of mucous tissues, in the gut, nose and pharynx. Haemorrhage and ulceration. Pus formation in chronic states. **Merc** is more for chronic, less purulent conditions where its slower action works well. **Other** salts have their own specialist niches, although are of lesser clinical significance.
CONSIDER	An especially important remedy. For acute, serious problems, with significant mucosal damage: • Dysentery, including colitis and IBD.

181

- Nephritis.
- Otitis externa.

Note destructive progression from inflammation to ulceration and haemorrhage.

POTENCY	6X – 12X. 30CH.

Merc

MERCURIUS SOLUBILIS
(Includes Merc-viv)
Quicksilver of mercury. Mineral

Polycrest. Anxious and restless, easily confused, they either withdraw and sulk or become hurried and dangerously angry

Painful **destructive** cellular degeneration in most body tissues. The slimy mucous in the mouth is an important pointer. Anaemia.

Exudates are offensive, yellow, and purulent. Significant antibacterial agent.

HEAD	Conjunctivitis: acrid, purulent, profuse. Eyelids swollen.
	Otitis externa and media.
ABDOMEN	Painfully swollen hepatitis.
GASTROINTESTINAL	**Gum:** abscess, jaundice, foul halitosis. Moist, spongy. PD. Salivation: bloody, slimy, and profuse.
	Teeth: loose.
	Tongue: teeth leave imprint on sides. Coated thick and yellow.
	Pharyngitis: rapid development of ulcers after weather change.
	Diarrhoea: bloody, flatulent, slimy, tenesmus. Coccidiosis.
UROGENITAL	Nephritis: albuminuria, haematuria, uraemia.
LAMENESS	Ataxia from extreme muscle weakness. Peripheral oedema.
JUVENILE	Viral Diarrhoeas: neonates: parvovirus.
SKIN	Dermatitis: eruptions: pimple, vesicle, ulcer.
FEVER	High, with restless. Profuse, foul-smelling sweating and shivering.
MODALITIES	Agg: extremes of temperature. Lying: on right side. Night. Perspiration. Warm room.
	Amel: dry heat, rest.
COMPARE	Other Mercuries. Kali-m Mez Phos Syph.
CONSIDER	This mercury salt has a profound influence on Acute, chronic, physical, and mental conditions:
	• Diarrhoea.
	• Hepatitis.
	• Mood swings.
	• Nephritis.
	• Otitis.
	Greenish, excoriating, and offensive exudates.
POTENCY	6X – 12X. 30CH.

Morb

MORBILLINUM
Measles nosode Animal

SKIN	Puppy mange with measles-like eruptions on abdomen.
CONSIDER	• Adaptive phase of Sarcoptic mange in puppies.
POTENCY	6X. 30CH.

Morph
MORPHINUM
Morphine Opium poppy Plant

CNS	Fits with hyperesthesia. Painful neuralgia. Vertigo from movement. Oversensitive and irritable after shock. From restless to hysterical. Prostration.
HEAD	Ptosis. Supraorbital neuralgia. Pruritus. Pupils: unequal. Strabismus. Otitis: left. Paroxysmal sneezing.
GASTROINTESTINAL	PD. Dry mouth. Anorexia. Tongue brown with a violet centre. Swallowing difficult. Constant vomiting of green fluid. Colic: acute, tympanitic. Rectum: bruised from severe constipation: dry, hard, knotted faeces. Fissures. Diarrhoea: dark, painful, watery.
RESPIRATORY	Lungs, heart: weak. Cough: exhausting, exudate: mucous, thin.
UROGENITAL	Paralysis of bladder. Chronic nephritis. Impotent male. Painful right spermatic cord. Prostatomegaly.
LAMENESS	Ataxia with muscles, jerking, twitching, and staggering.
SKIN	Livid purple spots. Elasticity lost. Pruritus.
MODALITIES	Agg: after sleep. Amel: heat.
COMPARE	Acid-oxal Cimic Grind Mez Op.
CONSIDER	• Nervous twitching • Neuralgia.
POTENCY	6X – 12X. 30CH.

Mosch
MOSCHUS
Musk gland secretion Animal

Epilepsy and other convulsive disorders with hysterical nervous spasms. Catalepsy and vertigo. Easily excited and hypersensitive to noise. Premature aging.

GASTROINTESTINAL	Anorexia. Nervous hiccough. PD variable. Tympanitic colic.
CARDIOVASCULAR	Arrhythmia. Palpitation. Weak.
RESPIRATORY	Asthma from anxiety. Acute constriction of larynx. Exudates are tenacious and mucous.
UROGENITAL	PU. Diabetes mellitus. Female genitalia: pruritis.

MODALITIES	Male: aggressive, impotent, oversexed. Agg: cold, open air. Amel: grooming. Massage.
COMPARE	Asaf Cast Ign Nux-m Samb Valer.
CONSIDER	Intense, severe asthma
POTENCY	12X. 30CH.

Dol
MUCUNA PRURIENS
Cowhage Dolichos Plant

GASTROINTESTINAL	Painfully swollen hepatitis. Colic: impacted, tympanitic. Swallowing is difficult.
SKIN	Intense pruritus with minor dermatitis. Right sided.
MODALITIES	Agg: night. Scratching.
COMPARE	Acid-nit Bell Hep Rhus-t.
CONSIDER	• Severe irrational pruritus.
POTENCY	6X – 12X.

Murx
MUREX PURPUREUS
Purple fish Animal

UROGENITAL	Anoestrous. Cystic ovaries. PU. Bloody chronic metritis. Prolapse. Excessive libido in sad individuals. Promotes female fertility.
COMPARE	Lil-t Plat Sep.
CONSIDER	• Anoestrous • Cystic ovaries • Metritis.
POTENCY	8X – 12X.

Myric
MYRICA CERIFERA
Bayberry Plant

GASTROINTESTINAL	Hepatitis. Bloody, jaundiced, spongy gums. Thick viscid saliva.
UROGENITAL	Chronic nephritis. Bilirubinaemia, frothy, urates.
COMPARE	Chel Nux-v.
CONSIDER	• Hepatitis with nephritis.
POTENCY	6X – 12X.

Myris
MYRISTICA SEBIFERA
Brazilian ucuba Plant

Encourages healing by promoting pus formulation. Antibacterial action.

GASTROINTESTINAL	Rectal fissure.
LAMENESS	Osteomyelitis, periostitis, sequestrum, trauma. Bacterial bursitis of digits.

SKIN	Bite wounds. Fistula. Foreign body. Ulcer.
COMPARE	Hep Sil.
CONSIDER	• Bacterial infection.
POTENCY	4X to promote formation of pus.
	12X. 30CH.

Naja

NAJA TRIPUDIANS

Cobra spp Animal

CNS	Sudden onset paralysis while conscious. Depressed.
	Fears: alone, rain.
HEAD	Ptosis. Otitis externa: exudate: black, fishy smell.
CARDIOVASCULAR	Acute, chronic endocarditis. Palpitation.
	Cough. Pain. Virus.
MODALITIES	Agg: stimulants.
	Amel: open air. Travel. Walking.
COMPARE	Crot-h Lach Spig Spong.
CONSIDER	• Heart failure of post viral endocarditis, infection.
POTENCY	4X – 12X.

Nat-c

NATRUM CARBONICUM

Sodium carbonate Mineral

Range from being cheerful to dull, sad and timid when influenced by disease or their fears: of men, people, thunder, and noise. A role in improving cellular metabolism by stimulating cellular function. Anaemia. Anxious and restless. Significant antibacterial agent.

HEAD	Rhinitis: chronic: watery exudate becomes mucous.
GASTROINTESTINAL	Chronically weak liver.
UROGENITAL	Infertility due to weak cervix in older mares.
	Acrid, offensive metritis.
LAMENESS	Ataxia with muscle weakness. Painful bog spavin.
JUVENILES	Neonatal indigestion with constipation or diarrhoea from milk substitute intolerance.
	Weak, floppy joints.
SKIN	Dry and cracked with vesicles.
MODALITIES	Agg: drafts. Heat. Music. Resting. Weather changes. Thunder.
	Amel: effort.
COMPARE	*Natrum arsenicosum* Nat-ars. Cough with crusty mucous nostrils. Dark purple oedema of throat. Distal oedema.
	Natrum salicylicum Nat-salic. Iritis. Retinal haemorrhage. Otitis interna with vertigo. Urticaria with plaques of oedema.
	Other Natriums. Caust Phos.
CONSIDER	• Severe anaemia.
	• Neonatal digestive upsets.
	• Neonatal flaccid joints.

| POTENCY | 6X – 12X. 30CH. |

Nat-hchls
NATRUM HYPOCHLOROSUM
Sodium hypochlorite Mineral

HEAD	Oedema. Conjunctivitis with epiphora and red, puffy eyelids. Sad.
GASTROINTESTINAL	Stomatitis: red, oedematous ulcers.
	Gastritis: vomit blood.
RESPIRATORY	Dyspnoeic cough with a frothy, pink exudate.
SKIN	Juvenile eczema with recurrent vesicles that form dry scabs covering whitish, oozing exudate.
COMPARE	Acid-nit Nat-s Rhus-t.
CONSIDER	• Dermatitis on face and front legs with vesicles.
POTENCY	12X.

Nat-m
NATRUM MURIATICUM
Sodium chloride Mineral

Polycrest. A similar, but more severe mental picture than the other *Nats*.
Anger in mild creatures. Company: averse to, so consolation aggravates and moves them from dull to excitable. Grief: suppressed anger but when this becomes overt, hurried, indifferent, and irritable signs become angry. Oversensitive, they startle easily. Anaemia with ascites, oedema, and leucocytosis. Significant antibacterial agent.

HEAD	Ophthalmia. Swollen eyelid. Cataract: incipient, senile.
	Coryza: acrid, initially flows freely then blocks.
GASTROINTESTINAL	Anorexia. PD. Tongue vesicles.
	Vomit: sticky, white.
	Constipation, diarrhoea: milk intolerance.
CARDIOVASCULAR	Anaemia from parasitism.
RESPIRATORY	Asthma: exudate: bland, copious, mucous.
UROGENITAL	Chronic nephritis. Anaemia, PU. SG low. Impotence.
LAMENESS	Stiff and uncomfortable. Hock: bog spavin. Achilles tendonitis.
COMPETITION	Tonic for debilitation from overwork.
JUVENILE	Digestive upsets from milk intolerance.
	Tendency to knuckle over on fetlocks in neonates.
SKIN	**Dermatitis.** Hair falls easily, pruritic in groin and periarticular. Urticaria when food changed.
MODALITIES	Agg: consolation. Draft. Summer heat. Resting. Stress. Thunder.
	Amel: fresh air. Exercise. Light. Lying on left.
COMPARE	Other Natrums. Caust.
CONSIDER	Prescribed in:
	• Anaemia. Acute. Babesiosis. Chronic parasitism.
	• Dermatitis: flea-bite allergy.
	• Eye disease of the elderly.

- Nephritis.
- *Never well since* syndrome.

POTENCY	6X. 30CH.

Nat-p
NATRUM PHOSPHORICUM
Sodium phosphate Mineral

HEAD	Tissue salt 10. Morning dullness.
	Eyes: one pupil dilated.
	Exudates: creamy, golden yellow.
GASTROINTESTINAL	Mouth: gingivitis, glossitis, creamy golden yellow.
	Vomiting is sour. Diarrhoea: greenish.
UROGENITAL	Sterility from metritis: exudate: acid, creamy yellow, or honey coloured, offensive.
POTENCY	12X.

Nat-s
NATRUM SULPHURICUM
Sodium sulphate Glaubers salts Mineral

Polycrest. Anxiety. Confusion. Fears: noise, thunder, and startle easily. Acute brain injury. Weakness from exposure. Anxiety. Confusion. Fears: noise, thunder. Startle easily. Significant antibacterial agent.

CNS	Brain injury. Haemorrhage. Oedema. Unconscious.
HEAD	Conjunctiva: dirty, yellow.
	Nasal exudate: bloody, catarrh, thick, yellow.
ABDOMEN	Hepatitis: chronic, painful, swollen. Vomit bile.
RESPIRATORY	Dyspnoea: chronic pneumonia.
	Cough: expectorant: green, ropy, thick.
UROGENITAL	Urine: bile, glycosuria, PU, red, sediment.
LAMENESS	Lymphadenitis.
MODALITIES	Agg: damp night air. Lying on left.
	Amel: change of position. Movement. Warm dry air.
COMPARE	*Natrum arsenicosum* Nat-ar. Grief. Suspicious. Noise sensitive Neonatal gastroenteritis. Merc-c Sulph Thuj.
CONSIDER	Of immense value in:

- Brain injury.
- Debility from exposure.
- Diabetes mellitus.
- Hepatitis.

POTENCY	6X – 12X. 30CH. 200CH.

Nep
NEPENTHE DISTILLATORIA
Pitcher plant

HEAD	Irritable, impatient and tire easily.
	Conjunctivitis. Atrophic rhinitis.
GASTROINTESTINAL	Mouth: gingivitis, glossitis, laryngitis, glossitis, rough, thick.
	Stomach: cancer, ulcer.

UROGENITAL	Ovaritis with genital pruritus.
LAMENESS	Back. left hip arthritis, painful, stiff, muscles.
MODALITIES	Agg: evening. Fresh air.
COMPARE	Arg-n Merc.
CONSIDER	• Cancer and ulcer of stomach.
POTENCY	12X.

Ner

NERIUM ODORUM

Rose laurel Plant

CNS	Ataxia and hemiplegia. Vertigo. Palpitation with great weakness.
HEAD	Face, ears: dermatitis: acrid, moist, red, rough, spots.
GASTROINTESTINAL	Hunger. PD. Colic: tympanitic. Vomit. Ineffectual urging: pruritus.
LAMENESS	Ataxia: polyarticular stiffness, weak.
SKIN	Dermatitis: bleeds, oozes, violently pruritic.
MODALITIES	Agg: friction of bandages, saddle etc. Rest.
COMPARE	Caust Con Lath Nat-m Rhus-t.
CONSIDER	• Paralytic weakness if combined with severe dermatitis.
POTENCY	3X – 12X. 30CH.

Nux-m

NUX MOSCHATA

Nutmeg Plant

Concentration: poor, confused, dull. Strange, ridiculous gestures. Startle easily. Severe mood swings. Vertigo.

HEAD	Unilateral venous epistaxis.
GASTROINTESTINAL	Colic: tympanitic. Faeces soft yet constipated.
CARDIOVASCULAR	Arrhythmia.
UROGENITAL	Postpartum haemorrhage, bloody metritis.
LAMENESS	Painful stiffness of right hip and stifle.
MODALITIES	Agg: cold, moist weather. Movement. Water. Amel: dry weather. Heat.
COMPARE	Asaf Ign Nux-v Puls Rhus-t.
CONSIDER	• Deteriorating behaviour with heart and joint disease.
POTENCY	2X – 12X.

Nux-v

NUX VOMICA

Strychnos nux vomica Poison nut Plant

Polycrest. Wide range of signs with behavioural and gastrointestinal effects significant.

Anger with violence, when they will bite and kick, sneaky. Anxiety: after food, after midnight. Confused, poor concentration and an aversion to company, leads to trembling anger. Also triggered by fears: approach, crowd, touch, work when they are impetuous, irritable, obstinate, and oversensitive, and easily offended. Hysterical.

Competition horses may be talented but need careful management. Often explains the dramatic improvement in individuals when moving to a fresh trainer. Significant antibacterial agent.

HEAD	Eyelids: red, swollen. Optic neuritis. Paralysis of ocular muscles. Photophobia.
	Sinusitis, snuffles: acrid, blocked indoors, head pressing. Exudate: bloody, diurnal, fluent, mucous.
ABDOMEN	Hepatitis: painful, swollen.
GASTROINTESTINAL	Eructation. Gums: bloody, swollen, white.
	Hunger is great. Jaundice. PD. Pharyngitis.
	Tongue: cracked, furred, yellow. Ulcers: bloody saliva. Vomit.
	Colic: irregular peristalsis, tympany. Hernia: inguinal, strangulated.
	Rectum: **constipation,** constriction, **i**mpaction. Alternates with diarrhoea: from inappropriate food, overeating. Tenesmus.
RESPIRATORY	Asthma: dyspnoea: bloody, hacking cough.
UROGENITAL	Nephritis, cystitis. PU. Spasm of sphincter. Labour effort weak. Oestrous: irregular cycle. Prolapse. Orchitis.
BREEDING	**Tonic** late in the breeding season modulates cycles, improves libido in both sexes.
LAMENESS	**Ataxia. Spinal neuralgia:** brachial plexus, sacro-iliac regions, painful.
COMPETITION	Overworked irritable horses in poor condition after a tough season. Liver enzymes high.
	Low grade abdominal pain.
FEVER	Always with gastric upset, widespread pain.
SKIN	Urticaria from digestive upsets.
MODALITIES	Agg: after eating. Morning. Rest. Warmth.
	Amel: cold, dry weather. Evening. Massage. Wet weather.
COMPARE	Bry Cup Graph Kali-c Lyc Sep Stry Sulph.
	Also remember **Grat** in females.
CONSIDER	An especially important remedy:
	• Colic with tympanitic including gastric dilatation.
	• Detoxification.
	• Diarrhoea from digestive upsets: overeating.
	• Gastric and duodenal ulceration.
	• Hepatitis and liver support.
	• IBD.
	Note the increasing general irritability and oversensitivity in overworked individuals.
POTENCY	12X. 30CH. 200CH. Often works better in evening.

Oci
OCIMUM CANUM
Brazilian alfavaca Plant

CARDIOVASCULAR	Lymphadenitis: right, inguinal, mammary.
UROGENITAL	Cystitis, urethritis, nephritis: blood, red to yellow, thick, turbid, urates.
	Female genitalia: pruritus.
	Left Orchitis.
COMPARE	Berb Hedeo Lyc Pareir Urt-u.
CONSIDER	• Urinary disease with urates.
POTENCY	6X – 12X.

Oena
OENANTHE CROCATA
Water dropwort Plant

CNS	Epilepsy, eclampsia preceded by stretching. From delirium to opisthotonos, unconscious. Desire to escape.
HEAD	Jaws locked: prolific foaming during fits.
UROGENITAL	PD PU. Chronic nephritis. Periparturient eclampsia.
MODALITIES	Agg: oestrous. Pregnancy.
COMPARE	Cic Kali-br.
CONSIDER	• Eclampsia.
	• Epilepsy from nephritis.
POTENCY	6X. 30CH.

Onos
ONOSMODIUM VIRGINIANUM
Onosmodium virginianum False cromwell Plant

CNS	Ataxia with muscle weakness, and vertigo. Confused.
HEAD	Hyperaemia of optic disc.
	Enlarged retinal vessels. Heavy eyelids.
	Chronis sinusitis with postnasal drip.
CARDIOVASCULAR	Arrhythmia with pain.
UROGENITAL	Pruritic nipples.
	Metritis: acrid, painful, profuse, yellow.
LAMENESS	Muscle: back, ataxia, shoulders, weak.
MODALITIES	Agg: bandaging. Jarring. Movement.
	Amel: drinking. Eating. Lying on back.
COMPARE	Gels Lil-t Nat-m Ruta.
CONSIDER	• Great muscle weakness.
POTENCY	12X. 30CH.

Orchi-e
ORCHITINUM EQUINUS
Testes nosode Animal

Male sexual deficiencies. HRT. Lazy, overweight, and quiet. Thin skinned pendulous abdomen.

UROGENITAL	Testes: small, soft, poor spermatogenesis.
BREEDING	Proven value for spermatogenesis in breeding males with low sperm counts.
SKIN	Thin and weak.

COMPETITION	Anabolic: geldings.
COMPARE	Avena Gins Orchi-c from canine testes. Test.
CONSIDER	• HRT: male. 6X daily, five days per week for months.
	• Low sperm counts need 6X twice daily for two months.
POTENCY	12X 30CH

Orni
ORNITHOGALUM UMBELLATUM
Star of Bethlehem Plant

GASTROINTESTINAL	Appetite; poor, eat lesser amounts often.
	Tongue: bloody, frequent vomiting.
	Stomach: full: fur ball, **pyloric stenosis.**
	Colic: chronic impaction.
COMPARE	Alum Aesc Bry Calc Nux-v Op.
CONSIDER	• Constipation: impacted colic.
	• Fur ball.
	• Pyloric stenosis.
POTENCY	2X twice daily in fur ball cases until resolved.
	6X daily for pyloric stenosis.

Osm
OSMIUM METALLICUM
Osmium Mineral

HEAD	Conjunctivitis. Glaucoma, Photophobia.
	Supraorbital neuralgia.
	Rhinitis: small mucous lumps. Irritable, restless at night.
RESPIRATORY	Laryngitis: cough: dry, hard, noisy, severe.
	Palate weak, floppy.
UROGENITAL	Albuminuria.
SKIN	Deformed hoof and nails. Pruritus smells of garlic.
MODALITIES	Agg: open air.
COMPARE	Arg-m Irid Mang Sel.
CONSIDER	• Early glaucoma.
	• Severe laryngitis.
POTENCY	6X. 30CH.

Ov
OVININUM
Nosode Oopherinum Ovarian extract Animal

HRT for behavioural and ovulation problems. Early aging with laziness and obesity Early aging with laziness and obesity.

ABDOMEN	Pendulous with thin, easily tented skin.
UROGENITAL	HRT after spaying. Promotes ovulation.
SKIN	Gradually deteriorates in quality, becomes dry and falls.
COMPARE	Aven Foll Gins Puls Sep.
CONSIDER	• HRT: female.
	• To improve ovulation.

191

POTENCY	6X – 12X.

OXYTROPIS LAMBERTI
Loco-weed Plant

Ataxia with diminished reflexes. Walk backwards. Desire to be alone. Averse to work. Vertigo.

HEAD	Dry mouth.
	Facial bones: painful.
	Ocular muscles: paralysis, pupils: non-reactive pupils.
GASTROINTESTINAL	Eructation. Anal sphincter relaxed and mushy faeces fall out.
UROGENITAL	PU PD. Pain. Nephritis. Impotence.
	Testes and spermatic cord pain.
LAMENESS	Painfully stiff muscular ataxia.
MODALITIES	Agg: alternate days.
	Amel: after sleep.
COMPARE	Astra-e Bar Lath Lol.
CONSIDER	• Painful ataxia.
POTENCY	4X – 12X. 30CH.

PAEONIA OFFICINALIS
Tree peony Plant

GASTROINTESTINAL	Severest, painful rectal fissures.
LAMENESS	Ataxia.
SKIN	Chronic, weeping ulcers on lower parts of limbs.
	Severe urticaria.
COMPARE	Acid-n Aesc Calc-fl Graph ham Sil.
CONSIDER	• Rectal fissures in the GSD.
POTENCY	4X and 30CH combined. Twice daily for months.

PALLADIUM METALLICUM
Palladium Mineral

Unhappy individuals. Irritable, obstinate, and easily offended, they need constant attention and reassurance. Weak, even exhausted, they may snap to life then slip back into tired phase. Ovarian infertility and female behavioural problems.

UROGENITAL	Anoestrous due to deficient ovaries.
LAMENESS	Right pelvic pain, front of the right sacroiliac joint: referred from ovary.
COMPETITION	Talented mares tire fast. Right sacroiliac pain.
COMPARE	Apis Arg-n Lil-t Ov Sep.
CONSIDER	Important and powerful:
	• Anoestrous from ovarian deficiencies.
	• Mood swings from ovarian pain.
	The behaviour and right sided pain are good pointers.
POTENCY	12X. 30CH. 200CH.

PANAX QUINQUEFOLIA
Ginseng Plant

Immune modulation. Tonic.

GASTROINTESTINAL	Tympanitic colic at the ileocecal junction.
RESPIRATORY	Persistent cough.
UROGENITAL	Studs: poor libido at the end of a long season. Orchitis.
LAMENESS	Stiff painful hindquarters: testicle **pinching during exercise.**
GERIATRIC	A good tonic.
COMPARE	Aven Coca Colos Eleuth Orchi-e (c) (combines well).
CONSIDER	• Chronic, nonspecific infections.
	• Enhances other remedies.
	• HRT with Orchi-e (c) in maturing studs.
	• Immune modulation.
POTENCY	2X – 4X.

Pancr
PANCREATINUM
Nosode Pancreas Animal

ABDOMEN	Support in pancreatic insufficiencies including Diabetes mellitus.
GASTROINTESTINAL	Faeces: bulky, greasy, pale, painless. Deficient in trypsin.
JUVENILE	Growth tonic in juvenile GSD. Poor feeders and look unthrifty.
COMPARE	*Trypsinum* Tryp. Similar, but not as good.
CONSIDER	• Pancreatic insufficiencies to reduce dependency on raw pancreas and hormones.
POTENCY	4X – 12X.

Op
PAPAVER SOMNIFERUM
Opium poppy Plant

Mood swings are great. From confusion to dull indifference. Excitable and oversensitive with anger, then extreme tiredness important. Ataxia.

Any disease associated with lethargy and absence of pain. Mood swings are great. From confusion to dull indifference. Excitable and oversensitive with anger. Tiredness is important. Ataxia.

CNS	Eclampsia: convulsions, opisthotonos. Unconscious.
HEAD	Eyes appear half closed. Pupils contracted, dilated, insensitive.
	Facial muscles: ptosis, spasmodic twitching.
GASTROINTESTINAL	Colic: severely **impacted colic** with vomiting. Impaction: great with tenesmus. Faeces: black balls, hard, small.
	Feline megacolon. Hair ball.
RESPIRATORY	Dyspnoea with cyanosis. Slow but marked snoring.
UROGENITAL	Eclampsia. The shock of foetal loss.

FEVER	Slow pulse. Sweating, snoring, thirst, and muscle twitching.
MODALITIES	Agg: heat. Sleep.
	Amel: activity. Cold.
COMPARE	Apis Bell Gels Nux-m.
CONSIDER	Important:
	• Constipation is severe.
	• Colic impacted for days.
	• Eclampsia and similar convulsions.
POTENCY	30CH. 200CH.

Pareir
PAREIRA BRAVA
Virgin vine Plant

UROGENITAL	Painful cystitis with chronically thickened bladder and urethral walls. Urine: bloody, thick, mucous.
COMPARE	Berb Chim Hydrang Oci.
CONSIDER	• Chronic cystitis.
POTENCY	4X – 12X.

Par
PARIS QUADRIFOLIA
One berry Plant

HEAD	May seem to have headache. Painful left neuralgia.
RESPIRATORY	Severe allergic coughing.
LAMENESS	Painful neuralgia of neck and withers.
UROGENITAL	Painful severe, chronic nephritis.
COMPARE	Berb Calc Chim Hydrang Oci Sil.
CONSIDER	• Nephritis.
	• Neuralgia.
POTENCY	4X – 12X.

Paro-i
PARONYCHIA ILLECEBRUM
Sanguinaria of Cuba Plant

HEAD	Encephalitis. Blepharitis and conjunctivitis.
	Otitis media, rhinitis. Purulent left sided sinusitis.
GASTROINTESTINAL	Mouth, lips, tongue: cracked corners, dry, saliva: dark yellow. PD.
	Colic, gastritis: tympanitic, vomiting.
	Rectal cancer. Diarrhoea: bloody, greenish, sour. Pruritus.
CARDIOVASCULAR	Myocarditis and pericarditis.
RESPIRATORY	Dyspnoea: intercostal pain. Expectoration tough.
UROGENITAL	PU. Glomerulonephritis. Dysuria. Incontinent. Prostatic adenoma and hyperplasia.
MODALITIES	Agg: movement.
COMPARE	Anac Anthr Ars Bapt.
CONSIDER	• Cancer and infection of rectum.

- Prostate disease.

POTENCY | 6X.

Passi
PASSIFLORA INCARNATA
Passionflower Plant

Insomnia in coughing or restless juveniles.

GASTROINTESTINAL	Flatulence after food. Diarrhoea: distresses.
RESPIRATORY	Cough is Kennel Cough-like. Nocturnal.
UROGENITAL	Eclampsia with atonic convulsions.
JUVENILE	All cases of insomnia and restlessness.
COMPARE	Coff (works well with) Daph. Ign.
CONSIDER	• Insomnia.
	• To settle new additions to family.
POTENCY	12X. 30CH.

Penic
PENICILLINUM
Antibiotic benzyl-penicillin Mineral

Allergies and immune modulation. Depressed and lethargic. Significant antibacterial agent. Exudates offensive and purulent.

HEAD	Allergic conjunctivitis.
GASTROINTESTINAL	Gingivitis, dental decay: right.
RESPIRATORY	Asthma, bronchitis, COPD, emphysema.
	Painful, dry cough.
LAMENESS	Acute bacterial arthritis. Myositis. Tendonitis.
SKIN	Benign cancer. Ringworm. Urticaria.
MODALITIES	Agg: cold. Damp. Movement.
	Amel: dry weather. Rest. Warmth.
COMPARE	Ars Bry Nat-s Puls Thuj.
CONSIDER	• Detoxify after drug therapy.
	• Modulate immune system.
	• Tonic for neonates born from dam's sick during pregnancy.
POTENCY	30CH.

Perh
PERHEXILIN
Perhexiline maleate Mineral

Glandular disease including Addison's. Paresis of face and left hind. Polyneuritis. Forgetful.

HEAD	Diplopia. Papilledema. Bilateral rhinitis.
GASTROINTESTINAL	Cirrhosis and hepatitis.
	Diabetes mellitus. Hypoglycaemia. Anorexia. PD.
	Gastritis with vomiting.
CARDIOVASCULAR	Arrhythmia and myocarditis.
UROGENITAL	PU Males with poor libido.
LAMENESS	Immune mediated polyarthritis. Left. Spondylitis.
SKIN	Alopecia. Contact dermatitis.

MODALITIES	Agg: flexion. Mornings.
	Amel: eating. Stretching.
CONSIDER	• Role in metabolic disorders.
COMPARE	Cob-n Kres Hydroph Karw-h Lath Merc Plb.
POTENCY	12X. 30CH.

Petr
PETROLEUM
Petrol Mineral

Angry, irritable, and confused. Fear of approach, of crowds. Easily upset. Pruritus.

HEAD	Eyelids, ears: dry, fissures, scurfy.
	Otitis media: deaf from mucous.
	Nostrils: bloody, cracked, ulcerated.
GASTROINTESTINAL	Diarrhoea: diurnal, profuse, watery.
UROGENITAL	Profuse albuminous metritis. Prostatomegaly.
LAMENESS	Distal dermatitis with cracked. Scabby lesions. Weak hooves.
SKIN	Greasy heel: blistered, cracked, dry, fissured, infected, moist.
MODALITIES	Agg: before thunder. Damp. Eating. Winter.
	Amel: dry, warm weather.
COMPARE	*Diesel oil* Dies. Similar. Anxiety, hypersalivation of travel sickness.
	Carb-v Graph Sulph Phos.
CONSIDER	• Offensive dermatitis of face and feet
	• Travel sickness.
POTENCY	6X – 12X.

Phenob
PHENOBARBITALUM
Phenylethylmalonurea Mineral

HEAD	Pruritic oedema. Sleepy.
GASTROINTESTINAL	Chronically swollen hepatitis.
SKIN	Allergies, urticaria: pruritic: severe.
	Exudate is honey-like.
MODALITIES	Agg: dairy. Fish. Heat.
	Amel: diet control. Rest.
COMPARE	Apis Bell Graph Kali-c Ran-b Rhus-t.
CONSIDER	• Barbiturate toxicity in epilepsy.
POTENCY	30CH.

Phos
PHOSPHORUS
Phosphorus Mineral

Polycrest. Fabulous creatures, best of company when well: high-spirited and energetic. Often described as *a glass of champagne*. But gradually fall apart when pressurized or ill. Anxiety in mornings when concentration is poor and need company.

Fears: irrational, noise, thunder, vets and become hypersensitive, indifferent, and irritable. Oversensitive. Startle easily. Timid. May threaten and be vocally aggressive, but not dangerous and rarely bite or kick. Significant antibacterial agent.

Severe inflammatory and degenerative effect on mucous membranes. Bone destruction and necrosis of liver. Great debility and emaciation.

CNS	Paralysis: ascending, motor, sensory.
HEAD	Facial paralysis. Periostitis. Cataract. Conjunctivae pale. Eyelid oedema. Glaucoma.
	Retinal degeneration and haemorrhage.
ABDOMEN	Hepatitis and pancreatitis: acute.
GASTROINTESTINAL	Gums: bloody, mucous. PD. Ulcer. Vomit after food.
CARDIOVASCULAR	Anaemia: destructive, severe. Pulse: fast, weak.
RESPIRATORY	Dyspnoea: pneumonia and congestion.
	Cough: dry, hard, painful.
UROGENITAL	**Cystitis, nephritis:** Acute, chronic. PU: albuminuria, bloody, brown, phosphaturia, red, turbid, sediment.
LAMENESS	Ataxia. Muscles weak, and tremble. DJD. Dysplasia. Osteomyelitis, osteoporosis. Periostitis: shins and splints. Joint pain. Sequestrum.
GERIATRIC	Ataxia and debility of premature aging.
SKIN	Haemorrhage is intermittent, excessive and punctiform.
MODALITIES	Agg: lying on left or painful side. Thunder. Touch. Twilight. Changeable weather. Work.
	Amel: chilly air. Drinking. Lying on right side. Sleep.
COMPARE	Ars Lyc Sil Tub Calc Chin-s.
CONSIDER	Has an enormous influence on:

- Anaemia is destructive: babesiosis.
- Bones: carpitis, shins, splints, spurs.
- Cataract if applied early, glaucoma, PRA, retinal trauma.
- Hepatitis.
- Nephritis.
- Pancreatitis.
- Pneumonia: acute.

Look out for these characteristics:

- Tall, slim individuals.
- Noise related anxieties.
- Enjoy work initially but soon tire.
- A 'sick looking' appearance.

POTENCY	12X. 30CH. 200CH.

Phys

PHYSOSTIGMA VENOSUM

Calabar bean Plant

Painful CNS and spinal conditions. Ataxia. Tetanic fits in epilepsy. Chorea. Meningitis. Irrational fears and startle easily.

HEAD	Glaucoma. Iritis. Profuse lachrymation. Night blindness Photophobia with contracted pupils.
	Rhinitis: acrid, blocked, fluent, ulcer
GASTROINTESTINAL	Tip of tongue is tender. Gastritis: painful after food. Constipation.

CARDIOVASCULAR	Fatty degeneration: feeble pulse, palpitation.
LAMENESS	Ataxia: jerking, twitching, trembling.
COMPARE	*Eserine* Esin. Blepharospasm with twitching eyelids.
	Contracted pupils. Palpitation. Con Cur Gels Oxyt Lol.
CONSIDER	• Meningitis with spinal irritation.
POTENCY	4X – 12X. 30CH.

Phyt
PHYTOLACCA DECANDRA
Pokeroot Plant

CARDIOVASCULAR	Lymphadenitis of axillary glands.
RESPIRATORY	Dry, hacking cough with a loss of voice. Intercostal arthritis.
UROGENITAL	Nephritis with dysuria.
	Mammary cancer: hard, purple, swollen, painful. Nipples cracked. Small pimples. Ovaritis.
	Orchitis: chronic, indurate, painful.
SKIN	Dry, poor, shrunken. Eczema: papules, pustules, slough.
FEVER	Alternates. Great weakness.
MODALITIES	Agg: exposure. Movement. Cold, damp weather. Getting wet.
	Amel: rest. Dry, warm weather.
COMPARE	Arum-t Bry Kali-c Merc Rhus-t Sang.
CONSIDER	Consider:
	• Lymph gland chronically swollen.
	• Mastitis.
	• Tonsillitis.
	Principle signs are pain, restlessness, and weak.
POTENCY	4X – 12X. 30CH.

Jab
PILOCARPUS PENNATIOFOLIUS aut microphyllus
Jaborandi Plant

HEAD	Hyperthyroidism. Iritis. Photophobia. Contracted unresponsive pupils. Otitis media with serous exudate.
GASTROINTESTINAL	Cyanosis. Dry. Hypersalivation.
	Diurnal free diarrhoea and vomiting.
CARDIOVASCULAR	Failure. Tachycardia.
RESPIRATORY	Bronchitis with oedema.
	Profuse foaming of serous exudate. AHS.
UROGENITAL	Scant urine. Tenesmus.
SKIN	Dry, one sided, widespread, persistent dermatitis.
COMPARE	Pilocarpinum hydrochloride aut nitricum aut purum
	Pilo. Meniere's disease. Haemorrhage.
	Profuse sweating.
CONSIDER	• Anhidrosis.
	• Hyperthyroidism.
	Metabolic disorders.

POTENCY	4X – 12X.

PIN-S
PINUS SYLVESTRIS
Scots pine Plant

GASTROINTESTINAL	Liver toxicity: sensitive to pine bedding.
RESPIRATORY	Mild bronchitis.
LAMENESS	Painful bursitis of digits.
SKIN	Widespread periarticular urticaria.
COMPARE	*Pinus montana* Pin-mo Mountain pine. Arthritis. Cartilage support. DJD. Osteoarthritis. Osteoporosis.
CONSIDER	• Allergies to pine products.
POTENCY	6X – 12X.

Plac-e
PLACENTA EQUINUS
Equine placenta Animal

CONSIDER	A potent tonic with a positive influence on protein metabolism. Weak muscled with separation anxiety.
COMPETITION	Anabolic for tired, thin athletes.
COMPARE	Species specific Plac remedies.
POTENCY	4X.

Plat
PLATINUM METALLICUM
Platinum Mineral

Polycrest. The pack leader. Cheerful, confident, haughty when outdoors. Confident. Fear of approach, crowds, men when they move from indifference to irritable.

Sad Females with marked tendency to oversensitivity and localised numbness. Hysterical spasms: pains increase and decreased gradually. Left sided.

CNS	Lead poisoning. Blindness, convulsions, head pressing.
HEAD	Eyelids twitch. Paralysis: right.
GASTROINTESTINAL	Great hunger. Faeces: clay-like, tenacious.
UROGENITAL	Nymphomania. Left ovaritis. Sterile. Post parturient: aggressive, hysteria. Poor mothering. Pruritus of vulva. Sexual development: excessive.
LAMENESS	Lumbar and sacroiliacs joints. Left, painful: referred from ovary.
COMPETITION	May improve action and temperament in difficult mares that experience mood swings and tend to leave sided back pain.
MODALITIES	Agg: evening. Sitting. Standing. Touch. Amel: exercise.
COMPARE	Lil-t Sep.
CONSIDER	• Lead poisoning. • Paralysis. • Parturient behavioural abnormalities.

199

Plect

PLECTRANTHUS FRUTICOSUS

Pink spur flower Plant

Nervous system disorders, bacterial and viral infections. Circulatory support.

GASTROINTESTINAL	Smooth muscle relaxant as an anti-spasmodic. Liver support.
UROGENITAL	Kidney tonic.
COMPARE	*Plectranthus barbatus* Plect-b in metabolic disorders.
POTENCY	6X.

Plb

PLUMBUM METALLICUM

Lead Mineral

Dull, apathetic, and timid, but being oversensitive they get angry. Fear in public. Emaciation, paralysis, and nephritis. Ataxia. Atrophy. Unconscious after epilepsy. Spinal paralysis.

HEAD	Glaucoma. Purulent ophthalmia. Optic neuritis. Contracted pupils.
GASTROINTESTINAL	Gums: blue margin, pale, swollen. Swallowing solids difficult. Constant vomiting.
	Colics: impacted, intussusception, strangulated, tympanitic.
	Constipation: black, hard, lumpy, painful.
CARDIOVASCULAR	Destructive anaemia. Superficial veins dilated.
UROGENITAL	Chronic nephritis: albuminuria, low SG, frequent and ineffectual: drops. Tenesmus.
	Habitual foetal loss.
	Genitalia hypersensitive. Indurate mammae.
LAMENESS	Ataxia from paralysis of muscle groups. Painful cramping.
SKIN	Dry hair with pigment change to brown or yellow.
MODALITIES	Agg: start of exercise. Night.
	Amel: exercise. Massage. Wrapping.
COMPARE	Alumn Plat Op Podo Merc.
CONSIDER	• Progressive ataxia.
	• Severe impacted colic.
POTENCY	12X. 30CH.

Podo

PODOPHYLLUM PELTATUM

Mandrake May apple Plant

GASTROINTESTINAL	Abnormal dentition. Grind teeth at night. PD chilly water.
	Diarrhoea: flatulent, green, gushes, offensive, pain level alternates.
	Ulcers, Constipation alternates with diarrhoea. Prolapse.
UROGENITAL	Pain in right ovary. Painful uterus postpartum. Prolapse.

LAMENESS	Ataxia of left side. Painful back and under right shoulder.
MODALITIES	Agg: early mornings. Hot weather. Teething.
COMPARE	Aloe Chel Merc Nux-v Sulph.
CONSIDER	• Diarrhoea when teething.
2X – 6X.	

Prim-o
PRIMULA OBCONICA
Primrose Plant

HEAD	Dermatitis over face and chin is moist and papular. Eyelid swollen.
ABDOMEN	Painful liver and spleen.
SKIN	Dermatitis: cracks, eruptions, excoriation, widespread. Worse over extremities and joints. Urticaria. Right. Agg: night.
COMPARE	*Rhus spp.*
CONSIDER	• Dermatitis of face and legs.
POTENCY	6X – 12X.

Laur
PRUNUS LAUROCERASUS
Cherry laurel Plant

CARDIOVASCULAR	Confused, dull and sad. Cyanosis from mitral valve regurgitation.
RESPIRATORY	Dyspnoea. Cough and exudates are variable: bloody, copious to dry, jelly-like.
LAMENESS	Hip, hock: painful. Horn: hard knotted, feet and nails.
COMPARE	Am-c Camph Sec.
CONSIDER	• Mitral valve disease with pulmonary oedema.
POTENCY	2X – 4X.

Prun
PRUNUS SPINOSA
Black thorn Plant

HEAD	Severe right ophthalmia. Vitreous flare. Nocturnal excitement.
GASTROINTESTINAL	Constipation: hard, knotted. Diarrhoea: painful, slimy.
RESPIRATORY	Severe palpitation with wheezing.
UROGENITAL	Painful Cystitis, urethritis. Ineffectual, slow urination.
LAMENESS	Strain and bog spavin.
COMPARE	*Prunus padusrheum* Prun-p. Bird cherry. Throat and rectal pain. *Prunus virginiana* Prun-v. Wild cherry. Heart and lung tonic.
CONSIDER	• Cystitis. • Neuralgia.
POTENCY	4X – 12X.

Psor

PSORINUM

Scabies mite nosode Animal

Polycrest. Miasm. Anxious and confused, this leads to May despair from itching. Irritable juveniles. Fears: crowds, thunder, travel when they become sad, obstinate. Dermatitis. Stimulate the body to react when the correct remedy cannot cure.

May be restless antibacterial agent. prophylactic against virus infection. Insomnia from itching. Significant antibacterial action

HEAD	Blepharitis. Conjunctivitis. Acrid. Ophthalmia; chronic, recurrent.
	Otitis with intolerable pruritus. Scabs: brown, chronic, moist, offensive, oozing, purulent, raw, red.
	Nostrils blocked. Coryza mucous.
GASTROINTESTINAL	Always hungry. Lips cracked in corners. Salivation: mucous, offensive, profuse, tenacious.
	Severe tonsillitis.
	Vomit during pregnancy.
RESPIRATORY	**Dyspnoea.** Asthma. Bronchitis. Weak heart.
	Cough: dry, hard, recurrent.
UROGENITAL	Mammae painfully swollen. Metritis: offensive.
JUVENILE	Retained meconium.
SKIN	**Dermatitis:** contact (wool) eczema. Crusty eruptions extensive. Coronary band. Swellings around the glands.
	Hair: dirty, dry, lustreless, matted, rough. Herpetic eruptions, especially on scalp and bends of joints. Intolerable pruritus. Pustules near hoof / nails.
	Sebaceous glands secrete excessively giving an oily skin. Ulcers heal slow. Urticaria after work.
MODALITIES	Agg: changeable weather.
	Amel: heat.
COMPARE	Sulph.
MIASM	Psor is one of the five **miasms.**
	Its sphere is:
	• Delayed recovery.
	• Minimal secretion.
	• Parasitism, including mange, worms, and blood parasites.
	• Promotes an active inflammatory response including liver and vascular problems.
	• Under function shows as delayed or reduced reaction to the correct remedy.
CONSIDER	A remedy with a justifiable reputation for revitalising where there is profound weakness.
	• Debilitated, dirty and smelly.
	• Hate cold.
	• Impression of sad, desperate cases.
	• Bronchitis is persistent, recurring and associated with chronic and purulent exudation.

- Diarrhoea, that is chronic and very offensive.
- Eczema is chronic and offensive.

POTENCY	12X. 30CH. 200CH.

Ptel
PTELEA TRIFOLIATA
Wafer ash Plant

GASTROINTESTINAL	Painfully enlarged liver. Sad and indifferent. Salivation is bitter and excessive.
	Tongue coated: brown or white, papillae red, obvious.
RESPIRATORY	Asthma. Dyspnoea.
MODALITIES	Agg: lying on left. Early morning.
	Amel: eating sour food.
COMPARE	Chel Mag-m Merc Nux-v.
CONSIDER	• Liver disease.
POTENCY	4X – 12X.

Pulx
PULEX IRRITANS
Human flea Animal

HEAD	Look prematurely aged, wrinkled. Impatient and irritable.
GASTROINTESTINAL	Offensive halitosis, Diarrhoea, and vomiting.
UROGENITAL	Painful Cystitis, urethritis. Dysuria.
LAMENESS	Painfully stiff back and shoulder muscles.
SKIN	Eczema: eruptive: small, red, widespread lesions.
MODALITIES	Agg: left side. Moving.
	Amel: lying down.
COMPARE	Psor.
CONSIDER	• Flea allergic eczema.
	• Cystitis.
POTENCY	12X. 30CH.

Puls
PULSATILLA VULGARIS
Pulsatilla nigricans Pasque flower Granadilla Plant

Polycrest. Abrupt, yet mild, affectionate, and anxious during fever. Carried, desire to be. Claustrophobia. Confused after eating when consolation ameliorates. Dull. Effeminate. Excitable.

Fear being alone, of crowds, dark, dogs. Hide. Hysteria. Impatient. Indifferent. Jealous. Mood swings: frequent, dramatic. Restless at night and when hot when can be sad, submissive, and suspicious.

Termed 'weathercock' for the changeable and contradictory nature of its signalment. Disposition and mental state are important.

Often tall, slim, fair-haired females. Significant antibacterial agent.

Often on the right side. Exudates are profuse, mildly purulent, and **bland**.

HEAD	Conjunctivitis. Eyelids agglutinated, inflamed. Hordeolum.
	Lachrymation: bland, mucous, profuse, thick, yellow.

	Ophthalmia in neonates. Veins of fundus enlarged.
	Otitis externa and media; exudate: bland, catarrhal, offensive.
	Pinna red, swollen.
	Nose: blocked: copious, offensive exudate, right, scaly.
GASTROINTESTINAL	Crack in middle of lower lip. Halitosis is offensive.
	Tongue covered in tenacious, white to yellow mucous.
	Colic; tympanitic colic.
	Diarrhoea: bloody, offensive, even dysentery.
RESPIRATORY	Cough: dry, often nocturnal.
	Expectoration: bitter, bland, greenish, thick.
UROGENITAL	Involuntary urination in juveniles and when coughing.
	Flatus, night, tenesmus.
	Metritis: acrid, creamy. Ovary: painful yet inactive.
	Orchitis and prostatitis.
LAMENESS	Back and large muscles: pain, stiff.
	Extremities: oedema.
COMPETITION	The wide application for this remedy in the management of behaviour shows a key role in females. Mood swings point to its reactions, particularly during ovarian: including silent heat, phases.
JUVENILE	**Neonatal ophthalmia.**
SKIN	Urticaria with diarrhoea from high protein over feeding.
MODALITIES	Agg: heat. Lying on left.
	Amel: gentle exercise in the open air.
COMPARE	Cycl Coff Kali-bi Kali-s Sulph.
CONSIDER	Of huge significance for its key role in the management of:

- Behaviour management in females.
- Conjunctivitis.
- Diarrhoea.
- Otitis.
- Ovarian disease.

	Remember. Principally a female remedy, but effective in effeminate, particularly juvenile, males. The desire for close contact, yet the ease with which they become irritable, is a significant sign. Always respond well to consolation.
POTENCY	12X. 30CH. 200CH.

Pyrog
PYROGENIUM
Rotting meat Animal

Septic, disgusting conditions. Restless and vocal.

GASTROINTESTINAL	Tongue: clean, dry, red, smooth. Vomit.
	Painless constipation.
UROGENITAL	Mastitis. Metritis. Retained foetal membranes. Septicaemia.

LAMENESS	Infected periarticular wounds and joints.
SKIN	Infected wounds.
MODALITIES	Agg: movement.
CONSIDER	The control of offensive bacterial infections:
	• Metritis.
	• Perineal sepsis.
	• Postoperative sepsis.
	• Purulent infected bite wounds.
	• Septicaemia.
POTENCY	12X. 30CH.

Querc
QUERCUS e glandibus
Acorn kernel Plant

Cushing's disease. Industrious workers before emotional breakdown.

ABDOMEN	Pendulous, thin skinned.
GASTROINTESTINAL	PD: dry mouth and pharynx. Constipation.
RESPIRATORY	Painful laryngeal cough with shortness of breath.
UROGENITAL	PU that is always worse at night.
LAMENESS	Painful stiffness of large back muscles.
SKIN	Widespread, mild dermatitis with slight itch.
COMPARE	Cortico Cortiso.
CONSIDER	• Cushing's disease in the dog responds well.
	• More difficult in the horse where the threat of associated laminitis is a factor.
	• Metabolic disorders.
	Works well alongside allopathic medication.
POTENCY	30CH.

Rad
RADIUM
Radium bromide Mineral

Apprehensive, depressed, and irritable. Enjoy company. Tire easily. Pruritus. Arthritis and cancer.

HEAD	Ataxia and other neuralgias: trigeminal.
GASTROINTESTINAL	Dry, painful throat. Eructation and vomiting.
	Colic: violent tympanitic. Constipation and Diarrhoea alternate.
RESPIRATORY	Dry persistent cough with low BP.
UROGENITAL	Nephritis: albuminuria, casts: granular hyaline. Chlorides. Enuresis.
LAMENESS	Muscles: back, large: painfully stiff. Arthritis.
	Brittle feet.
SKIN	Epithelioma. Erythema with necrotic, oedematous ulcers that heal slowly. Pruritus of digits.
MODALITIES	Agg: rising. Amel: open air. Grooming. Heat treatments.
COMPARE	Anac Ars Caust Puls Rhus-t Sep Uran-an X-ray.
CONSIDER	• Arthritis.
	• Nephritis.

- Skin cancer.
- Skin ulcers.

POTENCY	30CH. 200CH.

Raj
RAJANIA SUBSAMARATA
Raison seed Plant

CNS	Encephalitis. Meningitis. Severe mood swings. Acute conditions.
HEAD	Blepharitis and conjunctivitis. Pupils contracted, insensitive. Rhinitis and sinusitis: mucopurulent.
GASTROINTESTINAL	Mouth held open, jaw slack. Halitosis. Constipation followed by dysentery. Tympany.
RESPIRATORY	Pulmonary abscess. Weak, fast heart.
UROGENITAL	Metritis: profuse, sticky. Balanitis.
LAMENESS	Ataxia with slack muscles.
SKIN	Abscess. Cancer. Ulcers.
MODALITIES	Agg: movement. Amel: cool. Exudation.
COMPARE	Anthr Carb-v Lach Verat.
CONSIDER	• Diarrhoea. • Equine encephalitis. • Pyrexia of unknown origin.
POTENCY	4X − 12X. 30CH.

Ran-b
RANUNCULUS BULBOSUS
Bulbous buttercup Plant

HEAD	Herpes ulcers and vesicles on cornea. Day blindness. Photophobia. Irritable and oversensitive.
RESPIRATORY	Severe thoracic pain from damage to ribs and intercostal muscles.
SKIN	Eczema: blisters become pustules, vesicles: cracked, horny, thick.
MODALITIES	Agg: open air. Blanket touching skin. Evenings. Stormy wet weather. Amel: firm bandaging.
COMPARE	*Ranunculus glacialis* Ran-g. Reindeer flower. Bronchopneumonia. *Ranunculus flammula* Ran-fl. Lesser spearwort. Gangrene, ulcer. Bry Crot-t Euph-r Mez.
CONSIDER	• Corneal herpes ulcers. • Eczema with intense pruritus and vesicles. • Intercostal pain.
POTENCY	4X − 12X. 30CH.

Raph

RAPHANUS SATIVUS
Black radish Plant

HEAD	Oedema of lower eyelids.
	Pharyngeal mucous. Hysteria.
GASTROINTESTINAL	Liver and spleen painfully enlarged.
	Offensive eructation and vomit.
	Colic: tympanitic, severe.
	Diarrhoea: brown, copious, frothy, liquid.
UROGENITAL	Urine: copious, milk-like, turbid, yeasty sediment.
	Female genitalia: pruritus. Nymphomania: dislike females.
SKIN	Greasy. Pemphigus. seborrhoea.
COMPARE	Anac Arg-n Carb-v Lyc Uran-n.
CONSIDER	• Seborrhoea.
	• Tympanitic colic.
	• Tympanitic Diarrhoea.
POTENCY	4X – 12X. 30CH.

Rat
RATANHIA PERUVIANA
Mapato Plant

GASTROINTESTINAL	Severely painful rectal fissures.
COMPARE	Crot Dol Paeon Rauw Sang-n.
CONSIDER	• Anal fissures.
POTENCY	4X – 12X.

Rauw
RAUWOLFIA SERPENTINA
Rauwolfia Plant

HEAD	Ataxia. Vertigo. Rhinitis with dry ulcers. Excitable.
GASTROINTESTINAL	Aerophagy. Gastritis. Rectal fissure.
CARDIOVASCULAR	Arrhythmia. BP low. Bradycardia.
RESPIRATORY	Bronchitis and laryngitis: cough: bloody, mucous, sticky.
UROGENITAL	Cystitis. Dysuria. Reddish.
	Impotence, poor libido in both sexes.
LAMENESS	Arthritis of stifle.
SKIN	Cracks, fissures, and ulcers.
MODALITIES	Agg: after food. Evenings. Heat. Walking.
	Amel: fresh, open air. Arduous work. After Faeces.
COMPARE	Ars Aur Lach Nux-v Phos Rauw.
CONSIDER	• Addison's disease.
	• Pancreatitis.
	• Rectal fissures.
POTENCY	12X. 30CH.

Reser
RESERPINUM
Alkaloid of Rauwolfia Plant

Premature aging. Aggressive, excitable, and hyperactive. Short acting catalepsy.
Slow pulse.

GASTROINTESTINAL	Rhinitis. Pharyngitis and laryngitis.
	Stomach: cancer, ulcer.
UROGENITAL	Hypergalactia.
SKIN	Hair looks damp and dull.
COMPARE	Ars Aur Lach Nux-v Rauw.
CONSIDER	• Behaviour modification in aggressive individuals.
	• Cancer and ulceration of stomach.
POTENCY	30CH – 200CH.

Rham-cal
RHAMNUS CALIFORNICA
Californian coffee tree Plant

HEAD	Eyelids twitch.
	Poor hearing. Irritable, nervous, sad.
	Agg: evening.
LAMENESS	Weak hindquarters.
	Polyarthritis: bursitis, immune mediated, painful.
COMPARE	*Rhamnus cathartica* Rham-cath. European buckthorn. Muscle pains with gastroenteritis.
	Rhamnus purshiana Cas-c. (*Cascara sagrada*) Chronic constipation and gastritis.
	Acid-phos Cortiso Nat-m.
CONSIDER	• Immune mediated arthritis.
POTENCY	12X. 30CH.

Rheum
RHEUM PALMATUM
Rhubarb Plant

GASTROINTESTINAL	Variable appetite. Halitosis. Hypersalivation. Teething.
	Toothache: teething: diarrhoea: pain, pasty, sour. Mild tympanitic colic.
MODALITIES	Agg: after food. Movement.
COMPARE	Anth Hep Ip Mag-p Pod.
CONSIDER	• Teething problems.
POTENCY	3X – 6X.

Rhod
RHODODENDRON CHRYSANTHUM
Snow rose Plant

Fear of thunder. Painful, deformed arthritis of digits.

HEAD	Toothache amel by food and warmth.
RESPIRATORY	Severe pleural pain.
UROGENITAL	Orchitis with testicle drawn up: l > r. Hydrocele.
LAMENESS	Painful neck and shoulders. Digits: bursitis, fibrosis.
MODALITIES	Agg: early mornings. Night. Storms.
	Amel: after storms. Eating. Warmth.
COMPARE	Dulc Nat-s Rhus-t.

CONSIDER	• Arthritis of digits.
	• Fear of thunder, particularly terriers.
POTENCY	6X – 12X for arthritis. 200CH for fear.

Rhus-t
RHUS TOXICODENDRON
Poison ivy Plant

Sad at home but stimulated outside.

Fears: approach, irrational, irritable: Restless: juveniles at night. When well are often calm, easy to work with and train well. Significant antibacterial agent.

Remarkable healing effect on skin, muscles, and mucous membranes.

Exudates are profuse, acrid, offensive, and purulent.

Painfully swollen parts.

Fears: approach, irrational, irritable: Restless: juveniles at night. When well are often calm, easy to work with and train well. Significant antibacterial agent.

HEAD	Left parotid gland enlarged.
	Conjunctivitis. Iritis. Keratitis. Eyelids: oedema. Profuse purulent exudates. Ulcer. Lachrymation: acrid, profuse. Ophthalmia: flare. Cellulitis of orbit. Photophobia.
	Otitis: bloody, purulent, pinnae hot: swollen.
	Nose: bloody. Tip: red, sore, ulcerated.
GASTROINTESTINAL	Anorexia. Gums, chin, tongue: blisters, cracks, raw. PD. Jaw: dislocation.
	Tympanitic colic.
	Diarrhoea. Dysentery.
CARDIOVASCULAR	Arrhythmia, tachycardia. Hypertrophy from over work.
RESPIRATORY	EIPH: arterial.
UROGENITAL	PU: dark, scanty, sediment, white.
	Female genitalia: pruritis. Metritis: chronic, offensive, thin.
	Glans, prepuce, and scrotum swollen.
LAMENESS	Painfully swollen and stiff muscles of forearm and shoulder. Ligament and tendon strain. Condylar bone pains.
	Bursitis of carpal, hock, and digits.
COMPETITION	Assists horses to compete when affected by joint or muscle stiffness. Benefit from heat application before and after exercise, and warm bandaging. Heating pads and magnetopulse therapy over stiff loins.
SKIN	Cellulitis with intense pruritus: oedema, red, scaly, urticaria, vesicles.
MODALITIES	Agg: night. Rest. During sleep. Tired. After wet, rainy weather.
	Amel: open air. Warm bandaging and soaking. Exercise after a slow start. Massage. Physiotherapy. Stretching. Dry, warm weather.
COMPARE	*Rhus aromatica* Rhus-a. Fragrant sumach. Cystitis, nephritis: haematuria. Diabetes mellitus. Incontinence.
	Rhus glabra Rhus-g. Smooth sumach. Mouth ulcers. Tympanitic with disgusting flatus.
	Rhus venenata Rhus-v, Skin signs most severe.

209

CONSIDER	Acid-fl Bry Calc Phyt Rhus-v. Important: • Back problems, including sacro-iliac disease. • Joint stiffness, which is acute or chronic. • Muscle stiffness, particularly of the back. • Rectal abscess and fissures in initial stages. • Salmonellosis. In all conditions there is restless with stiffness. Improvement with warmth and exercise after being initially stiff.
POTENCY	6X – 12X for arthritis. 30CH for colic.

Ribes-n
RIBES NIGRUM
Black currant Plant

Chronic conditions associated with lethargy from depleted adrenal glands.
General anti-inflammatory and anti-allergic properties by exerting an improvement in the viability of endothelial cells. Significant antibacterial agent.

HEAD	Sinus, throat: chronic inflammation.
GASTROINTESTINAL	Control of inflammatory conditions associated with gram negative bacterial infection.
RESPIRATORY	Juvenile asthma, bronchitis, pleural oedema: chronic.
UROGENITAL	Diuretic in chronic nephritis.
LAMENESS	Muscle: generalised fatigue and stiffness.
SKIN	Direct influence on canine atopic dermatitis.
COMPARE	Cortiso Echi Eleuth Gins Rhus-t Rub-v Sil Tub. *Rubus chamaemorus* Rubu-c Cloudberry, may be more potent. *Rubus villosus* Rubu Blackberry. Anaemia and gastroenteritis.
CONSIDER	• Chronic inflammatory conditions of epithelium.
POTENCY	4X. 8X.

Rna
RIBONUCLEIC ACID
Rna nosode Animal

Leukaemia. Pancreatic insufficiency. Aggressive, dull, and sad.

UROGENITAL	Loss of libido in females.
LAMENESS	Spondylitis. Painful bursitis of shoulder and digits. Oedema.
SKIN	Chronic flaky dermatitis on digits.
MODALITIES	Agg: cold. Lying on back. Amel: lying on abdomen.
COMPARE	Cortiso Sil Tub.
CONSIDER	• Chronic eczema of digits. • Leukaemia. • Metabolic disorders. • Spondylitis.
POTENCY	12X. 30CH.

Ros-ca
ROSA CANINA
Dog rose Plant

HEAD	Otitis, rhinitis, sinusitis, upper respiratory viral infections: clear mucous. Headache.
RESPIRATORY	Bronchitis, tracheitis: cough: dry.
UROGENITAL	Cystitis: chronic.
COMPARE	Am-c Bry Kaliums Camph Phos Puls Rhus-t.
CONSIDER	• Respiratory congestion.
POTENCY	6X – 12X.

Rumx
RUMEX CRISPUS
Yellow dock Plant

HEAD	Dry rhinitis: exudate: copious, mucous. Restless.
GASTROINTESTINAL	Chronic gastritis. Hiccough. Meat intolerant. Flatus. Pruritus. Morning diarrhoea: watery brown.
RESPIRATORY	Bronchitis, tracheitis: cough: dry, insomnia. The initially frothy and watery exudate becomes stringy and tough.
SKIN	Severely pruritic eczema of digits. Urticaria. Agg: chilly air.
COMPARE	Bell Caust Sulph.
CONSIDER	• Irritating mucous cough. • Eczema.
POTENCY	6X – 12X.

Ruta
RUTA GRAVEOLENS
Common rue Plant

Polycrest. Lameness. Anxious, irritable, sad.

HEAD	Eye muscles strained.
GASTROINTESTINAL	Constipation: bloody, frothy, mucous. Carcinoma.
RESPIRATORY	Cough. Exudate: copious, thick, yellow.
LAMENESS	Lumbar pain that improves when ridden. **Bone pain:** periosteal: shin, splint. Ligament strains: achilles, annular, carpal, hamstrings: contracted, pain, stiff, tight. Carpal and hock ligaments: pain, strain, stiff.
COMPETITION	Huge influence in the management of ligament, periosteal and tendon problems. Prophylactic for 2-y-o's with a tendency to 'shins and splints'.
JUVENILE	**Tendon** contraction in neonates.
MODALITIES	Agg: cold, wet weather. Lying down. Morning.
COMPARE	Acid-fl Calc-fl Calc-p Thiosin.
CONSIDER	A huge remedy for athletes: • Injuries to bone and periosteum. • Ligaments: annular, carpal tunnel. • Tendonitis.

211

	• Periostitis, including shins and splints.
POTENCY	6X – 12X. 30CH.

Sabad
SABADILLA OFFICINALIS
Asagraea cevadilla seed Plant

HEAD	Allergies. Conjunctivitis, rhinitis, frontal sinusitis: exudate: acrid, copious, watery. Spasmodic sneezing. Chronic exudates become tough.
GASTROINTESTINAL	Chronic left sided pharyngitis. Diarrhoea: painful in juveniles.
SKIN	Inflammation and cracking of skin at junction of nails and hoof: deformed, horny, infected, thickened.
MODALITIES	Agg: cold and chilly water. Full moon. Amel: warm food and water. Wrapping.
COMPARE	Con Lach Lyc Puls Sep.
CONSIDER	• Seasonal allergies.
POTENCY	6X – 12X.

Sabal
SABAL SERRULATUM
Saw palmetto Plant

Promotes tissue building. Improves sexual debility. Dull and tire easily.

RESPIRATORY	Chronic bronchitis with mucous.
UROGENITAL	Mammae: underdeveloped. Ovaritis. Male cystitis. Epididymitis. Prostatic cancer and **hyperplasia.**
COMPARE	Acid-phos Acid-pic Apis Ferr-p Thuj.
CONSIDER	• Prostatic disease.
POTENCY	2X – 4X – 12X.

Sacch
SACCHARUM OFFICINALE
Cane sugar Sucrose Plant

HEAD	Corneal opacity with loss of vision.
GASTROINTESTINAL	Diabetes mellitus: fat, irritable juveniles with variable appetite, PD, PU, and anal pruritus.
CARDIOVASCULAR	Anaemia. Myocardial degeneration.
COMPARE	*Saccharum lactis* Sacch-l. Milk sugar. Diuresis and neuralgias. **Saccharum** Sacchin. Appetite lost. Diarrhoea. Weight loss.
CONSIDER	• Diabetes mellitus with heart weakness. • Metabolic disorders.
POTENCY	12X. 30CH.

Sal-ac
SALICYLICUM ACIDUM
Aspirin Salicylic acid Mineral

Sad with poor concentration. Excitable with vocalisation. Osteoarthritis and ulcers.

HEAD	Vertigo: fall to left. Retinal haemorrhage.
GASTROINTESTINAL	Stomatitis, pharyngitis: swallowing difficult. Vomiting. Gastroenteritis and ulcers.
LAMENESS	Spondylitis, sacroiliac disease: acute, chronic, painful. Carpus, hock: osteoarthritis, osteoporosis, spavin.
SKIN	Pruritic, pustular herpes. Urticaria.
MODALITIES	Agg: movement. Touch. Amel: scratching.
COMPARE	Acid-lact Chin Colch Urt-u.
CONSIDER	• Gastroenteritis.
	• Osteoarthritis.
	Ulcers.
POTENCY	12X. 30CH.

Salv
SALVIA OFFICINALIS
Sage Plant

Odd homoeopaths rarely use such a well-known for its regular employment as an antibacterial agent suggests it should be. Controls excessive seating and anxiety related conditions. Significant antibacterial agent.

HEAD	Right sided tearing pain in jaw, gums, and teeth.
GASTROINTESTINAL	Tympanitic colic. Diarrhoea: frequent, slimy, watery.
RESPIRATORY	Tickling to suffocative cough with bacterial involvement.
JUVENILES	Secondary bacterial infections with coughing.
COMPARE	*Chrysanthemum leucanthemum.*
CONSIDER	• Feline respiratory virus complex: acute.
	• Kennel Cough syndrome.
	Remember viral diseases, after purulent exudate.
POTENCY	6X – 12X. 30CH.

Samb
SAMBUCUS NIGRA
Black elder Plant

Anxiety with irritable whining in restless, easily startled individuals. Main sphere is mucous membranes, especially the respiratory organs. Snuffles and dry membranes in neonates.

HEAD	Dry, obstructed nose in juveniles. Snuffles.
GASTROINTESTINAL	Tympanitic colic. Diarrhoea: frequent, slimy, watery.
RESPIRATORY	Dyspnoea: snuffles: neonates: midnight, paroxysmal and suffocative. Nose: dry, obstructed.
UROGENITAL	Nephritis: acute. PU or scant.
LAMENESS	Cold oedema of extremities.
JUVENILES	Snuffles.
MODALITIES	Agg: rest. Amel: motion.
COMPARE	*Sambucus Canadensis* Samb-c Canadian elder. Diuresis.
CONSIDER	• Feline respiratory virus complex: acute.

- Kennel Cough syndrome.

Remember acute viral diseases, before purulent exudate.

POTENCY	6X – 12X. 30CH.

Sang
SANGUINARIA CANADENSIS
Blood root Plant

Exudates vary from dry to profuse. Offensive, string and yellow. Painful. Ulcerate.

HEAD	Pain in angle of jaw, Aural polyps. Chronic rhinitis.
GASTROINTESTINAL	PD. White tongue.
	Tonsillitis, pharyngitis, laryngitis. Ulcers.
	Diarrhoea: watery, yellow.
RESPIRATORY	Exudative asthma and pneumonia.
LAMENESS	Pain in right shoulder and left hip.
SKIN	Small sarcoid. Spring urticaria.
MODALITIES	Agg: motion. Touch.
	Amel: dark. Sleep.
COMPARE	Bell Ferr Iris Lach Meli Op Sang-n Sep.
CONSIDER	• Chronic respiratory disease with secondary infection.
POTENCY	4X – 8X.

Sang-n
SANGUINARINUM NITRICUM
Nitrate of sanguinary Mineral

Acute, chronic respiratory disease with secondary infection.
Exudates may be acrid, bloody, profuse, watery, and mucous. Hyperaemia.

HEAD	Lachrymation. Blocked nose. Turbinates swollen.
GASTROINTESTINAL	Ulcers on side of tongue. Painful rectal fissures.
RESPIRATORY	Bronchitis, pharyngitis, laryngitis: constricted, follicular.
COMPARE	Sanguinarinum tartaricum Sang-t. Exophthalmos. Arum-t Kali-by Psor.
CONSIDER	Acute, chronic rhinitis
	Rectal fissure.
POTENCY	4X – 12X.

Sanic
SANICULA AQUA
Water of Sanicula Springs Mineral

Exudates are dirty, mucous, ropy, and tenacious. Fear downward movement. Travel sickness.

HEAD	Photophobia.
GASTROINTESTINAL	Drink little and often. Vomit after eating.
	Constipation: heavy, large, offensive faeces.
RESPIRATORY	Exudative laryngitis and pharyngitis.
UROGENITAL	Metritis smells of fish or cheese.

SKIN	Brown, dirty, greasy, and wrinkled. Dandruff. Fissured. Digits.
COMPARE	Abrot Alum Calc Sil Sulph.
CONSIDER	• Constipation.
	• Travel sickness.
POTENCY	6X for constipation. 30CH for travel sickness.

Sarcol-ac
SARCOLACTICUM ACIDUM
Dextrum lacticum acidum Mineral

Easily annoyed and irritable after demanding work. PD. PU. Marked lameness from muscle weakness and exhaustion.

CARDIOVASCULAR	Myocardial strain: overexercise, virus. Vomiting.
UROGENITAL	Azoturia / myositis. Proteinuria with sediment.
LAMENESS	Acutely painful muscle cramping. Improves excretion of waste products from circulation during exercise. Aids recovery.
MODALITIES	Agg: exercise. Night.
COMPARE	*Lactis acidum* Lac-ac. Diabetes mellitus. Bursitis. Arn Berb Bry.
CONSIDER	• Early exhaustion.
	• Fitness programs.
POTENCY	4X – 12X for prevention. Combines well with Berb. 30CH and 200CH for treatment.

Saroth
SAROTHAMNUS SCOPARIUS
Scotch broom Plant

GASTROINTESTINAL	Tympanitic colic. PD.
CARDIOVASCULAR	Arrhythmia. Myocardial degeneration. Low BP.
UROGENITAL	Urethritis with diuresis and PU.
COMPARE	Dig Verat.
CONSIDER	• Heart disease with low BP.
POTENCY	2X – 6X.

Scel-t
SCELETIUM TORTUOSUM
Kanna Plant

Recent investigation into this South African species led to it gaining a reputation in behaviour modification. Anger. Restless. Anti-depressant.

COMPARE	Arg-n Coff Nux-v Scut.
CONSIDER	Management of severe behaviour problems in juveniles.
POTENCY	2X – 6X.

Scroph-n
SCROPHULARIA NODOSA
Knotted figwort Plant

Benign cancer of lymph glands mammae and skin. Dull, angry mornings. Orchitis. Vertigo.

HEAD	Photophobia. Eruptions, ulcers: ears.
SKIN	Small epithelioma. Lupus with ulcers.
MODALITIES	Agg: before and after food. Morning.
COMPARE	Astra-e Carc Con Lob-p Ruta.
CONSIDER	• Cancer of lymph glands and skin.
POTENCY	2X – 6X. 30CH.

Scut

SCUTELLARIA LATERIFOLIA
Skull cap Plant

Confused with poor concentration making them nervous and easily startled. A mild tranquiliser for neuritis with spasms in teething juveniles.

CNS	Chorea and other tremors.
GASTROINTESTINAL	Mild, tympanitic colic. Diarrhoea: pale.
CARDIOVASCULAR	Weak heart.
LAMENESS	Muscle twitching.
MODALITIES	Agg: movement.
COMPARE	Anth Coff Lyc Passi.
CONSIDER	• Chorea post distemper.
	• Mild tranquilisation in first aid situations.
POTENCY	4X – 12X. 30CH.

Sec

SECALE CORNUTUM
Claviceps purpurea Ergot Plant

Confused, dull and indifferent, but can be restless and suspicious.
Thin geriatrics with a poor circulation and a tendency to bleed.

HEAD	Hair: dry, falls easily, grey.
	Senile cataracts: female. Eye: dilated pupils, sunk.
	Sclera: prominent blue margin.
GASTROINTESTINAL	PD. Tongue bloody, coated viscid yellow, cracked.
	Tympanitic colic with offensive eructation.
	Diarrhoea: bloody, involuntary, olive-green, putrid.
	Anus may be wide open.
UROGENITAL	PU with dark, bloody urine. Geriatric enuresis.
	Nymphomania.
LAMENESS	Spinal neuritis.
	Distal circulation: poor: Navicular disease. Seedy toe.
SKIN	Even small wounds haemorrhage.
	Discharge: blood: black, oozes, offensive, watery.
MODALITIES	Agg: bandaging and wrapping. Heat.
	Amel: Chilly water hosing. Massage.
COMPARE	Ars Cinnm Colch Tab.
CONSIDER	• Navicular disease.
	• Poor distal circulation and healing.
	• Tendency to haemorrhage.
POTENCY	6X – 12X. 30CH.

Sel

SELENIUM
Selenium Mineral

Averse to company. Dull, lazy, and vocal. Sexual disturbances. Neurological complaints, including equine head shaking, related to cranial nerve irritation.
Mineral with wide ranging effects on nutrition and thus the body.

GASTROINTESTINAL	Abdomen: chronic, painful, swollen. Gums: bloody. Tongue: coated white, ulcerated. Constipation. Megacolon. Pruritus.
RESPIRATORY	Laryngitis. Hacking morning cough, lumpy mucous. Vocal, but hoarse.
UROGENITAL	Acetonuria, oxalates, phosphaturia. High SG. Dribble involuntary. Impotence with good libido. Prostatomegaly.
SKIN	Dry pruritus. Hair falling.
MODALITIES	Agg: after sleep. Heat. Mating. Morning. Amel: open air.
COMPARE	Acid-phos Agn Calad Kali-c Sulph Tell.
CONSIDER	• Impotence and prostatomegaly in debilitated geriatrics.
POTENCY	4X – 12X. 30CH.

Senec
SENECIO AUREUS
Golden ragwort Plant

ABDOMEN	Cirrhosis and **hepatitis**. Irritable and nervous.
GASTROINTESTINAL	A dry mouth with sour eructation and vomiting. Diarrhoea: dark, lumpy, pain, watery, tenesmus.
RESPIRATORY	Acute laryngitis with a loose, hoarse cough.
UROGENITAL	Nephritis and cystitis in irritable juveniles. Urine is bloody and hot with tenesmus. Painfully enlarged Orchitis and prostatitis.
COMPARE	*Senecio jacobaea* Senec-j. Stinking Willie. Has a similar action. Also, in meningitis. Alet Caul Sep.
CONSIDER	Cirrhosis, cystitis, and nephritis.
POTENCY	6X – 12X. 30CH.

Seneg
SENEGA
Snakewort Plant

HEAD	Left facial paralysis. Blepharitis. Healing after eye surgery. Exudates: excessive, watery mucous. Vitreous humor opaque. Eyelids: dry crusts. Rhinitis.
GASTROINTESTINAL	Vesicles in corners of lips.
RESPIRATORY	Asthma, bronchitis COPD, emphysema, laryngitis. Cough: hacking, hoarse, mucous, tough.
UROGENITAL	Chronic interstitial nephritis with mucous. Dysuria.
MODALITIES	Agg: rest. Slow walk outdoors. Amel: bend backwards. Sweating.
COMPARE	Am-c Calc Caust Nep Phos.

217

CONSIDER	• Geriatric respiratory disease.
	• Paralysis of face and eyelids.
	• Postoperative eye surgery.
POTENCY	2X – 6X. 30CH.

Sep
SEPIA SUCCUS
Cuttlefish Animal

Polycrest. Pre-eminently a female remedy. Hormonal swings with anger. Anger. Anxiety in evenings. Consolation aggravates. Dull. Fears: alone, thunder, travel, vets. Hysteria. Sad. Work averse to.

Impatient. Impulsive. Irritable. Oversensitive to noise.

Significant antibacterial agent. People: averse to. Restless when ovulating.

HEAD	Delayed closure of fontanelles.
	Tarsal tumours. Eczema of pinnae.
	Rhinitis and sinusitis: exudate: thick, greenish exudate.
ABDOMEN	Painfully swollen liver.
GASTROINTESTINAL	Crack in lower lip. Tongue: offensive white coating. Morning vomiting before food.
	Flatulence. Constipation: hard, large faeces. Tenesmus. Prolapse.
RESPIRATORY	Pleurisy. Laryngitis. Expectorant is profuse.
UROGENITAL	Cystitis, urethritis with red, sticky urine. Lithiasis.
	Metritis: green to yellow. Uterus, vagina: prolapse.
LAMENESS	Painfully stiff and twitching muscles of lower back. Pain and stiffness of small joints.
COMPETITION	An especially important remedy for working females with a tendency to anger and muscular stiffness during oestrous.
SKIN	Inferior quality and hair falls. Offensive Ichthyosis. Roots are sensitive. Ringworm-like lesions during spring. Urticaria when outdoors.
MODALITIES	Agg: cold. Damp. Evenings. Left side. Mornings. Music. Before thunder. Washing.
	Amel: Hot bandaging. Exercise. Pressure. After sleep. Cold washing.
COMPARE	Lil-t Murx Nat-m Phos Sil Sulph.
CONSIDER	Valuable in the management of:
	• Anxiety around parturition.
	• Behavioural problems related to oestrous.
	• Metritis.
	• Uterine prolapse.
POTENCY	12X. 30CH. 200CH.

Seq-g
SEQUOIA GIGANTEA

	Giant redwood tree Plant
UROGENITAL	Male: prostate: hyperplasia. Libido, poor.
COMPARE	Sabal Gins Lyc
CONSIDER	• Prostate disease.

POTENCY	4X – 12X.

Ser-ang
SERUM ANGUILLAE
Eel Animal

CARDIOVASCULAR	Mitral valve insufficiency.
UROGENITAL	Acute, chronic nephritis. Albuminuria, anuria, oliguria. Oedema.
COMPARE	Lach Vip.
CONSIDER	• Nephritis with heart disease.
POTENCY	6X – 12X. 30CH.

Sil
SILICEA TERRA
Flint Mineral

Polycrest. Anxious, mild creatures when well.

Concentration is difficult and leads to confusion making them hurried, irritable, and oversensitive, during which consolation aggravates. Dull. Exhaustion. Hurried.

Fears: injections, public.

Wide action centres on defective, present, or historical nutrition. Wide ranging from bones to epilepsy. Post vaccination problems. Suppuration. Fistula.

Significant antibacterial agent.

Ripens abscesses since it promotes suppuration. Deep and slow in action. Where problems have a historical basis silica takes time to work.

CNS	Fits preceded by confusion
HEAD	Corneal abscess, opacity. Hypopyon. Lachrymal duct swollen. Ophthalmitis.
	Noise sensitive. Otitis externa, media: purulent. Crusts: bleed, dry, hard, itchy.
	Nasal bones: sensitive, perforated.
	Chronic osteomalacia.
ABDOMEN	Liver abscess.
CARDIOVASCULAR	Lymphadenitis of inguinal glands.
RESPIRATORY	Pneumonia: chronic: cough: bloody daytime cough, lumpy, thick, purulent. Slow healing.
UROGENITAL	Urine is bloody, passed involuntary, and has a red or yellow sediment.
	Metritis: acrid, milky. Mammae: fistula: hard, lumpy, ulcerous. Sensitive vaginal and vulvar cysts.
LAMENESS	Coccyx, sacroiliac: injury. Spondylitis.
	Tire easily when exercised and muscles of forearm and hamstrings are weak.
	Hooves, nails: cracked, crumble, deformed. Seedy toe and white line disease.
GERIATRIC	Premature aging: tissue degeneration, chronic infection.
SKIN	Unhealthy. Abscess, boils, cracks on toes, fistulae, and foreign bodies. Injuries: readily become purulent, easily develop tracts, ulcers.
	Fibrosis. Scar tissue. Tumours: hard, indurate.

MODALITIES	Agg: Morning. New moon. Noise. Washing.
	Amel: summer. Warmth. Humid, wet weather.
COMPARE	Acid-fl Acid-pic Calc Gunp Hep Kali-p Phos Sanic Thuj.
CONSIDER	A remedy with a profound influence on chronic conditions:
	• Abscess and pus anywhere.
	• Anal fistulae in the GSD.
	• Blindness from corneal opacities.
	• Scar tissue.
	• Sinusitis that is chronic and neglected.
	• Tumours that are hard and indurate.
	Remember that silica is a slow acting remedy. Just when ready to change the prescription it works.
POTENCY	6X – 12X. 30CH. 200CH.

Card-m

SILYBUM MARIANUM

Carduus marianus St Mary's thistle Plant

Angry, easily startled with liver and metabolic disease. Fall backwards in vertigo.

ABDOMEN	Painful ascites, cirrhosis, and hepatitis.
GASTROINTESTINAL	Halitosis. Vomit: acrid, green, watery.
	Faeces: alternate, constipation to bright yellow diarrhoea.
RESPIRATORY	**Dyspnoea:** of asthma, aggravated by movement.
UROGENITAL	Urine: deep yellow to golden, sweet smelling.
	Enhances metabolism during demand for heavy milking.
LAMENESS	**Pain** over large muscles referred from abdominal disease.
MODALITIES	Agg: movement.
COMPARE	Aloe Bry Chel Chin-s Merc Podo.
CONSIDER	• Acetonemia.
	• Hepatitis.
	• Metabolic disorders.
POTENCY	2X – 6X – 12X.

Sol

SOL

The sun's energy

Skin problems, particularly those caused by or aggravated by the sun. Exhaustion.

CARDIOVASCULAR	Fast, weak pulse.
SKIN	Melanoma. Sunburn. Warts.
COMPARE	Acon Bell Cund Nat-c Staph X-ray.
CONSIDER	Essential in management of:
	• Melanoma in grey horses.
	• Heat and sunstroke.
POTENCY	30CH. 200CH.
	Prevention of melanoma. 30CH every two weeks.

Dulc
SOLANUM DULCAMARA
Bittersweet Plant

Polycrest. Bossy, hurried, impatient, indifferent, irritable, sad, restless. Keynote is aggravation brought on by weather changes. Significant antibacterial agent.

CNS	Localised paralysis.
HEAD	Ringworm: crusts: bloody, brown, pruritus. Conjunctivitis: allergic, granular, profuse, thick, watery, yellow. Otitis media: mucous. Nostrils: blocked, bloody, crusts, mucous, neonate, thick, yellow.
GASTROINTESTINAL	Anorexia. Saliva: profuse, soapy, tenacious. Vomiting: mucous, tenacious, white. Colic with diarrhoea: bloody, green, mucous, slimy, watery: especially in summer.
CARDIOVASCULAR	Lymphadenitis: inguinal and parotid glands.
RESPIRATORY	Dyspnoea. Asthma. Dry, hoarse cough after exercise.
UROGENITAL	Cystitis: mucous, purulent, sediment, thick. Mammae: engorged, painful.
LAMENESS	Muscle: neck, wither, and shoulder: stiff with great weakness. Shin soreness. Weak distal circulation.
COMPETITION	Prophylactic for athletes during adverse weather.
SKIN	**Dermatitis:** crusts: bloody, brown to yellow, crusts, pruritic, red spots. Warts: face, feet: large, palmer, smooth. Urticaria.
MODALITIES	Agg: night. Cold, damp, rainy weather. Amel: active. Warmth.
COMPARE	Bry Bar-c Calc Cimic Nat-s Rhus-t.
CONSIDER	A remedy to consider in condition markedly affected by the typical weather changes: • Coughing. • Diarrhoea. • Dermatitis. • Joint and muscle stiffness. • Warts. How conditions worsen in poor weather worth noting.
POTENCY	4X – 12X. 30CH.

Sol-n
SOLANUM NIGRUM
Black nightshade Plant

CNS	Epilepsy and meningitis. Widespread tetanic spasms. Delirium. Restless and may be violent.
GASTROINTESTINAL	Pupils: contract and dilate alternately. Rhinitis: acute: mucous, profuse, watery.
RESPIRATORY	Thick, yellow exudate on larynx.

UROGENITAL	Bell.
CONSIDER	• Epilepsy.
	• Meningitis.
POTENCY	12X. 30CH.

Solid
SOLIDAGO VIRGAUREA
Golden rod Plant

HEAD	Allergic conjunctivitis: epiphora: water, pruritis.
RESPIRATORY	Asthma, bronchitis: cough: exudate: bloody, mucopurulent.
UROGENITAL	Cystitis, urethritis, nephritis. Urine: brown to clear, calculi, profuse, sediment. May be scant and thick. Dysuria.
COMPARE	Ars Seneg.
CONSIDER	• Allergic respiratory conditions.
	• Urethral blockage.
	• Painful urinary tract disease.
POTENCY	2X – 6X – 12X.

Spig
SPIGELIA ANTHELMIA
Pinkroot Plant

Heart disease. Angry and confused. Fear approach, injections, and touch. Oversensitive, irritable, and suspicious. Sad.

HEAD	Neuralgia. Photophobia. Dilated pupils.
GASTROINTESTINAL	Painful fissure on tongue. Halitosis. PD. PU.
CARDIOVASCULAR	Arrhythmia. Violent palpitation. Dyspnoea.
MODALITIES	Agg: motion. Noise. Touch. Turning. Washing.
	Amel: lying on right. Holding head high.
COMPARE	*Spigelia marylandica* Spig-m. Mania. Vertigo.
	Acon Arn Cact Cimic Cina Naja Sabad Spong Teucr.
CONSIDER	• Painful cardiac disease.
POTENCY	6X – 12X.

Spong
SPONGIA TOSTA
Roasted sponge Animal

Great exercise intolerance. Anxiety after midnight and during sleep. Concentrate poorly. Dull, timid, and sad. Startle easily. Irrational, inconsolable fears.

HEAD	Epiphora: mucous to watery, tenacious.
GASTROINTESTINAL	PD / PU. Hiccough. Great hunger. Tongue: brown, dry, vesicles.
CARDIOVASCULAR	Thyroid enlarged. Heart failure. Right sided hypertrophy. Palpitation after midnight.
RESPIRATORY	Dyspnoea: asthma and tracheitis: cough: harsh, suffocating, expectorant: dry to profuse, mucous.
UROGENITAL	Epididymitis and Orchitis.
SKIN	Lymphadenitis with oedema and pruritis.

MODALITIES	Agg: after sleep. Climbing.
	Amel: hold head down.
COMPARE	Acon Brom Iod Lach Merc-i-r.
CONSIDER	• Right sided heart failure with tracheitis.
POTENCY	2X – 8X.

Stann

STANNUM METALLICUM

Tin Mineral

Dull, sad, and suspicious. Irritable, and fears of crowds, men, agg: pregnancy means they may become angry and violent. **Great debility.**

GASTROINTESTINAL	Painful abdomen responds to pressure.
RESPIRATORY	Bronchitis, COPD, emphysema, pneumonia: dyspnoea. Cough: dry, painful, exudate: greenish, mucopurulent, tenacious.
UROGENITAL	Metritis.
LAMENESS	Front legs: spasmodic trembling of large muscles. Bursitis: digits, hock.
MODALITIES	Agg: lying on right. Amel: coughing. Firm pressure.
COMPARE	Bac Calc Caust Helon Sil Tub.
CONSIDER	• Any chronic respiratory condition with a profuse mucopurulent exudate.
POTENCY	12X. 30CH.

Staphyloc

STAPHYLOCOCCINUM

Bacteria of *Staphylococci spp* Animal

HEAD	Chronic bacterial conjunctivitis. Photophobia. Meibomian cysts.
CARDIOVASCULAR	Immune mediated thyroiditis. Chronic hepatitis. Endocarditis.
LAMENESS	Septic arthritis. Neonatal infections.
SKIN	Acute, chronic, allergic, immune mediated problems. Pedal dermatitis. Lupus. Pyoderma.
COMPARE	Echi Eleuth Streptoc.
CONSIDER	• Bull terrier dermatitis.
	• Allergic and bacterial skin infections.
	• Lupus and other immune mediated conditions.
	• Mastitis: individual and herd health.
POTENCY	12X. 30CH.

Stict

STICTA PULMONARIA

Lungwort Plant

Restless and nervous, they may become hysterical.
Acute viral infections with mucous exudates.

| HEAD | Conjunctivitis, rhinitis, sinusitis: atrophic, chronic. |

GASTROINTESTINAL	PD / PU. Diarrhoea: frothy, morning, profuse.
RESPIRATORY	Laryngitis, tracheitis: cough: hacking, nocturnal.
LAMENESS	Bursitis and muscle pains: neck, with, right shoulder.
MODALITIES	Agg: light, noise, and sudden temperature changes.
COMPARE	Dros Rumx Samb.
CONSIDER	• Viral infections with mucous exudate and joint pain.
POTENCY	2X – 6X – 12X.

Streptoc
STREPTOCOCCINUM
Mixed *Streptococcal spp* Animal

A direct application in any condition associated with these bacteria. Exudates are chronic and purulent. Autoimmune conditions.

HEAD	Meningitis. Conjunctivitis.
GASTROINTESTINAL	Liver abscess. Hepatitis.
	Neonatal omphalophlebitis.
CARDIOVASCULAR	Endocarditis. Lymphadenitis. Strangles.
UROGENITAL	Cystitis, nephritis. Mastitis.
LAMENESS	Traumatic and iatrogenic septic arthritis.
SKIN	Allergic and bacterial dermatitis. Immune mediated.
COMPARE	Echi Eleuth Staphyloc.
CONSIDER	• Arthritis that is septic.
	• Mastitis.
	• Strangles.
POTENCY	12X for treatment. 30CH for prophylaxis.

Stront
STRONTIUM METALLICUM
Strontium Mineral

Postoperative haemorrhage control. Lameness. Restless. Insomnia.
Oedema of extremities.

HEAD	Otitis externa: chronic, crusty, pruritic
GASTROINTESTINAL	Anorexia. Oesophageal stenosis.
	Diarrhoea: chronic, painful, morning.
LAMENESS	Bursitis: chronic, hock, femur, right shoulder, sacroiliac.
SKIN	Dermatitis: chronic, moist, pruritus.
MODALITIES	Agg: cold. Start of exercise. Weather changes to damp.
	Amel: heat.
COMPARE	Arn Bar-c Carb-v Dulc Ruta Sil.
CONSIDER	• Chronic lameness aggravated by weather changes.
	• Postoperative haemorrhage and shock.
POTENCY	12X. 30CH.

Stroph-h
STROPHANTHUS HISPIDUS

Kombe seed Plant

CARDIOVASCULAR	Arrhythmia with a fast pulse. Mitral valve insufficiency. Heart muscle weak: oedema, pain.
RESPIRATORY	Asthma: oedema, pulmonary congestion. Oedema.
UROGENITAL	PD / PU. Albuminuria.
SKIN	Chronic urticaria.
COMPARE	Other *Strophanthus spp*. Acid-phos Dig.
CONSIDER	• Heart disease with oedema.
POTENCY	2X – 6X.

Strop-s

STROPHANTHUS SARMENTOSUS

Arrow poison *Apocyanaceae sp* Plant

CARDIOVASCULAR	Anxiety and irrational fears.
	Acute, chronic heart disease. Prolonged P-R interval. Ventricular failure. Violent palpitation.
UROGENITAL	Cystitis. Pale urine smells of horse or fruit. Pale.
LAMENESS	Arthritis. Myositis.
MODALITIES	Agg: excitement. Exercise. Standing.
	Amel: lying down. Rest.
COMPARE	Other *Strophanthus spp*. Acid-sarc Acon Bry Kali-c Lach.
CONSIDER	• Severe heart disease.
POTENCY	4X – 6X – 12X.

Sulfa

SULFANILAMIDUM

Antibiotic sulphanilamide Mineral

Apathy, confused with poor concentration. Mood swings from being happy to sad. Left sided. Heart, skin, and nerves.

CNS	Chronic encephalopathy.
	Muscle atrophy: begins at extremities, bilateral, progressive.
HEAD	Chemosis, conjunctivitis. Eyelids: yellow pustules. Hordeolum. Cloudy lens. Optic neuritis. Retinal haemorrhage.
	Atrophy auditory nerve.
	Papules, pustules on pinnae and nostrils.
ABDOMEN	Diabetes mellitus. Enlarged painful liver.
GASTROINTESTINAL	Anorexia. Cyanosis. Gastric ulcer. Vomit.
CARDIOVASCULAR	Arrhythmia. Agranulocytosis, aplastic and haemolytic anaemia, leukaemia, leukopenia. Asthma.
UROGENITAL	Cystitis, nephritis. Anuria, calculi, haematuria, porphyrins.
	Paralysis with slow passing of urine.
	Male infertility: weak spermatogenesis.
LAMENESS	Polyarthritis. Painful stiffness of sacroiliac.
SKIN	Burns, sunburn, and photosensitization.
	Dermatitis with papules. Pityriasis. Psoriasis. Vesicles.

MODALITIES	Agg: exudates. Hot treatments.
COMPARE	Ars Cic Kres Sulfonam.
CONSIDER	<ul><li>Anaemia and leukaemia.</li><li>Cancer of blood and lymphoid.</li><li>Heart weakness with arrhythmia.</li><li>Poor spermatogenesis with anaemia.</li><li>Chronic, progressive nephritis.</li></ul>
POTENCY	12X. 30CH. 200CH.

Sulfon

SULFONALUM

Derivative from coal tar Mineral

CNS	Ataxia, chorea, paralysis, vertigo. Apathy and confusion. Irritable with mood swings.
	Bloodshot eyes. Ptosis.
RESPIRATORY	Pulmonary congestion. Dyspnoea.
UROGENITAL	Cystitis, nephritis: albuminuria, bile pigment, blood, casts, tenesmus.
LAMENESS	Ataxia with loss of reflexes and twitching.
SKIN	Erythema, purpura, pruritus.
CONSIDER	<ul><li>Viral ataxia.</li></ul>
POTENCY	4X – 12X. 30CH.

Sulfonam

SULFONAMIDUM

Antibiotic sulphonamide Mineral

Polyneuritis with behavioural changes. Aggressive and averse to company, movement, work. Disobedient. Sad and indifferent. Oversensitive to noise. PD / PU. Left sided.

HEAD	Conjunctivitis with heavy eyelids and pustules.
	Night blindness.
	Otitis externa: painless, purulent pustules.
GASTROINTESTINAL	Hungry. Dry mouth. Tongue: red spots on the side.
	Painfully enlarged liver. Jaundice. Vomit.
	Faeces: soft, yellow, forced in a jet.
CARDIOVASCULAR	Tachycardia. Haemolytic, hypochromic anaemia from poor nutrition. Parotid salivary gland lithiasis.
UROGENITAL	Cystitis. Urethritis. Acrid, cloudy, concentrated, haematuria. Enuresis.
	Female genital pruritus. Mucous, white metritis.
LAMENESS	Muscles painfully stiff.
SKIN	Acne-like exfoliation. Folliculitis. Papules. Pruritus. Chronic, benign, hereditary pemphigus. Vesicles.
	Early morning urticaria.
MODALITIES	Agg: exertion. Evening.
	Amel: pressure. Rest.
COMPARE	Eup-p Nat-m Sulfa Tub.
CONSIDER	<ul><li>Behaviour modification.</li><li>Lithiasis of parotid salivary gland.</li><li>Pemphigus.</li></ul>

| POTENCY | 30CH. 200CH. |

Sulph-i
SULPHUR IODATUM
Sulphur iodide Mineral

HEAD	Parotid lymphadenitis.
GASTROINTESTINAL	Thickened tongue. Tonsils: enlarged, red.
UROGENITAL	Hard mammary cancer.
SKIN	Lupus: papules and pruritus.
	Ear, nose, urethral meatus.
COMPARE	Sulph.
CONSIDER	• Chronic offensive and resistant dermatitis.
	• Lupus.
	• Pododermatitis.
POTENCY	12X. 30CH.

Sulph
SULPHUR LOTUM
Sublimate of sulfur Mineral

Polycrest. Animals that respond to sulphur can be wholesome fun and cheerful until ill when always irritable, depressed, thin, and weak, even with good appetite.

When anxious they are confused in mornings, dull, hurried impatient and restless: at night. Oversensitive. Timid. Work: averse to. Epilepsy, Particular affinity for skin. When carefully selected remedies cannot act, especially in acute diseases, rouses the reactionary powers of the organism. Significant antibacterial agent.

HEAD	Conjunctivitis: acute, chronic. Cornea: acute ulceration. Eyelids: ulcers on margins
ABDOMEN	Liver: enlarged, pain.
GASTROINTESTINAL	Anorexia is excessive. Eructation: putrid. Lip dry, bright red, burning. PD.
	Colic after drinking: gastric, duodenal ulcers.
	Constipation: frequent, hard.
	Rectal prolapse, pruritus, red.
RESPIRATORY	Dyspnoea: nocturnal, pain, rales.
	Exudative cough: green, morning, purulent, soft, sweet.
UROGENITAL	Cystitis: colourless, enuresis, frequent, mucous, purulent.
	Metritis: acrid, pruritus. Nipples cracked, pruritus.
LAMENESS	Left shoulder and wither pain.
SKIN	Unhealthy. Dry, excoriated in folds, infected, pimples, scaly.
MODALITIES	Agg: damp. Eleven am. Rest. Scratching. Spring. Washing.
	Amel: dry, warm weather.
CONSIDER	Significant actions include;
	• Behaviour poor when ill
	• Dermatitis
	• Stimulate unresponsive healing
COMPARE	Acon Aloe Calc Lyc Puls Psor Sep.
POTENCY	12X. 30CH.

Symph
SYMPHYTUM OFFICINALE
Comfrey Bone knit Plant

HEAD	PU / PD with great weight loss. Diabetes mellitus. High SG.
GASTROINTESTINAL	Gastric and duodenal ulcers with pruritus of rectum.
UROGENITAL	Oedema of prepuce.
LAMENESS	Non-union of fractures. Penetrating wounds to periosteum. Periarticular exostoses. Ringbone. Painful, chronic, calcification, ligaments, tendons.
COMPARE	Arn Calc-fl Calc-p Ruta.
CONSIDER	<ul><li>Eye injuries.</li><li>Gastric ulcers.</li><li>Injury to bone, ligaments, periosteum, and tendons: Acute, chronic.</li></ul>
POTENCY	2X – 6X – 12X.

Syph
SYPHILINUM
Nosode of syphilis Animal

Miasm. An important miasmic remedy with a role in chronic and destructive conditions. Emaciation
may be great. Despair. Dull. Fear: dark. Memory: poor. Significant antibacterial agent.

HEAD	Eye: cornea: chronic lymphoid inflammation, lachrymation: profuse, ulcer. Eyelid: painfully swollen at night.
GASTROINTESTINAL	Salivation excessive. Teeth decay at gum edges. Tongue: coated, cracked, indent of teeth. Ulcers: painful. Rectal fissure.
RESPIRATORY	Dyspnoea of asthma. Cough: dry, hard, nocturnal. Laryngitis is painful on palpation.
UROGENITAL	Female genitalia: pruritic, ulcers. Ovaritis. Metritis: acrid, profuse, watery.
LAMENESS	Contracted muscles of sacroiliac region, back and shoulders. Pain is nocturnal
SKIN	Dermatitis with interdigital eruption. Reddish brown eruptions. Falling hair.
MODALITIES	Agg: night, seashore, summer. Amel: day, inland, mountains, slow exercise.
COMPARE	Acid-nit Alum Aur Kali-i Merc.
CONSIDER	Its main actions are in.<ul><li>Asthma.</li><li>Eczema.</li><li>Keratitis.</li></ul>Chronicity, disgusting exudates with emaciation lead to Syph.
POTENCY	12X. 30CH. 200CH.

Syzyg
SYZYGIUM JAMBOLANUM
Jambol seeds Plant

GASTROINTESTINAL	PU / PD with great weight loss. Diabetes mellitus. High SG.
COMPARE	Ins.
CONSIDER	• Diabetes mellitus.
POTENCY	6X – 12X.

Tab
TABACUM
Nicotiana tabacum Plant

Death-like collapse with vomiting. Anxious, apprehensive, dull, and sad.
Fear being alone and travelling on water.

CNS	Great vomiting and collapse of travel sickness.
HEAD	Blindness: atrophy of optic nerve.
GASTROINTESTINAL	Pharyngitis with a morning cough.
CARDIOVASCULAR	Arrhythmic and weak.
JUVENILE	Collapse with diarrhoea, vomiting of parvovirus infection.
MODALITIES	Agg: rhythmic movement.
	Amel: lying flat out. Uncovering.
COMPARE	Ars Camph Verat.
CONSIDER	• Diarrhoea of the most severe kind.
	• Parvovirus.
	• Seasickness: treatment and prevention.
POTENCY	12X for prevention of travel sickness.
	30CH for treatment of Diarrhoea.

Tama-g
TAMARIX GALLICA
Tamarisk Plant

CARDIOVASCULAR	Anaemia: to stimulate erythrocyte and platelet production. Bruise: easily.
COMPARE	Bapt Calc-p Chin Ferr Kali-ars Nat-m.
CONSIDER	• Anaemia from parasitism.
POTENCY	2X – 6X.

Tarax
TARAXICUM OFFICINALE
Dandelion Plant

GASTROINTESTINAL	Painfully swollen hepatitis. Tympanitic colic.
MODALITIES	Agg: lying down. Rest. Sitting.
	Amel: touch.
COMPARE	Bry Hydrc Nux-v.
CONSIDER	• Hepatitis.
POTENCY	2X – 6X.

Tarent-c

229

TARENTULA CUBENSIS
Cuban spider Animal

LAMENESS	Pain over lumbar area. Great restlessness.
SKIN	Painful abscess and necrosis, sepsis, toxaemia.
MODALITIES	Agg: night.
COMPARE	Ars Anthr Apis Bell Crot Echi Tarent.
CONSIDER	• Painful sepsis.
POTENCY	6X. 30CH.

Tarent-h

TARENTULA HISPANICA
Spanish spider Animal

Extremely restless nervous system with chorea and hysterical epilepsy. Disobedient, destructive, and violent. Hurried, restless and odd movements include dancing to music. OCD: box walking.

UROGENITAL	Oversexed. Ovaritis: genital pruritus.
LAMENESS	The most severe jerking and twitching.
MODALITIES	Agg: contact. Movement. Noise.
	Amel: soft music. Flashing lights. Massage. Open air.
COMPARE	Agar Ars Cupr Mag-p Tarent-c.
CONSIDER	• Box walking and weaving.
	• Chorea.
POTENCY	6X. 30CH. 200CH.

Tell

TELLURIUM METALLICUM
Tellurium Mineral

HEAD	Conjunctivitis: purulent. Entropion, eczema.
	Otitis externa: chronic, purulent, lesions behind ear.
ABDOMEN	Hepatitis.
LAMENESS	Severe right sided pain over lower back and sacroiliac.
	Painfully contracted, stiff joints.
SKIN	Dermatitis of small flea-bite-like pimples.
	Lupus erythematosus. Ringworm. Urticaria with vesicles.
COMPETITION	Older, stiff backed show jumpers.
COMPARE	Ars Alum Caps Psor Sec.
CONSIDER	• Lupus.
	• Spondylitis.
POTENCY	12X. 30CH.

Ter

TEREBINTHINIAE OLEUM
Turpentine Mineral

A widespread action, but notable for its association with bleeding mucous surfaces. Significant antibacterial agent.

HEAD	Intensely painful right eye.
ABDOMEN	Pelvic peritonitis.
GASTROINTESTINAL	Dry tongue with prominent papillae.

	Colic: tympanitic, severe. Vomiting.
	Dysentery. Helminthiasis.
CARDIOVASCULAR	Rapid, weak pulse.
RESPIRATORY	Dyspnoea with haemoptysis.
UROGENITAL	Secondary nephritis. Urine: scant, smells of violets. Tenesmus.
	Puerperal metritis, peritonitis.
	Male urethritis: painful erections.
LAMENESS	Back pain referred from kidney.
SKIN	Erythematous eruptions are pustular, vesicular, and pruritic.
COMPARE	Acid-nit Alumn Sec Canth.
CONSIDER	• Colic with severe tympany.
	• Nephritis with great pain.
POTENCY	2X – 8X.

Teucr
TEUCRIUM MARUM VERUM
Cat-thyme Plant

HEAD	Excitable, oversensitive. Conjunctivitis with swollen eyelids. Tarsal tumour.
	Rhinitis: blocked, crusty, hard, mucous. Offensive. Polyps.
GASTROINTESTINAL	Halitosis. Hiccough. Vomit.
	Evening anal pruritus: helminths.
RESPIRATORY	Dry cough with profuse expectoration.
LAMENESS	Arthritis of digits. Seedy toe, white-line disease.
SKIN	Dry, pruritic dermatitis.
COMPARE	Cina Ign Sang Sil.
CONSIDER	• Feline, chronic upper respiratory disease.
	• Hoof problems.
POTENCY	2X – 8X – 12X.

Thala
THALAMUS
Thalamic nosode Animal

GASTROINTESTINAL	Dull, best when alone. Painful hepatitis and pancreatitis.
UROGENITAL	Poor libido.
LAMENESS	Neuralgia of shoulder and spine. Spondylitis. Weak hooves.
MODALITIES	Agg: cold. Heat.
	Amel: exercise outdoors.
POTENCY	30CH.

Thal
THALLIUM metallicum aut aceticum
Thallium acetate Mineral

Acts on endocrine glands, adrenals, and thyroid. Hyperthyroidism. Hepatitis. Emaciation with great weakness. Anxious and irrational. Right.

231

HEAD	Purulent conjunctivitis and iritis.
CARDIOVASCULAR	Parasitic anaemia. Capillary fragility. Fast weak pulse. Cyanosis.
RESPIRATORY	Dyspnoea. COPD. Emphysema. Pleurisy.
UROGENITAL	Acute glomerulonephritis. Urine: casts, dysuria, haematuria, involuntary, pain, proteinuria.
LAMENESS	Arthritis and spondylitis of large joints. Paralytic trembling and weakness. Chronic painful myositis.
SKIN	Alopecia. Dry. Pigmented. Pododermatitis. Weak hooves.
MODALITIES	Agg: night. Palpation. Amel: exercise.
COMPARE	Aran Arg-n, Caust Cedr Lath Plb.
CONSIDER	• Adjunct in Babesiosis. • Metabolic disorders. • Myositis.
POTENCY	12X. 30CH.

Thiopen
THIOPENTONUM
Sodium thiopental Mineral

The reversal of specific anaesthetic overdose and destructive, iatrogenic phlebitis.

COMPARE	Lach Vip.
POTENCY	30CH.

Thiop
THIOPROPERAZINUM
Majeptil Mineral

Behavioural and neurological problems. Awkward and fearful at night with morning anxiety on awakening. Confused. Desire to be alone but need company in evenings. Restless and nervous they experience severe and dramatic mood swings. Often right sided. Hypothyroidism.

CNS	Chorea. Epilepsy. Hypertonia. Opisthotonos. Torticollis. Vertigo.
HEAD	Choroiditis. Dacryocystitis. Pruritus of ear and deafness. Rhinitis, sinusitis: acute, chronic, crusts, dry, mucopurulent. Frequent nocturnal sneezing.
GASTROINTESTINAL	Voracious hunger, but morning anorexia. Bloody Gingivitis, stomatitis. Vomit. Tympanitic colic. IBD. Rectum: painful fissures. Constipation: hard, nocturnal. Megacolon. Faeces: pasty, not sticky, smell of rancid oil.
CARDIOVASCULAR	Arrhythmia. Bradycardia. Incomplete right heart block. Ventricular and supraventricular extrasystoles.
RESPIRATORY	Dyspnoea. Chronic laryngitis, bronchopneumonia. Abscess. Dry.
UROGENITAL	Oliguria. Poor libido.

LAMENESS	Left sided arthritis and spondylitis.
SKIN	Folliculitis. Lupus. Photosensitization. Pigmentation. seborrhoea. Spots on face lips and nose.
MODALITIES	Agg: afternoon. Evening. At rest. Bending backwards. Stimulation.
	Amel: car travel. Heat treatment.
COMPARE	Aqua-m Ars Chlorp Halo Kres Levo Nat-m Sep Tub.
CONSIDER	• Anal fissures.
	• Behaviour modification.
	• Heart disease.
	• IBD.
	The great weariness and depression are important. Mood swings.
POTENCY	12X. 30CH.

Thiosin

THIOSINAMINUM

Oil of mustard seed Plant

HEAD	Corneal opacity, scarring and ectropion.
LAMENESS	The rehabilitation of strained tendons and ligaments.
COMPETITION	May prolong usefulness where chronic thickening of any tendon or ligament reduces function.
SKIN	**Adhesions and scarring.**
COMPARE	Caust Graph Ruta.
CONSIDER	Essential:
	• Adhesions in tendon sheaths.
	• Chronic ligament, tendon strains.
	• Scar tissue resolution.
POTENCY	2X – 4X.

Thlas

THLASPI BURSA PASTORIS

Shepherd's purse Plant

HEAD	Haemorrhage during nasal surgery. Vertigo on rising.
UROGENITAL	Cystitis, urethritis: blood, calculi, chronic, sediment with severe colic.
	Painful spermatic cord and testes.
	Pain during work referred during work.
COMPARE	Clem Croc Mill Trill Urt-u.
CONSIDER	• Cystitis with blocked urethra.
	• Colts that trap testicle during work.
	• Ethmoid hematoma.
POTENCY	4X – 12X.

Thuj

THUJA OCCIDENTALIS

***Arbor vitae* The tree of life Plant**

Polycrest. Angry, anxious, confused, dull, excitable, fears: approach, strangers. Hurried, irritable, obstinate, sad. Vaccinosis. Action on the skin particularly warts and soft tumours. Has antibacterial and immune modulation properties. Significant antibacterial agent.

HEAD	Conjunctivitis: eyelids agglutinated. Iritis, tarsal tumours.
	Otitis: externa and media: chronic, purulent.
	Nose: bloody, chronic, green, mucous, purulent, ulceration.
GASTROINTESTINAL	Anorexia. Dental decay. Ranula. Tongue has painful blisters.
	Colic with Diarrhoea and tympany.
	Rectal fissures. Warts. Constipation: violent tenesmus.
RESPIRATORY	Asthma, laryngitis: juveniles: cough: afternoon, dry, dyspnoea.
UROGENITAL	Urethritis. Metritis; greenish, profuse, thick. Ovaritis: left, severe pain.
	Inflammation of prepuce and glans. Orchitis: chronic, indurate. Prostatomegaly.
LAMENESS	Achilles tendonitis with hock pain. Myositis: twitching, trembling, weakness. Hoof: brittle, distorted, shoe-slip, soft.
COMPETITION	Vaccinosis in athletes is a severe problem.
SKIN	Dirty, greasy, unhealthy. Dandruff, dry, hair falls, scaly, wart, white.
GERIATRIC	Improves elderly small dogs with obesity. Small skin cysts and tumours
MODALITIES	Agg: after breakfast. Cold, damp air. Music. Night. 3a.m. and 3p.m. Vaccination.
COMPARE	Ars Nat-m Nat-s Sabin Sil Vac.
CONSIDER	• Detoxification.
	• Hoof and nail conditioner.
	• Metabolic disorders.
	• Skin cancer and warts.
	• Vaccination reactions.
POTENCY	12X. 30CH. 200CH.

Thymol
THYMOLUM
Thyme-camphor Plant

GASTROINTESTINAL	Helminthiasis with irritability and weakness.
UROGENITAL	PU. Cystitis: acrid, urates.
	Priapism. Prostatitis.
COMPARE	*Carbon tetrachloride* Carbn-t. Hookworm.
CONSIDER	• Helminthiasis and male sex problems.
POTENCY	6X – 12X.

Thyr
THYROIDINUM
Nosode of Ovine thyroid gland Animal

Hyper and hypothyroidism. Thyroiditis. Epilepsy. Aggression in males that does not respond to castration. Sad. Stupor alternates with restlessness and then irritability leads to rage.

GASTROINTESTINAL	Pharyngitis left side: congested, dry, raw. Tympanitic colic.
CARDIOVASCULAR	Exercise intolerance.
	Tachycardia with palpitation. Dry cough.
UROGENITAL	PU. Albuminuria. Glycosuria. Neonatal Monorchidism.
LAMENESS	Arthritis with cold extremities. Obese.
	Distal oedema.
SKIN	Pruritic dermatitis is dry and widespread.
COMPARE	Calc Fuc Lyc Spong.
CONSIDER	• Behavioural problems.
	• Dermatitis.
	• Glandular weakness.
	• Metabolic disorders.
	• Monorchidism.
	• Obesity.
	• Thyroid imbalance.
POTENCY	2X – 6X – 12X. 30CH.

Trib
TRIBULUS TERRESTRIS
Ikshugandha Plant

An underutilised remedy with widespread actions in male sexuality, arthritis, and pain control. Anxiety and restlessness. Urinary gravel in small ruminants.

LAMENESS	Joint: arthritis and bursitis.
	Anabolic, general athletic support.
CARDIOVASCULAR	Blood pressure, vessel, and cardiac support.
UROGENITAL	Tonic for athletes on high protein diets.
	Male: improved sexual health and performance.
COMPARE	Eleuth Gins Rhod.
CONSIDER	• Athletic support.
POTENCY	2X – 4X.

Trif-p
TRIFOLIUM PRATENSE
Red clover Plant

HEAD	Rhinitis, sinusitis: allergic: exudate: mucous, profuse, watery. Pharyngitis: harsh cough.
LAMENESS	Painfully stiff neck.
SKIN	Dry, crusty dermatitis.
COMPARE	*Trifolium erectens* Trif-e. White clover. Salivation. Swollen glands. Merc Syph.
CONSIDER	• Acute oral and nasal exudates.
POTENCY	2X – 4X.

Tril
TRILLIUM PENDULUM
White beth root Plant

235

HEAD	Arterial gum, nasal haemorrhage after exercise.
RESPIRATORY	Laryngitis. EIPH. Expectoration: bloody, copious purulent.
UROGENITAL	Fibroids. Threatened foetal loss.
	Severe arterial postpartum haemorrhage. Metritis: bloody, copious, stringy, yellow. Prolapse.
LAMENESS	EIPH if associated with URT disease. Combine with Cinnm and Mill.
COMPARE	Cinnm Fic Ham Ip Lach Mill Sab.
CONSIDER	• EIPH.
	• Postpartum haemorrhage.
POTENCY	2X – 6X. 30CH.

Tnt
TRINITROTOLUENUM
Trinitrotoluene Mineral

CNS	Coma fits and vertigo. Averse to company. Sad.
GASTROINTESTINAL	Jaundice. Vomit. Constipation followed by Diarrhoea.
CARDIOVASCULAR	Severe, degenerative anaemia. Arrhythmia. Palpitation. Tachycardia.
RESPIRATORY	Dry, paroxysmal cough.
UROGENITAL	Mild cystitis with dark urine.
SKIN	Pruritus: subcutaneous haemorrhage, oedema.
COMPARE	Ars Cina Phos Plb Zinc.
CONSIDER	• Degenerative anaemia: Babesiosis.
POTENCY	12X. 30CH.

Tritic
TRITICUM REPENS
Couch grass Plant

UROGENITAL	Cystitis, nephritis, pyelitis: acute, chronic. Urine: acrid, crystals, dysuria, incontinent, mucopurulent, tenesmus. Frequent snorting.
COMPARE	Chim Pop Sen Uva.
CONSIDER	• Cystitis.
POTENCY	4X – 10X.

Tub
TUBERCULINUM bovinum kent
Tubercular abscess Nosode *Animal*

Miasm. Evening anxiety in juveniles.

Dull. Fears: animals, dogs, irrational. Irritable. Careless, offended easily, they often injure themselves.

Wander: tend to. Work: averse to with severe fatigue from movement.

Signs constantly change, and often employed as an adjuvant when well selected remedies cannot improve a condition. Illness from the slightest exposure.

Rapid emaciation. Extreme wasting. Significant antibacterial agent.

CNS	Meningitis.
HEAD	Otitis media, externa: chronic, offensive.

GASTROINTESTINAL	Tonsillitis, diarrhoea: chronic, juveniles.
RESPIRATORY	Bronchopneumonia: cough: dry, hard, juveniles, nocturnal.
UROGENITAL	Cystitis, nephritis: chronic. Benign mammary tumours.
SKIN	Dermatitis: chronic, severely pruritic.
JUVENILE	Diarrhoea: chronic, juveniles, offensive, purulent. Respiratory disease.
MODALITIES	Agg: early morning. Movement. Music. Sleep. Before storms.
	Amel: open air.
MIASM	One of the five miasms with special roles:
	• Grief.
	• Tissue destruction with pus and then fibrosis.
COMPARE	*Tuberculinum avis* Tub-a Avian TB. Post viral bronchopneumonia. Bry Calc Chin.
CONSIDER	Important in juvenile situations:
	• Bronchitis and pneumonia.
	• Tonsillitis.
	Always fatigue and weight loss.
POTENCY	30CH. 200CH.

Dam
TURNERA APHRODISIACA
Damiana Plant

UROGENITAL	Incontinence. Prostatomegaly. Geriatrics. Oestrous delayed in juveniles.
COMPARE	Con
CONSIDER	• Urinary debility in geriatrics
	• Delayed puberty in juvenile females.
POTENCY	2X – 6X.

Uran-n
URANIUM NITRICUM
Uranium nitrate Mineral

Polycrest. Emaciation. Ascites. Dry skin. Angry and sad.

HEAD	Conjunctivitis with agglutinated lids.
ABDOMEN	Diabetes mellitus. Hepatitis.
GASTROINTESTINAL	Ravenous appetite with gastric ulcers.
	PD, and vomiting.
	Colic: tympanitic: flatus.
UROGENITAL	Diuresis, glycosuria, incontinence, PU.
COMPARE	Acid-lact. Acid-phos. Arg-n. Ars. Kali-bi. Lyc. Phos. Uran. Syzyg.
CONSIDER	PU with severe tympanitic.
	• Diabetes mellitus.
	• Flatulence.
	• Gastric ulceration.
	• Metabolic disorders.
POTENCY	8X – 12X.

Urt-u
URTICA URENS
Stinging nettle Plant

Agalactia, lithiasis and urticaria with restlessness.

UROGENITAL	FLUTD. Agalactia and inappropriate lactation. Mammary oedema. Metritis is acrid. Uterine haemorrhage.
	Scrotal eczema.
BREEDING	Encourage milking with low potency.
	Dry off with high potency.
MODALITIES	Agg: chilly air. Water. Touch.
CONSIDER	• Improve lactation with 2X – 4X. Works well with Alf.
	• Dry-off milk with 200CH.
	• Urticaria with 30CH to 200CH.

Ust
USTILAGO MAYDIS
Corn smut Plant

HEAD	Depressed, oversexed males with excessive lachrymation.
UROGENITAL	Postpartum arterial haemorrhage. Metritis: bloody, clotted, stringy.
SKIN	Alopecia. Copper coloured spots. Dry. Pruritus. Pimples. Sunburn.
MODALITIES	Agg: movement. Touch.
	Amel: rest.
COMPARE	Sab Sec Viol-t.
CONSIDER	• Oversexed males.
	• Postpartum haemorrhage.
POTENCY	2X – 6X.

Uva
UVA URSI
Bearberry Plant

Cystitis, pyelitis and urethritis. Urine is bloody, calculi, clotted, mucopurulent and slimy. Tenesmus. Involuntary.

POTENCY	2X – 6X.

Vac
VACCININUM
Nosode from vaccine Animal

May reverse side effects from vaccination reactions. Desire carried. Impatient. Irritable. Skin cancers at the actual site of vaccination

COMPARE	Maland Thuj: combines well here. Var.
CONSIDER	• Prophylactic. Three days before and after a specific vaccination where history suggests reaction.

- Combine with specific nosode.
- Reversal of vaccination reactions.

POTENCY	30CH. 200CH.

Vacc-v
VACCINUM VITUS IDAEA
Cowberry Plant

GASTROINTESTINAL	Colic. Constipation. Diarrhoea: coliform. IBD.
UROGENITAL	Female: HRT.
COMPARE	Agn Oest Puls Sep
CONSIDER	• Diarrhoea: bacterial
	• HRT: female.
POTENCY	2X – 6X.

Valer
VALERIANA OFFICINALIS
Valerian Plant

Pre-competition relaxant but never lower than 8X, for fear of a positive swab test.
Caution, for the natural substance may cause ataxia with injury possible.
Sensitive, irritable, and nervous individuals that may become hysterical.

LAMENESS	Painful stiffness of the large muscles of lower back and hips. May jerk and twitch.
MODALITIES	Agg: dark.
	Amel: exercise outdoors.
COMPARE	Asaf Croc Ign.
CONSIDER	• Behavioural problems.
POTENCY	6X. 30CH.

Vanad
VANADIUM METALLICUM
Vanadium Mineral

Immune system modulation where anaemia and inflammation are problems. Sad. Hysteria.

HEAD	Appear to go blind. Conjunctivitis.
GASTROINTESTINAL	PD. Liver: fatty degeneration. Diabetes mellitus.
CARDIOVASCULAR	Destructive anaemia. Fatty degeneration of heart.
RESPIRATORY	Paroxysmal dry cough with a bloody exudate.
UROGENITAL	PU. Cystitis, nephritis: albuminuria, casts, glycosuria.
COMPARE	Ars Phos.
CONSIDER	Severely debilitating conditions:
	• Anaemia.
	• Metabolic disorders.
	• Widespread inflammation.
POTENCY	12X. 30CH.

Variol
VARIOLINUM
Nosode of smallpox Animal

HEAD	Swollen eyelids. Conjunctivitis.
RESPIRATORY	Cough: exudate: bloody, mucous, viscid.
LAMENESS	Painful stiffness of large joints and muscles.
SKIN	Dry, hot pustules.
COMPARE	Apis combines well. Thuj Vac.
CONSIDER	• Vaccination reactions
POTENCY	30CH. 200CH.

Verat
VERATRUM ALBUM
White hellebore Plant

Polycrest. Foolish actions during episodes of hysterical rage with violence.
Sad, vocal Collapse with extreme coldness, cyanosis, and weakness.
Postoperative shock with a rapid, feeble pulse.
The profuse, violent retching and vomiting is most characteristic.
Excessive dryness of mucous membranes.

GASTROINTESTINAL	**Appetite** is voracious. Coprophagia. PD/PU: thirst for chilly water but vomited as soon as swallowed. Tympanitic colic.
	Diarrhoea is copious, watery, and evacuated forcefully. There is fear, pain, and prostration.
	Constipation: neonates with retained meconium, particularly if associated with wintry weather. Faeces: large: strain until exhausted. Cold sweat.
CARDIOVASCULAR	**Palpitation:** anxiety, rapid audible respiration.
	Pulse: feeble, irregular.
RESPIRATORY	**Bronchitis:** chronic, geriatric, mucous, rales. Cough on coming inside from chilly air.
UROGENITAL	Puerperal mania. Both sexes are oversexed.
LAMENESS	Large muscles of lower back and shoulder are painfully stiff.
JUVENILE	Severe constipation and diarrhoea with collapse.
MODALITIES	Agg: cold wet weather. Night.
	Amel: exercise and warmth.
COMPARE	Acon Bapt Bell Ferr-p Gels.
CONSIDER	Can save lives in:
	• Behavioural problems at parturition: 'Gilt fear syndrome.'
	• Death imminent with cyanosis, prostration, and shock.
	• Heart stimulant.
POTENCY	2X – 12X. 30CH. 200CH.

Verat-v
VERATRUM VIRIDE
American hellebore Plant

Anxious, irritable, suspicious, and aggressive when ill. Significant antibacterial agent.
Fits and delirium from meningitis and sunstroke. Heart disease.

HEAD	Facial chorea. Bloodshot eye. Pupils dilated.
GASTROINTESTINAL	Hiccough. Hypersalivation. PD.

	Tongue: red streak, yellow to white.
	Oesophagus: constricted, spasms.
CARDIOVASCULAR	BP low. Pulse irregular, slow, weak. slow.
	Incompetent valves.
RESPIRATORY	Pneumonia, congestion: cough: harsh, paroxysmal.
UROGENITAL	Scant, cloudy urine. Rigid os.
	Postpartum sepsis.
LAMENESS	Painful stiffness of large joints and muscles.
SKIN	Pruritic eczema with fits.
MODALITIES	Agg: cold. Evening. Sun's heat. Movement.
	Amel: holding head down. Massage.
COMPARE	Acon Bapt Bell Ferr Gels.
CONSIDER	• Bacterial fevers.
	• Heart disease.
POTENCY	2X – 6X. 30CH.

Verb
VERBASCUM THAPSUS
Mullein Plant

CNS	Neuralgia: neck, painful.
HEAD	Neuralgia: jaw left. Eardrum: deaf: scales.
GASTROINTESTINAL	Colic: lower abdomen.
RESPIRATORY	Asthma: dyspnoea: cough: harsh, nocturnal.
UROGENITAL	Cystitis. Dribble constantly. Enuresis.
LAMENESS	Neuralgia of right digits.
MODALITIES	Agg: barking. Biting. Day. Sneezing. Weather changes.
COMPARE	Caust Plat Rhus-a.
CONSIDER	• Painful neuralgia.
POTENCY	4X – 12X.

Verbe-h
VERBENA HASTATA
Blue vervain Plant

Anxious, irritable, and restless. Depression. Mild relaxant. Moody.
Painful arthritis. Ovaritis.

RESPIRATORY	Bronchitis, tracheitis: cough: harsh.
UROGENITAL	Agalactia. Ovaritis.
LAMENESS	Digits: neuralgic arthritic pain.
COMPARE	Apis.
CONSIDER	• Arthritis.
	• Ovaritis.
POTENCY	12X. 30CH. 200CH.

Vesp
VESPA CRABO
European hornet Animal

Anxious, irritable, and restless. **Pain.**

HEAD	Chemosis and oedema.
UROGENITAL	Acute urethritis. Erosion of cervix. Left ovaritis.

SKIN	Acute, allergic erythema with wheals and pruritus. Bites and stings.
MODALITIES	Agg: direct heat. Amel: chilly water. Vinegar.
COMPARE	Apis.
CONSIDER	• Allergic reactions. • Ovaritis.
POTENCY	6X. 30CH. 200CH.

Vib
VIBURNUM OPULUS
High cranberry Plant

Cramping of smooth muscle. Sad restless creatures that become hysterical.

CNS	Vertigo. Fall backwards.
GASTROINTESTINAL	Colic: acute, spasmodic. Constipation: hard, large, balls.
UROGENITAL	Painful cystitis. Urinate while walking. PU: pale coloured. Threatened foetal loss in cats and mares. Infertility: ovarian insufficiency. Metritis: exudate: acrid.
LAMENESS	Stiff, painful back muscles.
MODALITIES	Agg: evenings. Night. Lying down. Warm room. Amel: firm massage. Open air. Rest.
COMPARE	*Viburnum lantana* Vib-l Viburnum Grape vine for painfully deformed arthritis of digits. DJD. *Viburnum prunifolium* Vib-p. Black haw. Habitual foetal loss. Cancer of the tongue. Uterine tonic. Caul Cimic Sep Xan.
CONSIDER	• Habitual foetal loss.
POTENCY	2X – 4X.

Vinc
VINCA MINOR
Lesser periwinkle Plant

HEAD	Sad, confused. Vertigo. One nostril blocked. Upper lip, base of nose: seborrhoea.
GASTROINTESTINAL	Diphtheria: cough: frequent, hacking.
UROGENITAL	Uterine fibroids: passive haemorrhage.
SKIN	Dermatitis: acute dermatitis: face, head: exudate: offensive, pustular, pruritic. Hair matted.
MODALITIES	Agg: anger. Walking. Amel: moving outdoors.
COMPARE	Ner Staph
CONSIDER	• Moist, offensive dermatitis.
POTENCY	4X – 8X.

Viol-o
VIOLA ODORATA
Blue violet Plant

Clever, excitable, can be hysterical. Vertigo. Right side.

HEAD	Anorexia. Otitis: deaf, painful. Sinusitis.
RESPIRATORY	Cough: dyspnoea: dry, short, spasmodic. Palpitations.
UROGENITAL	Enuresis: milky, strong, in nervous juveniles. Fibroids.
LAMENESS	Painful stiffness of joints and muscles.
	Carpal / metacarpals.
MODALITIES	Agg: cool air.
COMPARE	Apis Aur Caul Ign Puls Sep Vesp.
CONSIDER	• Insect stings and bites.
	• Right sided otitis.
POTENCY	4X – 8X.

Viol-t
VIOLA TRICOLOR
Pansy Plant

Anxiety during fever. Disobedient. Indifferent. Irritable.

UROGENITAL	PU: offensive, smells of cats. Balanoposthitis.
SKIN	Dermatitis: face, head: cracks, Juvenile, nocturnal, pruritic, purulent, tenacious.
MODALITIES	Agg: night. Winter.
COMPARE	Calc Lyc Rhus-t Sep.
CONSIDER	• Disgusting juvenile dermatitis.
POTENCY	4X – 8X.

Vip-a
VIPERA ASPIS
European adder *Vipera beris* Animal

CNS	Ascending polyneuritis with paralysis. Confused and sad.
GASTROINTESTINAL	Liver: enlarged, painful. Jaundice.
	Lips, tongue: dry, livid, protruded, swollen.
CARDIOVASCULAR	Dyspnoea. Heart failure. Larynx, extremities: oedema.
UROGENITAL	Haematuria.
LAMENESS	Muscles: distal: painful, swollen, stiff.
SKIN	Boils, pimples: peel in flakes.
MODALITIES	Agg: touch. Weather changes.
	Amel: raise affected limb.
	Bitis arietans Bit-a. Puff adder. Similar.
CONSIDER	• Phleg leg.
	• Snake bite.
POTENCY	30CH.

Visc
VISCUM ALBUM
Mistletoe Plant

Overstimulation of vagus nerve. Cancer. Sad and very dull but easily angered.

CNS	Epilepsy: mild. Face: chorea. Vertigo: persistent.
CARDIOVASCULAR	BP low. Cardiac insufficiency from valvular hypertrophy. Pulse: palpitation, weak.

LAMENESS	Neuralgia: spinal: pains may alternate from hip and hock to shoulder and elbow.
	Thighs: pruritus. Extremities: oedema.
CANCER	Cytotoxic and immune system modulating activities. Protects against drug toxicity.
	Shows great promise in cancer management.
MODALITIES	Agg: lying on left side. Movement. Cold, stormy weather.
COMPARE	Bry Cad-m Conv Hed Puls Rhod Sec.
CONSIDER	• Cancer.
	• Heart failure.
	• Neuralgia.
POTENCY	4X – 12X. 30CH. 200CH.

Agn
VITEX AGNUS CASTUS
Chaste tree Plant

Sad, indifferent creatures with poor concentration. Weak sexual function.

HEAD	Orbital dermatitis. Photophobia. Dilated pupils.
ABDOMEN	Ascites. Painfully swollen spleen.
GASTROINTESTINAL	PU yet thirstless. Mouth and gum ulcers.
UROGENITAL	Agalactia. Sterility: chronic metritis: exudate: yellow to white. Placental retention.
	Balanitis and impotence. Tonic.
COMPETITION	Tonic, particularly in the older athlete. Works well with Alf and Gins.
COMPARE	Acid-phos Alf Camp Gins Lyc Sel.
CONSIDER	• As a breeding tonic.
POTENCY	4X – 12X.

Vitis-v
VITIS VINIFERA
Grape vine Plant

On skeleton to develop healthy bone.

LAMENESS	Arthritis: digits: deformed and painful. Regulates bone metabolism. Bone cancer.
COMPETITION	Tonic, particularly in the older athlete. Works well with Alf and Gins.
COMPARE	Acid-phos Alf Arg-m Camp Gins Lyc Pin-mo Sel.
CONSIDER	• Arthritis: chronic.
	• Bone metabolism in osteoporosis of dysplasia and physis.
	• Metabolic disorders.
POTENCY	4X – 12X.

Wye
WYETHIA HELENOIDES
Poison weed Plant

GASTROINTESTINAL	Pharyngitis: follicular, nervous, sad.

	Diarrhoea: nocturnal.
RESPIRATORY	Asthma, bronchitis, laryngitis: dyspnoea: cough: dry, hacking. Epiglottis: oedema. Follicular nodes.
LAMENESS	Pain along spine and carpus.
COMPETITION	2-Y-O with follicular pharyngitis.
MODALITIES	Agg: afternoon. Exercise. Massage.
COMPARE	Arum-t Lach Sang.
CONSIDER	• Follicular pharyngitis.
POTENCY	4X – 8X.

Xan
XANTHOXYLUM FRAXINEUM
Prickly ash Plant

GASTROINTESTINAL	Mouth: dry with hypersalivation.
	Jaw: neuralgia: injury: hemiplegia.
	Pharyngitis, gastritis: from overeating.
	Dysentery.
CARDIOVASCULAR	Sluggish capillary refill time. Aphonia. Cough: constant, dry.
LAMENESS	Neuralgia: left.
POTENCY	6X – 12X.

X-RAY
X-RAYS
Energy

GASTROINTESTINAL	Anorexia. Constipation. Diarrhoea.
CARDIOVASCULAR	Anaemia. Leukaemia. Leukopenia. Thrombocytopenia
UROGENITAL	Low sperm count due to atrophy.
SKIN	Hyperkeratosis. Sarcoid. Melanoma of grey horses.
MODALITIES	Agg: cold. Movement.
	Amel: heat.
COMPARE	Cadm-s Merc Phos Sec Sol.
CONSIDER	Melanoma.
POTENCY	• 30CH.

Zinc
ZINC METALLICUM
Zinc Mineral

A disturbed nervous system with seriously reduced vitality.

CNS	Epilepsy and hydrocephalus. Roll head from side to side.
HEAD	Chorea-like twitching. Paresis.
	Conjunctivitis: medial canthus: pruritic. Ptosis. Roll eyes. Squint.
GASTROINTESTINAL	Gums: bleed, halitosis. Dentition: difficult.
	Diarrhoea: painful, neonatal: green, mucous tenesmus.
CARDIOVASCULAR	Anaemia: haemolytic, parasitism, severe.
RESPIRATORY	Asthmatic-type bronchospasm: cough: debilitating, harsh, juveniles, painful.
UROGENITAL	Ovary: left painful.

LAMENESS	Erections: violent. Orchitis: retracted: painful. Neuralgia: spinal, neck, wither to sacroiliac: extreme pain.
MODALITIES	Chorea-like twitching: fears touch. Agg: touch. Between 5 and 7pm. Amel, when eating. Production of exudate.
COMPARE	*Zinc carbonicum* Zinc-c. A direct role on enzyme systems.
CONSIDER	• Haemolytic anaemia from parasitism. • Neuritis. • Orchitis due to retracted testicle. • Weak respiratory system.
POTENCY	6X – 12X.

Zinc-val
ZINC VALERIANICUM
Valerianate of zinc metal

Ovaritis. Hysterical from pain. Severely painful neuralgia.

UROGENITAL	Painful ovulation.
LAMENESS	Neuralgia: spinal: pain. Cannot sit still.
COMPETITION	Working mares: difficult behaviour: ovarian pain.
COMPARE	Anth Kali-bi.
CONSIDER	• Severest neuralgia and ovarian pains.
POTENCY	12X. 30CH for months.

Zing
ZINGIBER OFFICINALE
Ginger Plant

HEAD	Irritating, debilitating, and severely pruritic rhinitis. Pimples. Significant antibacterial agent.
GASTROINTESTINAL	Vomiting of travel sickness. Tympanitic colic. Anus: painful during pregnancy: relaxed sphincter. Diarrhoea: food poisoning: flatulent.
RESPIRATORY	Asthma without anxiety. Cough: dry, hacking.
UROGENITAL	Cystitis, nephritis: tenesmus. Balanitis.
LAMENESS	Polyarticular weakness.
COMPARE	Calad.
CONSIDER	• Adjunct in debility. • Travel sickness.
POTENCY	2X – 6X. 30CH.

THE BOWEL NOSODES
Introduction: The Bowel Nosodes form a group of eleven homoeopathic remedies. Originally the brainchild of Dr Bach: of Flower Remedy fame, John, and Edward Paterson completed his work.

Origin: Developed from gram-negative, non-lactose fermenting bacteria found in the intestine of human patients. They studied how these gut bacteria grew along clinical pathways that led to them concluding they grew as a healing clinical response in patients with a disturbed vital force.

Different to them causing disease. An interesting case of the body recognising a need for useful bacteria and initiating steps to grow them. This rings an obvious chord with modern approach of adding helpful bacteria to feeding regimes.

The main Bowel Nosodes are.

Bacillus 7, Bacillus 10, Coccal Co, Dysentery Co, Faecalis, Gaertner Bach, Morgan Gaertner, Morgan Pure, Mutabile, Proteus and Sycotic Co.

May combine Morgan Pure, Gaertner and Bach.

Treatment: Usually given infrequently in the 6X or 30CH potency. Combine with or follow synergistic or associated remedies.

Bac 7
BACILLUS 7 BACH
Citrobacter spp. Enterobacter spp.

INTRODUCTION	Chronic mental and physical debility, often tired or lazy creatures. Premature senility.
GASTROINTESTINAL	Flatulence.
CARDIOVASCULAR	Pulse and BP low.
RESPIRATORY	Asthma. Mucous: Kali-c like.
UROGENITAL	Urine output low. Impotent: both sexes.
LAMENESS	Chronic arthritis: often fibrotic changes, stifle.
MODALITIES	Agg: cold, damp, draft, movement: initially.
	• Amel: exercise, rest, warmth: heat treatments.
RELATED	Brom Kali-c Iod.

Bac 10
BACILLUS 10 Paterson
Enterobacter spp.

INTRODUCTION	Poor appetite associated with bloody, spongy gums. Diarrhoea: mornings. Anal sac disease with pruritus.
RESPIRATORY	Cough: choking, mornings.
UROGENITAL	Urine: fishy smell.
LAMENESS	Hindquarters: left sided pain and stiffness. Stifle.
SKIN	Sarcoid: distal, flat.
RELATED	**CALC-FL.**

Dys Co
DYSENTERY CO
Salmonella spp.

INTRODUCTION	Fears: anticipatory, people, strange places.
HEAD	Facial muscles: chorea.
	Colic: flatulent. Diarrhoea: nervous.
GASTROINTESTINAL	Indigestion: chronic.
	Faeces: frequent, mucous
SKIN	Dermatitis: crust, dandruff, dry, sticky.
MODALITIES	Agg: mornings: early. Stuffy atmosphere. 3am- 6am, crowds.
RELATED	Ars-a Anac Arg-n Cadm-m Chin-ars Kalm Tub.

Gaert
GAERTNER Bach

Salmonella spp

INTRODUCTION	Impaired nutrition and malnutrition in emaciated juveniles with good appetite. Detoxification. Weaning.
BEHAVIOUR	Hypersensitive, Fear: heights.
GASTROINTESTINAL	Gastro-enteritis: chronic, IBD, helminthiasis, salivation, vomit: chronic.
SKIN	Dermatitis: face and head: pustule. Mange: infected. Otitis externa: teething.
RELATED	**ARS MERC PHOS SIL** Bac Calc-p Calc-s Kali-p Nat-p Nat-s Phyt Puls Syph Zinc-p.

Morg
MORGAN *Bach*
Morganella, Proteus and Salmonella Spp.

INTRODUCTION	Combination of Morgan Pure and Morgan Gaertner.
BEHAVIOUR	Depressed. Irritable. Restless. Company: averse to but may also show separation anxiety.
HEAD	Conjunctivitis. Dermatitis: crack, dry, hot. Nasal Exudate: clear, white, thin.
ABDOMEN	Liver pain.
GASTROINTESTINAL	Congestive states Glossitis, lip: cracked and dry. Pharyngitis, vomiting. Borborygmi: obvious. Constipation: offensive, painless. Faeces: bloody, mucous, offensive, passed easily. Perianal pruritus.
RESPIRATORY	Cough: dry. Bronchopneumonia, bronchitis, tracheitis: congestion of all mucosae.
UROGENITAL	Cystitis: tenesmus. Urine: glycosuria, offensive. Ovarian pain with irritability in mares.
LAMENESS	Arthritis: fibrous swelling. Shoulder: pain.
SKIN	Dermatitis: pruritus. Feet: cracked, dry and hot.
MODALITIES	Agg: bathing, heat.
RELATED	Graph **MED PSOR SULPH.**

Prot
PROTEUS *Bach*
Proteus spp. Edwardsiella spp.

INTRODUCTION	A strong affinity with the Muriaticums. Often acute conditions. May influence chronic diseases including epilepsy where these may be stress related.
BEHAVIOUR	Aggressive: bite and kick without warning. Irritable. Resistance. Tantrums.
GASTROINTESTINAL	Problems follow stress. Vomit: allergic, bloody. Colic: flatulent, IBD: allergic. Malena.
LAMENESS	Azoturia, cramp, muscles: twitch.
SKIN	Dermatitis: pruritus, vesicle.
MODALITIES	Agg: cold mornings, fever, night, storms, sun. Amel: eating, rest.
RELATED	**NAT-M** Am-m Apis Bar-m Con Cupr.

Syc-co
SYCOTIC CO Paterson
Acinetobacter spp. Streptococcus spp.

INTRODUCTION	Weak, anaemic, and irritable individuals. Exudates are thick, yellow.
BEHAVIOUR	Fears: being alone, dark.
CNS	Meningitis.
HEAD	Conjunctivitis: tacky and yellow. Eyelid: blinking. Photophobia, sinus: pain.
GASTROINTESTINAL	Generalised inflammation, constipation, Diarrhoea, gastritis.
RESPIRATORY	Cough: Acute, chronic: mucous, irritable at night.
UROGENITAL	Kidney pain: urine offensive.
LAMENESS	Movement is stiff and weary. Lumbar and sacroiliac pain. Shins and splints in weak individuals. Sensitive soles.
SKIN	Cysts, dermatitis: post vaccination with erythema, pustules, or vesicles. Oily, warts: on mucocutaneous structures.
MODALITIES	Agg: cold, damp, eggs, movement: initially. Night. Amel: coast, exercise, when persisted with. Heat.

ISOPATHY

Definition: Isopathy is the art of treatment by utilising material from the actual organism, or disease products, implicated in an illness. Preparations thus obtained are termed nosodes.

Cover the debate on whether homoeopathy is distinct from isopathy, in the second volume of this work.

Healers have used medicines for a long time and after proving them, earned right as remedies with the following list indicating where they earned a place in materia medica.

MAJOR NOSODES

Ambra Grisea
Anthracinum
Bacillinum
Carcinosin
Cartilago spp
Corticotrophin
Cortisone
D.N.A.
Epihysterinum
Folliculinum
Hippomanes
Hippozaeninum
Hirudin
Histaminum
Hydrophobinum
Hypophysis
Hypothalamus

Lac caninum
Malandrinum
Medorrhinum
Morbillinum Influenzinum
Oopherinum
Orchitinum spp
Pancreatinum
Parathyroidinum
Scarlatinum
Streptococcus
Thalamus
Thyreotrophic hormone
Thyroidinum
Trypsinum
Tuberculinum aviare
Tuberculinum Bovinum

Vaccininum
Variolinum

MODERN NOSODES

This list gives examples of nosodes produced directly from microbiological agents and used for disease control, either against the specific disease, or against a similar family of diseases. Thus, *Streptococcus equi* is of value in the management not only of equine strangles but also against other Streptococcal disorders.

Produce nosodes against any disease involving microbiological agents: bacteria, fungi, viruses. The following good examples are in use.

AVIAN

E. coli spp

Fowl Pest

Marek's Disease

Salmonella spp

CAPRINE

Mastitis

CANINE

Canine Distemper

Hepatitis

OVINE

Scrapie

PORCINE

Streptococci spp

Mycoplasma spp.

BOVINE

Brucella abortus

Colibacillosis

Husk: *Dictyocaulus arnfieldi* (lungworm)

Foot-rot

Mastitis

Mucosal Disease

Pasteurella spp

FELINE

Chlamydia

Coronavirus

Herpes virus

Infectious peritonitis

Leukaemia

REPERTORY

MIND

Capitalised remedies are the ones recommended as being first to consider in all diagnoses.

ABANDONED: feels	ACID-PHOS ARG-N ARS AUR CALC KALI-BI IGN LACH LIL-T PHOS PSOR PULS Anac Caps Coff Mag-m Stram Anac Bar-c Calc-s Cann-i Cann-s Carc Cycl Hell Mez Plat Rhus-t Sep Valer Verat
, juveniles	ACID-PHOS IGN Caps Coff Puls
ABUSED: violence from	ARN CARC COFF STAFF Anac Aur Bry Hyper Led Nat-s Op
ACRAL lick granuloma	ANTH CAPS IGN NAT-C NUX-V PHOS PULS PSOR Acid-phos Bell Hyos Kali-c Lyc Sil Agar Bor Ther
ACTIVITY: desire for	AUR TARENT Bar-c Hyos Ign Lach Op Sep Coff Passi Puls
AEROPHAGIA	ANT-T ARG-M ARS MED NUX-V PLAT PULS STRAM Allox Bell-p Hyos Rauw Tarent Tell
, behaviour, odd	MED STRAM Hyos Tarent
, behaviour, reasonable	ANT-T ARS NUX-V PLAT
AFFECTIONATE: excessive	PULS Ars Carc Croc Ign Nat-m Nux-v Phos Plat Puls
AGGRESSION / ANGER	ACID-NIT ANTH BELL BRY CAUST DULC KALI-B LACH LYC MERC NUX-V PALL PLAT SEP STRAM SULPH Anac Apis Aur Cina Coloc Hep Hyos Kali-i Lil-t Merc Nat-c Staph Tarent Thyr
, dangerous	ACID-NIT ANTH BRY MERC-C NUX-V STRAM Anac Tarent
, dominance	ARN BRY CUPR NUX-V PALL PLAT SULPH Anac
, fear, from	ACON ARN BELL IGN PULS Carc Cina Phos Puls Stram Aur
, food related	ANTH ARN BRY CUPR NUX-V PALL PLAT SULPH Anac Kali-c
, inter-animal	ACON ANTH APIS IGN LACH NAT-M NUX-V PLAT SEP Cina
, juvenile	CHAM CINA PHOS Anac Calc-p Nux-v Tub
, maternal	ACON ANTH APIS PALL PLAT PULS SEP Bell Carc Cina Foll Grat Lil-t Nux-m Nux-v Ars Bry Ign
, pain, from	ACON ANTH ARN ARS AUR BELL CUPR IGN KALI-BI NAT-M NUX-V PLAT PULS Acid-nit Ant-t Bry Carc Cina Dulc Hep Lach Lyc Sep Staph Ars-i Caps Col Hyos Kali-c Kali-s Mag-c Merc Nat-c Phos Rhus-t
, play induced	ANTH CALC-P PHOS Anac Cina Nux-v Tub Tarent
, predatory	ANAC Caust Hyos Lach Med Merc Stram
, pregnancy, during	NUX-M SEP
, redirected	ANTH LACH NUX-V Anac Caust Ign Plat Puls Thuj Tub
, territorial	ARN BRY CUPR NUX-V PALL PLAT SULPH Acid-nit Anac Ant-t Hep Ars Caps Caust Kali-c Mag-c Rhus-t

251

, time, evenings	LYC Am-c Bry Calc Kali-c Croc Op Petr
, training, during	ANAC ANTH AUR IGN LYC NUX-V SEP Bry Ferr Ferr-ars Hep Lach Thuj Verat
, violence, with	ACID-NIT ACON ANAC ANTH AUR HEP LACH NUX-V STAPH TARENT Apis Ars Bell Bry Calc Caust Chel Croc Graph Hyos Lyc Nat-m Nux-v Plat Sep Staph Carb-v Kali-c Lyss Petr Tarent
AGORAPHOBIA	GELS LYSS Acon Arg-n Levo Kali-ars Phos Sep
ANOREXIA	Acid-phos Hyos Ign Kali-chl Phyt Tarent Verat Viol-o
ANTISOCIAL	Anac Caust Lach Med Stram
ANXIETY	ACON ANAC ANTH ARN ARS BELL BRY CINA CUPR IGN NAT-M NUX-V OP PALL PLAT PULS SULPH Acid-nit Ant-t Ars-i Aur Bell Caps Caust Coloc Dulc Hep Hyos Kali-bi Kali-c Kali-s Lach Lyc Mag-c Merc Nat-c Phos Rhus-t Sep Staph Tarent Bov Calc-s Petr
, air, open, amel	CANN-I KALI-S Bry Crot-t Lyc Mag-m Puls Rhus-t Sulph
, destructive behaviour	ANAC ARS CAUST Acid-nit Cupr Hep Kali-c Lach
, eating, during	Kali-c
, fear, with	ACON ANAC ARS CAUST IGN PSOR SEC Acid-nit Aeth Alum Aur Bism Calc Canth Chin Cocc Coff Cupr Dig Graph Hep Kali-c Lach Lil-t Lyc Nat-m Nux-v Phos Plat Puls Rhus-t Sep Spig Stront Verat
, feather plucking, with	ANAC ARS CAUST IGN PSOR Acid-nit Aur Calc Canth Cocc Coff Cupr Dig Hep Kali-c Lach Lil-t Lyc Nat-m Nux-v Plat Puls Rhus-t Sep Verat Canth Coff Cupr Graph Phos Spig
, juveniles	ANTH CINA Calc-p Coff Phos Tub Kali-c Passi
, noise, agg	Aur Caust Phos Sil Acon Bor
, separation, agg	ARG-N ARS PULS RHUS-T Anth Bell Bor Halo Hyos Kali-c Lyc Sil Bism Agar Ther
, sleep, after	STAPH
, thunder, before	NAT-C PHOS
, during	ACID-NIT CAUST GELS LYC NAT-C PHOS SEP
, time, afternoon	IGN NATRUMS
, training, apathy to	ACID-PHOS BAR-C CALC IGN PULS RHUS-T Apis Arg-n Arn Ars Aur Aur-i Bapt Cimic Gels Kali-bi Nat-m Op Phyt Sep Sil Stram Sulph Aloe Cinch Ham Hell
BITE: will	ACID-NIT ANTH ARG-N ARN ARS AUR BELL LACH LYC MERC-S NAT-M STRAM Anac Cina Hyos Kali-c
, dangerous	ACID-NIT ARS MERC Kali-c
, fear from	ANTH ARS ARG-N AUR LYC Kali-c Acon Nat-m
, malicious	LACH MERC-C NAT-M STRAM Anac
, pain, teeth	ANTH Calc Chin-s Cocc Rhod
, self, pruritus from	ANTH ARS Cina
BORED: easily	LYC MED MERC SULPH TUB Bar-c Caps Clem Con Nat-c Nux-v Plb Alum Spig
CARRIED: desire to be	ANTH ARS BRY PULS Coff
, constant	ANTH

, restless, with	ARS BRY IGN PULS Coff
CAUTIOUS	ARS Cupr Ign Lyc Puls
CHEERFUL: excessive	CANN-I CANN-S CIC COFF CROC HYOS LACH NAT-C Acid-fl Acid-nit
CHEWER: fabric / furniture...	ANTH ARS FRAG HYOS MED NUX-V PULS Anac Arg-n Calc Carc Ign Nat-m Nat-s Plat Sil Staph
COMPANY: needs	ANTH GELS IGN NAT-M NUX-V STAPH Alum Anac Bar-c Carb-an Cic Con
, geriatrics, in	BAR-C CARB-AN CON
, rehoming, when	IGN NAT-M
COMPANY: averse to	ALUM ANAC ANTH ARG-N ARS GELS IGN LYC NAT-M NUX-V STAPH Acid-phos Ant-t Aur Bar-c Bufo Calc-p Caps Carb-an Carb-v Cimic Clem Coloc Con Cupr Cycl Ferr Hyos Kali-bi Kali-br Kali-c Kali-p Lac-c Lach Lyc Nat-c Nat-p Nat-s Pall Plat Puls Rhus-t Sil Sep Stram Staph Sulph Tarent Thuj Tub Verat X-ray
, desire for	ARG-N ARS BISM HYOS KALI-C LAC-C LYC PHOS PULS Calc Camph Con Gels Ign Lil-t Mez Nat-c Nux-v Pall Stry Apis Elaps Kali-ars Kali-p Sep Stram
CONCENTRATION: poor	ACID-PHOS ANAC BAR-C CARB-S CARB-V CARC CAUST GLON GRAPH LACH LYC NAT-A NUX-M NUX-V PHOS SEP SIL Apis Arg-m Calc Calc-fl Cann-i Carb-an Cimic Cocc Con Cupr Dulc Gels Hell Hyos Kali-c Lac-c Lil-t Merc Nat-c Nat-m Plat Puls Sel Stram Sulph Syph Tab Thuj Zinc
CONFIDENCE: low	CALC-FL CARC LYC NAT-M SIL STRAM Bar-c Lac-c
, juvenile	BAR-C Aeth Carc Phos Sil
, performance anxiety	ARG-N GELS LYC Carc
CONFUSED	ACID-PHOS CAPS IGN NAT-C NAT-SIL PHOS PULS PSOR Acid-phos Aur Calc-c Calc-p Calc-s Caust Gels Hyos Kali-c Lyc Nat-m Puls Sep Sil Stram Sulph
CONSOLATION: agg	CARC NAT-M SEP SIL Ign Lyc Nat-m
, inconsolable	ACON CHIN IGN NUX-V Anth Ars Caust Lyc Nat-m Petr Plat Puls Spong Stann Verat
COPROPHAGIA	ARS HYOS MED NUX-V PULS Bapt Calc Carc Crot-h Cupr Ferr-ars Ferr Nat-m Nat-s Phos Plat Sil Staph Anac Arg-n Ign
DEFIANT	CAUST IGN LACH NAT-M NUX-V SEP SIL Anac Hep Tub
, training, to improve	IGN NAT-M NUX-V
DEMANDING	ANTH LACH LYC NUX-V Anac Caust Ign Nat-m Nux-v Plat Puls Thuj Tub
DEMENTIA: senile	ARG-M CON PHOS Bar-c
DESTRUCTIVE	BELL LYC NUX-V STAPH STRAM CUPR Anac Agar Hyos Lil-t Tub
DISOBEDIENT	MERC NUX-V TUB Acid-nit Am-c Chin Dig Lyc Guai Lyc Tarent Viol-t
DULL: head injury, after	ARN HELL NAT-S Cic Hyper Merc Rhus-t
EFFEMINATE	LYC PULS Calc Plat Sil Thuj
ELIMINATION DISORDERS	FOLL LYC OEST OV STAPH TEST UST Acid-phos Agn Bar-c Calc Con Oest Plat Sep Sil Thuj
, juveniles	LYC PULS TEST Acid-phos Calc Oest Plat Sep Thuj

253

, submissive	BAR-C CALC-FL CARC LYC NAT-M SIL STRAM Aur Calc-c Kali-c Nux-v Psor Thuj
, female, neutered, in	FOLL OEST OV Agn
, males	LYC PULS TEST Bufo Calc Plat Sil Thuj
EROTOMANIA: females	CALC-P LACH PLAT SABIN ZINC Aster Canth Med Stram
, males	BUFFO CANN-I CANTH MED MERC NUX-V PHOS PLAT SIL STRAM Acid-fl Agar Alum Calc Graph Hyos Kali-br Kali-c Lach Lyc Nat-c Nat-m Orig Plb Thuj Tub Verat
ESCAPE: desire to	ANTH ARS BELL BRY STRAM VERAT Aesc Agar All-s Anth Bry Chel Cic Cocc Crot-h Cupr Dig Glon Hell Ign Iod Lach Lil-t Merc Nux-v Oena Phos Plb Ran-b Rhus-t Verat
EXCITABLE	ACID-NIT ACID-PHOS ACON ANAC ANTH APIS ARG-N AUR BELL CARC CAUST COFF COLL GRAPH HEP HYOS KALI-BR KALI-I LAC-C LACH MAG-P MOSCH NAT-M NUX-V OP PHOS PULS STRAM STAPH ZINC-P Arn Ars Aur-m Bry Calc-p Calc-s Camph Cann-i Cann-s Canth Cic Cimic Colch Cupr Dig Ferr Ferr-p Gels Ign Iod Kali-ars Kali-p Kali-s Lyc Mag-m Merc Mez Nat-c Petr Plat Podo Psor Sep Sil Spig Spong Stann Sulph Tarent Verat Zinc
, adults	ACON ARG-N MAG-P NUX-V PHOS
, exercise, amel	RHUS-T SEP Calc Carc Ign
, juvenile	ACID-PHOS ACON ARG-N PULS Coff Passi
EXTROVERT	Bell Carc Ign Lach Phos Puls Staph
FEAR	ANTH ARG-N ARN ARS BELL GELS LACH LYC NUX-V PHOS PULS SEP SIL STRAM Bar-c Bor Cann-i Cic Graph Hyos Kali-c Lyss Mand Nat-a Nat-c Plb Rhod
, alone, of being	ARG-N ARS CROT-C HYOS KALI-C LYC PHOS STRAM Apis Arist-cl Camph Clem Con Crot-c Elaps Gels Kali-p Lac-c Lyss Puls Sep
, animals, of	BELL CALC Chin Tub
, anticipation	ARG-N ARN GELS LYC PHOS PULS SEP SIL Graph
, approached, being	ARN Ambr Bell Cupr Ign Lyc Stram Thuj
, cars, of	BOR BRY COCC GELS SANIC Bar-c Calad Dies Ferr Gels Petr Puls
, carried, being	BOR SANIC Bry
, dark, of	CANN-I PHOS STRAM Acon Apis Arg-n Ars Calc Camph Carb-a Carb-v Caust Cupr Hyos Lyc Med Puls Rhus-t Sang Stront Valer
, exertion, of	ARG-N CALC KALI-C NUX-V SIL SULPH Anth Aur-i Graph Hyos Iod Kali-p Nat-m Nat-p Ran-b Sel
, men, of	BAR-C CIC LYC NAT-C Anac Aur Bell Hyos Ign Kali-bi Lach Plat Puls Sel Sep
, motion, of	BRY
, noise, of	NUX-V PHOS Bor Mand
, parturition, during	ACON Anth Plat Puls Sep
, water, rushing	BELL HYOS LYSS STRAM Canth Lach Verat
, thunder, of	ACON GELS HYOS NAT-C PHOS RHOD Acid-nit Bor Elect Sep Sil

, transport, of	DIG HYOS LACH NAT-C Acon Berb Bor Bry Cocc Gels Kali-i Mag-c Mand Nat-c Stann Stram Verat (vomiting)
, vets, of	ACON BAR-C CIC GELS IOD LYC NAT-C SIL All-s Ars Aur-m Bar-c Carc Lach Sep Staph
, water	BELL HYOS LYSS STRAM Canth Lach Verat
FEARLESS	AGAR OP Anth Berb Bov Calad Calc-s Caust Dros Ferr-p Ign Merc
FEAR: take fright easily	ARG-N ARS BAR-C BELL BOR GRAPH LYC NAT-A NAT-C NUX-V PHOS PULS SEP STRAM Acon Ant-c Aur Bufo Calc Calc-p Cann-i Caps Carb-an Carc Caust Clem Cocc Coff Dig Glon Hyper Ign Lach Lil-t Mag-c Merc Nat-m Plb Psor Samb Sil Sulph Ther
GESTURES: odd, makes	HYOS Bell Cocc Mosch Sep Stram Tarent
, automatic / rhythmic	ANT-T ARS HYOS MED NUX-V PULS STRAM TARENT Acid-phos Anac Arg-n Bell Calc Carc Cupr Ign Lach Mosch Nat-m Nat-s Plat Sep Sil Staph
GRIEF	ACID-PHOS AUR CAUST IGN LACH NAT-M NUX-V PHOS STAPH Astac Bov Hist Led Prim Rhus-v Urt-u
, from physical problem	ACID-PHOS IGN NAT-M PHOS
, mental problem	IGN NAT-M PHOS STAPH Carc
GROOM: self, excessively	ARS HYOS MED NUX-V PULS Anac Arg-n Calc Carc Ign Nat-m Nat-s Plat Sil Staph
HEAD SHAKING equine	APIS ARS CORTISO SEL Astac Bov Hist Led Prim Rhus-v Urt-u
, acute	APIS ARS CORTISO
, chronic	RHUS-T SEL Hist
HOMESICK	ACID-PHOS BRY CAPS CARB-AN IGN MAG-M MERC Acid-nit Aur Bell Caust Clem Cocc Coff Crat Hell Kali-p Nat-m Phos Sil Staph
, rehoming, juveniles	ACID-PHOS Caps
, rehoming, adults	IGN NAT-M Caps
HURRY: work, constantly	ACID-SUL KALI-C LIL-T NUX-V STRAM TARENT SULPH Acon Arg-n Ars Bell Camph Cann-i Coca Coff Merc Viol-t
HYPERACTIVE generally	ARS COFF HYOS IGN MED STRAM TUB Anac Ars-i Calc-p Cina Iod Nux-v Passi Thuj Verat
, juvenile	Coff Passi Tub
HYPERSENSITIVE	ACID-NIT ACON ANTH ARG-N BELL BRY CALC CHIN HEP IGN LYC NAT-M NUX-V PHOS PULS SIL SULPH
HYPERSEXED	GELS LACH PHOS PLAT STRAM Acid-pic Anh Bufo Canth Grat Hyos Med Orig Tub
, female	PLAT Anh Grat Orig
, juvenile	PULS Acid-pic Bufo Canth
, male	LACH PHOS Canth Tub
, mentally unstable	STRAM Anh Hyos
, mounting behaviour	Acid-pic Bufo Tub
HYSTERIA	ACON ARG-N CUPR GELS IGN PHOS STRAM Ergot Kali-ars Hyos Tarent Thyr Val
, chronic	IGN Thyr
, post trauma	GELS IGN Valer

IMPATIENT	ARG CARC IGN IP MED NUX-V SEP SIL SULPH Acid-nit Acid-sul Acon Anac Apis Ars Bry Calc Cina Coloc Dulc Hep Hyos Iod Kali-bi Kali-c Kres Lach Lyc Nat-m Plan Plat Psor Puls Rhus-t Staph Tarent
, adult	CORTISO IGN NUX-V PULS SEP STRAM Tub Verat
, hot, when	Anth Ip Nat-m Nux-v Puls Viol-t
, juvenile	ARG-N IGN SIL Carc Tub
IMPETUOUS	ACID-NIT HEP NUX-V SEP Anac Anth Bry Carb-v Kali-c Nat-m Staph Sulph Zinc
, mental instability, with	IGN MED STRAM Hyos
IMPULSIVE	ARG-N IGN PULS Ars Aur Cic Med
INDIFFERENT	ACID-PHOS CADM-MET CARB-V STAPH THYR Acid-pic Chin Cimic Cina Gels Hell Ign Lyc Merc Nat-m Nux-v Op Phos Plat Puls Rheum Sep
, constantly	Carb-v Op Thyr
, juveniles	ACID-PHOS Thyr
, loved ones, to	HELL PHOS, SEP Acid-fl Acid-phos Acon Syph
, neonates, own to	PHOS SEP Acon Lyc
, opposite sex, to	SEP Puls
INSANE: parturition, after	Aur Bell Camph Cann-i Chlol Cimic Cupr Hyos Kali-bi Lyc Nux-v Plat Puls Sec Stram Sulph Verat
IRRATIONAL: jump window	ARG-N AUR Aeth Arg-m Ars Bell Camph Carb-s Chin Glon Thea Thuj Verat
IRRITABLE	ANTH BRY NUX-V SEP SIL STAPH Caps Cina Croc Mag-c Rheum Syc-co Tub
, consolation, agg	NAT-M NUX-V SEP SIL Acid-nit Bell Cact Calc-p Plat
, dentition, during	ANTH RHEUM Calc-p
, eating, during	Bor Bry Hydr Kali-c Nat-c Nat-m Puls
, illness, during	BRY SIL Mag-c
, juvenile	ANTH SIL Caps Cina SIL Tub
, mornings	STAPH Acid-nit Calc Carb-s Iber Lach Mang Merc-i-r Nat-m Nat-s Petr
, pain during	BRY ANTH Acid-nit Ars Aloe Colch Coloc Hep Op
, parturition, during	ANTH CINA MAG-C
, pregnancy, during	ACON Anth Sep
, thunder, before	NAT-C
, trifling things	ACID-NIT ANTH NUX-V Ars Bell Calc Caust Cimic Cina Clem Hep Med Mez Nat-m Phos Plat Ptel
JEALOUSY	APIS HYOS LACH NUX-V Calc-s Caust Cench Kali-c Lyc Med Plat Puls Staph Stram
, females, fighting	APIS
, rage	HYOS Lach
, adult	ACID-NIT MERC-C Hep
KICKS	ACID-NIT ANTH BELL Lyc Merc Stram Sulph
KILL: desire to	HEP HYOS Alum Ars Ars-i Bell Iod Lach Merc Nux-v Petr Phos Plat Staph Stram
, neonates, own	NUX-V PLAT Ars Ars-i Hep Merc Tarent

LAZY	CALC-P CAUST GELS SULPH Carb-v Foll Mag-c Oest Test Thyr
, evenings	SULPH Agar Calc-p Coca Mag-m Nat-m Pall Plb
, food, after	Acid-phos Agar Anac Ant-c Bar-c Chel Chin Kali-c Lyc Nat-m Phos Plat Plb Thuj Zinc
, HRT needed female	Oest Plac
, HRT needed male	Orchi-e (c) Plac
, thyroid, hyper	Thyr
LIGHT: averse to	BELL CON GELS STRAM Acon Am-m Calc Stront-c
LOOK AT: cannot bear	ANT-C ARS NAT-M TUB Anth Ant-t Chin Cina Iod
MALICIOUS	ANAC LACH NAT-M STRAM Acid-nit Anth Ars Aur Bel Bor Calc Cupr Hep Hyos Lac-c Led Lyc Nat-c
MANIA	BELL LACH LYC STAPH STRAM Anac Carc Hyos
, chronic mental problem	BELL STRAM Hyos
, vocalisation, with	Bell Cocc Stry-m Tarent Verat
MASTURBATION / MOUNTING	ANAC ARN ARS BRY CUPR HYOS MED NUX-V PALL PULS PLAT SULPH Acid-nit Ant-t Arg-nit Calc Carc Caust Hep Ign Kali-c Mag-c Nat-m Rhus-t Staph
MOANING: dentition	ANTH Podo
, epilepsy, during	IGN Sil Tub
, fever, during	PULS Arn
, juveniles	ANTH Cina Podo
, pain, from	Coff Coloc Eup-per Hydr Nux-v
MOODY	ALUM BELL BOV CARC FERR IGN STRY-M IOD LYC PLAT PULS SARS ZINC Acid-sul Acon Bar-c Carb-an Cench Chin Croc Dros Ferr-p Graph Kali-c Naja Nat-m Nux-v Phos Sulph
, mood swings	CARC LACH STAPH Anac Con Hyos Med Nat-s
, parturition, at	Cann-i Cimic Hyos Stram
MUSIC: aggravates	ACON GRAPH NAT-C NUX-V SEP Acid-phos Aloe Ambr Anac Calc Anth Coff Croc Dig Lyc Nat-s Phos Sabin
NERVOUS	Arg-n Bor Bufo Gels Mag-c Mag-p Phos Tarent
NYMPHOMANIA	GRAT HYOS LACH ORIG PLAT STRAM Med Bell Cann-i Kali-br Lil-t Lyc Staph Bar-m Canth Merc
OBSTINATE	ALUM ANAC ARG-N BAR-C BELL BRY CALC CALC-P CHIN CINA IGN SIL SULPH TARENT TUB Acid-nit Acid-phos Acon Ant-c Ars Calc-s Caps Caust Crot-h Hep Hyos Kali-c Kali-p Lyc Mag-m Pall Psor Sanic Spong Staph Thuj
, geriatric	CALC-P Alum Anac Bar-c Con Tub
, juveniles	CALC CALC-P Bar-c SIL Tub
OCD	ARS HYOS MED NUX-V PULS Anac Arg-n Calc Carc Ign Nat-m Nat-s Plat Sil Staph
OVERSENSITIVE	ACID-NIT ACON ANTH ARG-N BELL BRY CALC-P CUPR IGN LYC NAT-M NUX-V PHOS PULS SIL SULPH Colch Hep Hyos Kali-ars Kres Rhod
, constant	ACID-NIT ARG-NIT LYC

257

, geriatric	ANTH CALC-P NAT-M NUX-V Hep
, illness, during	ACID-NIT ANTH BELL
, juvenile	ANTH CALC-P LYC
PAIN: vocal	ACON ANTH Apis Ars Bell Coloc Plat
PAINLESS: unexpected	OP STRAM Hell
PANIC DISORDER	ACON ARG-N GELS KALI-ARS PHOS STRAM Anth Cann-i Carb-v Cocc Cupr Cupr-ars Hyos Lyc Sulph Tab
PERFORMANCE; anxiety	ARG-N GELS LYC NAT-M Acon Ars Carb-v Sil Thuj
PICA	ARS HYOS MED NUX-V PULS Anac Arg-n Bapt Calc Carc Crot-h Cupr Ferr Ferr-ars Ign Nat-m Nat-s Phos Plat Sil Staph
RAGE	AGAR ANAC BELL CANTH HYOS LAC-C LACH LYC MOSCH OP STRAM NUX-V VERAT Acon Aeth Arn Ars Camph Carb-s Colch Cupr Hell Lol Nat-m Phos Puls Sec Sol-n Staph Sulph Tab
RESTLESS	ACON ANAC ANTH ARG-N ARS ARS-I BELL BAPT CALC CALC-P CAMPH CARC CIMIC CIC COFF COLOC CUPR CUPR-ARS FERR FERR-ARS HELL HYOS IGN LYC MED MERC PLB PULS PYROG RHUS-T SEC SEP SIL STAPH STRAM SULPH TARENT
, evenings	CAUST KRES Alum Am-c Ars Calc Carb-v Merc Nat-c Rumx
, juveniles	ARS MERC RHUS-T RHEUM Anac Anth Arg-n Carc Med Tarent Tub Verat
, nocturnal restlessness	ARS CAUST HYOS KALI-ARS KRES LYC MERC PULS RHUS-T Ant-t Arg-m Arg-n Ars-i Bell Calc Carb-v Caul Caust Cic Cupr Cycl Ferr Ign Iris Kali-br Lac-c Mag-m Med Nat-a Phos Podo Ran-b Sep Teucr Valer
, parturition, at	ANTH SEP Acon Camph
, pregnancy, during	Colch Nux-v
, thunder, before	Gels Psor Rhod
, during	Gels Psor Rhod
RUN AWAY: desire to	HYOS STRAM TUB VERAT Iod Nux-v Orig Tarent
SCREAMING: fit, before	CIC CUPR HYOS Amyl-n Apis Bell Bufo Ip Kali-br Lach Lyc Oena Op Stram Sulph Zinc
, fit, during	HYOS OP Amyl-n Apis Art-v Camph Caust Cic Cina Crot-h Cupr Ign Ip Lach Lyc Merc
SENSITIVE: fireworks, to	ACON BELL COFF NAT-C PHOS Bor
, juveniles	ANTH CARC IGN NAT-M PHOS Acon Ant-c Bell Calc-p Cina Kali-p Nux-v Puls Scut Staph Teucr Tub
, light, to	BELL NUX-V PHOS Acon Ars Colch Kali-p Nat-m
, looked at, being	CALC
, noise, to	ACON AGAR BELL BOR CHIN CHIN-A COFF CON IGN KALI-C NUX-V OP PHOS SEP SIL THER TUB ZINC ZINC-P Acid-fl Anth Arg-n Arn Ars Ars-i Aur Bar-c Bry Calc Carb-s Carb-v Carc Caust Cocc Ferr Ferr-ars Ferr-p Ip Kali-p Lac-c Lach Lyc Lyss Mag-c Mag-m Man Med Merc Nat-c Nat-m Nat-s Plat Puls
, voices, loud, to	LACH Bell Hyos
, water, splashing	ACID-NIT LYSS

SHOCK	ACON ARN CAMPH CARB-V OP VERAT
SHY	IGN PULS SIL STAPH SULPH Bar-c
, female	PULS STAPH
, juvenile	IGN SIL
STARTLE: easily	BELL NAT-M NAT-S NUX-V PHOS SIL STRAM VERAT Bor Hyos Kali-c Kali-p Nat-c Acid-n Anth Camph Cocc Ign Kali-br Psor Scut Sep Tarent Ther
, constantly	Bor Hyos Kali-c Nat-c
, illness, during	BELL NUX-V PHOS SIL Kali-p Verat
, juvenile	NAT-M PHOS SIL Bor Nat-c
STEREOTYPIC	ANT-T ARS HYOS PULS STRAM TARENT Med Nux-v Anac Arg-n Bell Cupr Plat Sep Staph Acid-phos Calc Ign Lach Lyc Nat-a Op
STRIKING: air, empty, at	BELL HYOS Kali-c Nat-c Stram
SUSPICIOUS	ACON ANAC ARS BAR-C BRY CANN-I CAUST CENCH CIC DIG KALI- ARS LACH LYC PULS RHUS-T SULPH Arn Aur Bapt Bar-m Bar-s Bell Bor Calc-p Cimic Cocc Crot-h Cupr Dros Hell Hyos Kali-p Lycps Med Merc Morph Nat-a Nat-c Nux-v Op Phos Plb Sep Spig Stram Verat-v
, illness, during	ACON PULS SULPH CAUST Dig
, juvenile	PULS RHUS-T Anac Bar-c
, overwork, from	BRY LACH SULPH Anac
THUNDER: enjoys	Carc Sep
TRAVEL: enjoys	CALC-P CARC Hipp Iod Merc
, prevention	Cocc Coca Ip Petr Sanic Scut Tab
, sickness	ANT-T BRY IGN TAB VERAT Apom Bor Coca Cocc Dies Ip Mag-c Nat-c Petr Sanic Scut
, treatment	Cocc Ip Tab
VEHICLES: chases	ANAC ARN BELL BRY CUPR HYOS NUX-V PALL PLAT STRAM SULPH Acid-nit Ant-t Ars Caps Caust Hep Kali-c Lach Mag-c Op Rhus-t Sec
VIOLENCE: tendency to	ANAC AUR BELL CIC HEP HYOS NUX-V STRAM TUB Anth Ant-t Bry Carb-s Carb-v Iod Kali-i Kali-p Lach Led Nat-m Petr Phos Sep Sulph Tarent Verat Visc
, pain, agg	ANTH AUR HEP
VOCALISE: excessively	ACON CALC HYOS IGN KALI-C LYC STRAM Alum Anth Aur Bell Bufo Canth Chin-s Cic Cocc Esin Phos Ran-b Stram Verat-v
, boredom	ARG-N ARS LIL-T SEP Foll Sulph Thal
, fearful	ARG-N Kali-c Hyos
, loneliness, from	ACID-PHOS CAPS IGN PHOS SEP Psor Puls
, seeking company	ACID-PHOS ARG-N SEP Caps
, territorial	SEP STRAM Lil-t
WALK: odd / rhythmic	ANT-T ARS MED PULS STRAM THUJ Hyos Tarent
, circles, in	Stram Thuj
, CNS disease, during	STRAM Hyos

, stereotypic	ANT-T ARS MED Tarent
, wander, desire to	BRY TUB VERAT Calc-p Elat Kali-br
WORK: amel	SEP Camph Con Croc Cupr Cycl Ferr Hell Helon Iod Kali-br Lil-t Merc-i-f Nat-c Nux-v
, bad attitude to	AUR CALC LYC NAT-M SEP SIL SULPH
, averse to	AUR SEP SIL Graph
, geriatric	NAT-M SIL Con Graph
, juvenile	CALC LYC NAT-M SULPH

CENTRAL NERVOUS SYSTEM

ATAXIA	ACON ALUM BOR CALC CAUST CHLORPR COCC CON GELS PHOS RHUS-T Agar Bry Cic Cupr-ac Dros Hell Hyos Kres Nat-m Stram Sulfon Tarent-h Zinc
, circling, to left	RHUS-T
, to right	CAUST
, head shaking, after	Con
, to left	NAT-M Con Zinc
, to right	ACON CAUST
, injury, concussion	ARN HYPER NAT-S Cocc Hell
, infection, after	CALC GELS PHOS Chlorpro
, fall, backwards	RHUS-T Acid-phos Bry Calc Carb-an Caust Chin Kali-c Nux-v Sil Spong
, forwards	NAT-M RHUS-T Acid-phos Alum Calc-p Camph Caust Cic Elaps Ferr Graph Lach Nux-v Podo Ran-b Sabin Sil Sulph
, left	CON NAT-M ZINC Aur Bell Bor Calc Caust Eup-per Eup-pur Lach Sulph
, right	ACON CAUST Calc Sil Zinc
, geriatrics	PHOS Alum Con Syph
, move downhill, amel	BOR
, agg	BOR CALC FERR Con Kali-bi Plat Sanic Sulph
, recumbency, amel	COCC
, staggering	GELS
, wobbler, equine	Arn Alum Caust Con Gels
CANCER cns	CON PHOS VISC Ars Ars-i Bar-c Calc Carb-an Croc Kali-i Kres Lach Plb Sil Thuj Tub
CEREBRAL haemorrhage	ACON ARN BELL BOTH COCC COLCH GELS IP LACH OP Aur Bar-c Camph Chin Coff Cupr Crot-h Ferr Hyos Lyc Nat-m Nux-m Nux-v Phos Puls
CHOREA	AGAR CALC CAUST CIC CINA CUPR LACH LAT-M MYGALE STRAM TARENT Zinc
, facial	Caust Cupr Mygal
, left sided	Cimic Cupr Rhod
, one sided	Calc Cocc Croc Cupr Nat-s Phys
, viral	CALC Agar Mygal Tarent

COMA	ACON BELL IGN LACH NUX-V PULS Bar-c Cann-i Cocc Hell Hyos Mosch Nux-m
,anaesthetic emergency	**NOSODE** ARN Cocc Hell
CONCUSSION	ARN NAT-S HYPER Cic Op
CUSHINGS DISEASE	ARN CALC CORTISO HYPER LYC NUX-V PHOS Colos Cortico Chlorpro Ins Querc Syzyg Tarax
DIABETES INSIPIDUS	ACID-PHOS CORTISO URAN-N Acid-acet Alf Apoc Cann-i Cortico Eup-pur Sel
ELECTRIC SHOCK	ARG-M ARN ARS Cic Verat
ENCEPHALITIS / 'losis	ACON ARG-M PHOS Alum Astrag Nosode Raj Sulpha
EPILEPSY: fits	ANTH ARG-M ARG-N BELL CALC CAUST CUPR GELS IGN MAG-P NAT-S NUX-V PLAT SEP SIL SULPH Bar-m Bufo Camph Cic Con Ferr-cy Hyos Kali-Br Petr Plb Prot-b Rauw Stry Thyr Visc Zinc
, body, thrown back	Camph
, forwards	CUPR
, collapse, after	SIL SULPH Cic
, confused, after	LACH
, cyanotic, during	BELL CUPR Oena
, excitement, before	IGN MAG-P PHOS KALI-Br Zinc
, foaming, mouth, during	ANTH CUPR SIL Bufo Cic Cina Hyos Oena Aster Caust Glon Hyos Lach Op Sil Stry
, lethargy, after	KALI-Br
, male, hyper sexed	GELS NUX-V Bufo Con
, parasites, intestinal	CINA Anth Bell Cic Hyos Ign Kali-br Sabad Sil Spig Stann Stram Sulph Tanac Ter
, screaming, during	HYOS SIL Bufo Cic Oena
, sleep, during	ARG-N BELL CAUST CUPR GELS HYOS IGN KALI-C LACH SIL STRAM SULPH Cic Op
, status epilepticus	Acon Aeth Bell Cocc Oena Plb Zinc
, sudden onset	Bell Verat-v
, teeth, ground, during	Bufo Hyos
, tetanic spasms	CIC HYPER NUX-V PETR PLAT SEP STRY Acid-hydr Am-c Anac Ant-t Arn Atro Bell Calc Camph Canth Cocc Con Cupr Hyos Ign Ip Kali-br Lach Laur Led Lob Lyc Lyss Mag-p Merc Mosch Oena Op Phys Phyt Plb Puls Rhus-t Sec Stram Ter Tetanus nosode
, thunder, during	GELS Agar
, trauma	ARN HYPER NAT-S Chlol Cic Cur Hell Led Nux-v
, uremic	KALI-BR Acid-carb Cupr Dig Kali-s Mosch Op Plb Ter Verat-v
, urination, during	Bufo CAUST Hyos Oena Plb
, profuse, after	CUPR LACH CAUST
, vaccinosis	SIL Apis Ant-t Bell Cic Thuj Vac-nosodes
, vertigo, with	CAUST HYOS LACH SULPH Plb Tarent
, vomiting, after	ARS CALC CUPR

261

, during	CUPR Ant-c Ip
, waking, on	IGN Bell Lyss
HYPERMETRIA	Acon Agar Cupr Naja Verat-v
MENINGITIS	APIS BELL HELL RAJ STRAM ZINC Acid-hydr Acon Agar Bry Calc Calc-p Cic Cocc Cupr-ac Cup Gels Glon Hippoz Hyos Kali-br Lach Merc Nat- m Op Phos Plb Rhus-t
, leptospirosis	Acid-hydr Acon Agar Apis Bell Bry Calc Calc-p Cic Cocc Cupr-ac Cupr Gels Glon Hell Hippoz Hyos Kali-br Lach Merc Nat-m Op Phos Plb Raj-s Rhus-t Sil Stram Sulph Nosode
, painful and active	BELL STRAM Hell
, depressed / inactive	Hell Raj Zinc
NARCOLEPSY	ANT-T Allox Nux-m Op
NEURALGIA	ACON BELL BRY CALEN HYPER MAG-P NAT-S PHOS Bell-p Beryl Chlorpro Coff Mag-s Op Thal
, brachial	BRY HYPER Flav Kalm Rhus-t Thala
, dental	HYPER CALEN
, oedema	ARN NAT-S Apis Hyper Cic Coff Op Stram
, extremities	HYPER
, facial	PHOS Beryl Mag-s
, sciatica	Thal
, trauma	BRY HYPER PHOS
, trigeminal	Bell-p Chlorpro Thal
NEURITIS	ACON BELL COFF HYPER PHOS Arn Ars Cic Coca Gels Hell Hep Hyos Ip Kalm Kali-p Led Lob Merc Nat-s Nat-m Nux-v Op Puls Rhus-t Sil Stram Teucr
PARALYSIS	ACID-PHOS ACON APIS ARS CALC-FL CAUST GELS LACH NUX-V PHOS PLB RHUS-T SIL SULPH Acid-oxal Aesc Agar Alum Am-c Astrag Bufo Cann-i Cocc Con Crot-c Dig Graph Hyos Ner Pexid Zinc
, acute	ACON BELL PHOS Acid-oxal
, geriatric	CAUST PHOS Acid-oxal Alum Con
, hemiplegia, left	APIS CAUST LACH NUX-V RHUS-T Con Pexid
, right	CAUST RHUS-T Crot-c Plb
, injury, after	ARS CAUST LACH NUX-V RHUS-T
, lead poisoning	Alum Op Plb
,myelopathy degenerative	ACID-OXAL ARS CANN-I CAUST CON LATH NUX-V PLB RHUS-T Acid-pic Alum Gels Led Lyss Mang Sec
, peri parturient	PHOS RHUS-T
, radial	ACON PLB Carb-s Cur Hipp Merc Ruta Rhus-t
, slow to develop	CAUST PHOS Alum Con Zinc
, sphincters	CAUST
, toxicity	Apis Ars Gels Lach
TETANUS	BELL CIC HYPER LED NUX-V OP STRY Acon Ang Arg-n Calen Camph Caust Cedr Cocc Crot-c Cupr

, prophylaxis	Cupr-ac Gels Glon Hep Hyos Laur Lyc Mosch Nux-m Oena Plat Plb Sec Stram Upa Verat HYPER LED Myris Nosode

HEAD
EYES EARS NOSE

ABSCESS	ACON ARN BELL CALC LYC HEP SIL Myris
, attitude, depressed	CALC Hep
, bone, osteomalacia	ACID-NIT AUR PHOS SIL Acid-fl Acid-phos Arg-m Asaf Hep Nat-m Staphyloc
, chronic	CALC SIL
, painful	Hep LYC
, prevention	ACON ARN BELL CALC LYC HEP SIL Myris
CANCER	ARS AUR PHOS Colos Kali-s
, painful	AUR Colos Kali-s
, tiredness, with	ARS Colos PHOS
DANDRUFF	NAT-M PHOS SULPH Canth Carb-s Graph
, anger	NAT-M SULPH Canth
, sadness	Carb-s Graph
DISCOLOURED	ARS CALC FERR LYC MED SEP THUJ Tub
, affectionate	ARS THUJ
, hair, lighter	ARS CALC FERR LYC MED SEP TUB Acid-nit Acid-phos Arg-m Chel Clem Crot-h Kali-c Mag-m Mang SEP THUJ Oest Orchi-e (c)
, neutering, after	
, tiredness	CALC FERR MED
ECZEMA / Dermatitis	CALC DULC HEP PSOR RHUS-T Sars SULPH Cic Crot-t Graph Mez Petr Tub
, pruritus little	Cic
, scabby	Cic Mez
, smelly	SULPH PSOR
, wet	DULC PSOR RHUS-T SULPH Graph Mez Sars Tub
HORNS	ARN HYPER SIL Cast-eq Led Myris
, injury	ARN HYPER
, juveniles	Cast-eq
LUPUS	ACID-FL APIS ARS CORTISO SEP SULPH Cortico Hydrc Kres Mand Tell
PAIN	BELL BRY HYPER MERC NUX-V PULS Chel Spig Verb
, acute	BELL HYPER NUX-V Spig Verb
, bone	Caps Chin-s Cimic Hep Merc Phos Phyt Sil
, malar	Aur Calc-p Kali-bi
, chewing, when	Anth Bell Bism Bry Nat-m Staph
, chronic	BRY MERC-C PULS Chel

263

, cold, agg	MAG-P RHUS-T SIL Bell Carb-s Colch Dulc Mag-c Merc Rhod
, amel	KALI-S All-c Puls
, eating, after	MEZ
, exertion / movement, after	BRY Cact
, eyes, below	Acon Arg-n Ars Bell Gels Nux-v Sil
, time, diurnal	SPIG Cimic Stann
, evening	Chin-s Mez Phos Plat Puls Sulph Thuj Verb Zinc
, morning	Chin-s Cupr Nux-v
, night	MERC Acon Calc-p Caust Cocc Con Glon Guai Lach Mag-c Mag-p Mez Phyt Sep Sil Sulph
, unilateral	Caust Kali-bi
PARALYSIS	CAUST GELS PHOS Zinc-pic
, acute, left	PHOS
, right	CAUST
, chronic	GELS PHOS
RINGWORM	CALC DULC SEP Bac Nosode Tub
, dirty looking	CALC DULC SEP
, immune suppression	Bac Tub
, nutrition, poor	As above plus Colos
SEBACEOUS CYSTS	HEP Graph Kali-c
, chronic	Graph
, painful	Hep Kali-c
URTICARIA	APIS ARS Chlol Cop Nosode
, acute	APIS
, bladder disease, with	Cop
, liver disease, with	Chlol
, vaccinosis	APIS Nosode
VEINS	HAM LACH THUJ Nosodes
, distension	CHIN LACH THUJ Ferr Glon Op Plat Sulph
, painful, left side	LACH
, tiredness, with	Chin
WARTS	ACID-NIT CAUST DULC
, behaviour, difficult	ACID-NIT
, smooth	DULC
, tiredness, with	CAUST

EARS

ABSCESS	AUR HEP SIL CALC Calc-s
DEAFNESS	CAUST HEP LYC MERC-S PSOR PULS SIL Verat-v

, geriatric	MERC-S Cic
, otitis media, from	MERC-s PSOR PULS SIL
EXUDATE	ACID-NIT AUR CALC HEP KALI-BI LYC MERC PSOR PULS SIL SULPH THUJ Calc-s Cist Crot-h Graph Hydr Kali-c Kali-p Kali-s Tell Tub Zinc
, acrid	SULPH Tell
, bloody	PSOR SIL Calc-s Crot-h
, left	Graph Zinc
, offensive	AUR CALC KALI-BI LYC PSOR PULS Calc-s Cist Hep Kali-p Tub
, right	ACID-NIT LYC SIL THUJ
, thick	CALC KALI-B Calc-s Hydr
, watery	PULS Cist Graph Kali-s
ECZEMA / DERMATITIS	CALC CAUST LYC PSOR STAPH SULPH Bar-c Graph Petr Staphyloc Zinc
OTHEMATOMA	ACON ARN CALC-FL HAM Thiosin
, acute	ACON ARN HAM
, chronic	HAM CALC-FL Thiosin
OTODECTIC MANGE	PSOR Ars-i Graph Maland Tell
, exudate	Ars-i
, dry and scaly	Maland
, honey-like	Graph
, purulent	PSOR Tell
OTITIS: MED & INTERNA	ACID-FL ANTH ARS AUR BELL BRY CALC CAUST GELS HEP KALI-BI LACH MERC-C MERC PSOR PULS RHUS-T Ars-i Calc-s Caps Cist Elaps Graph Ins Kaliums Malan Scroph-n Tell
, externa	ACID-PHOS ANTH BELL KALI-BI LACH MERC-C Canth Hep
, interna, acute	ANTH BELL KALI-BI MERC-C Hep
, chronic	CALC LYC Calc-s Hep
, neurological signs	BRY CAUST GELS MERC NAT-M RHUS-T Con Hep

EYES

BLEEDING	PHOS Both Crot-h Led Symph
, clotting defects	Both
, retinal	PHOS
, vitreous	Crot
BLEPHARITIS	ANT-C ARG-M ARG-N APIS CALC-S CARB-S GRAPH LYC MED MERC PETR RHUS-T STAPH SULPH TELL
, oedema	APIS
, eyelids raw	NAT-M MERC-C Ant-c
, hordeolum / sty	LYC STAPH
, injury	APIS ARG-N STAPH

, purulent	ARG-N RHUS-T Calc-s Tell
, skin disease, with	Tell
CANCER	CALC LYC PHOS Kali-i Nosodes Sol Visc Zinc
, bone, orbit	CALC Kali-i Visc Zinc
, cystic	Acid-benz Calc Calc-fl Graph Merc Sil
, epithelial	LACH COLOS
, left sided	LACH
, sarcoma	PHOS
, sun related	PHOS Sol
, tarsal	ZINC Kali-i Puls Sep Sil Staph Thuj
CANTHI	ARG-N ARS CALC LYC MERC NAT-M SIL
, cracks	GRAPH LYC Nat-m Sulph
, chronic	SIL
, pus	ARG-N
, absent	MERC-C
CATARACT	CALC CALC-FL CAUST PHOS SIL SULPH CALEN Mag-c
, diabetic	CALC PHOS SULPH Mag-c
, geriatric	CALC-FL CAUST SIL
, injury	PHOS CALEN
CHEMOSIS	APIS ARG-N RHUS-T Kali-i
, acute	APIS RHUS-T
, chronic	Kali-i
CHERRY EYE	APIS ARG-N CALC RHUS-T Kali-i
, acute	APIS RHUS-T
, chronic	Kali-i
CONJUNCTIVITIS	ACON ALL-C ALUM APIS ARG-N ARS BELL CALC-S CARB-S EUPHR RHUS-T SABAD STAPH SULPH
, granular	ARG-N Alum Apis Calc Euphr Ham Kali-bi Merc Petr Phyt
, acute	ACON APIS BELL All-c Euphr
, chronic	SULPH
, exudate, acrid	NAT-M RHUS-T SULPH
, bland	All-c Euphr
, clear	ACON BELL
, purulent	ARG-N Calc-s Symph
CORNEA; generally	ACON APIS ARG-N ARN ARS AUR CALC KALI-BI SIL STAPH SULPH Acid-sul Calen Con Euphr Led Sol
, abrasion / injury	ACON APIS ARN STAPH CALEN Led
, 'blue-eye,'	NOSODE Acid-nit Calc Calc-fl Can-s Kali-bi Led Phos Ruta Sil
, burns	CANTH

, chlamydial infection	NOSODE Acid-nit Arg-n Colos Graph Kali-bi Hipp Lem-m Phos
, fistula	Apis Merc-s Sil
, foreign body	ACON ARN LED SIL Calen Merc-s Puls Staph Sulph
, herpes virus	NOSODE Acid-nit Calc Calc-fl Can-s Kali-bi Led Phos Ruta Sil
, keratitis	CAL SULPH Acid-sul Con Euphr
, KCS	LYC NAT-M SULPH Alum Lith-c Mez Sol Zinc
, opacity acute	ACON APIS ARG-N SIL
, chronic	SIL Cadm-s
, pannus / pigmentation	ARG-N AUR MERC-S SULPH Abr Sol
, ulcer	APIS CALC EUPHR Acid-nit Arg-n Ars Aur Bar-c Calc-p Calc-s Cann-s Chin Clem Con Crot-t Form Graph Hep Ip Kali-bi Kali-c Lach Merc Merc-s Merc-i-f Nat-c Nat-m Psor Puls Rhus-t Sang Sanic Sil Sulph Thuj
EXUDATE, acrid	Anth Carb-s Euphr Graph Hep Sulph
, bloody	Carb-s Caust Hep Kali-c Merc Puls
, thick	Chel Euphr Hep Hydr Kali-bi Lyc Nat-m Puls Sil
, yellow	PULS SIL Agar Arg-n Calc Calc-s Euphr Kali-bi Lyc Merc Sep Sulph Thuj
ECCHYMOSIS	ARN CACT LED Acid-sul Acon Bell Chlol Con Crot-h Cupr-ac Glon Ham Kali-chl Lach Lyc Nux-v Phos
EYELIDS	ARG-M ARG-N CAUST NAT-M SEP THUJ Bor Graph Petr Tub
, ectropion / entropion	ARG-M ARG-N Bor
, eczema / dermatitis	THUJ Graph Tub
, excoriation	ARS
, paralysis	ARG-N CAUST
FOREIGN BODY	ACON ARN LED SIL STAPH SULPH
, acute & surgical	ACON ARN STAPH Led
, chronic	SIL SULPH
GLAUCOMA	ACON BELL GELS PHOS RHUS-T Abel Asarum Atrax Cortico Osm
, acute	ACON BELL
, chronic	GELS PHOS RHUS-T
, painful, very	BELL Osm
HERPES	APIS CAUST MERC NAT-M PSOR Graph Nosodes Tub
, acute	Nosodes MERC-C PSOR
, chronic	APIS CAUST NAT-M Tub
HORDEOLUM	LYC PULS SEP STAPH SULPH Carb-s Con Graph
INJURY	ACON ARN CALEN STAPH Led
, direct blow	ARN Led Symph
, tear & surgery	ACON CALEN STAPH
LACHRYMATION excess	APIS ARG-N ARS CALC MERC NAT-M NUX-V PULS All-c Euphr Kali-c Sabad Squil Tell Verat Zinc

267

, acute	ARG-N ARS All-c Euphr
, chronic	APIS CALC NAT-M
, ducts blocked	ARG-M PULS SIL Acid-fl
, tear staining	ACID-PHOS RUTA SEP Nat-c. Wash with mild bicarbonate solution.
MEIBOMIAN GLAND	STAPH Aeth Clem Colch Con Phyt Staphyloc Sulph
NEW FOREST DISEASE	ARG-N CADM-S CALC CON SIL SULPH Cann-s Kali-i Merc-s
OPHTHALMIA	ACON ALL-C APIS ARN ARS BELL CALC CALC-S EUPHR LYC MERC NAT-M PSOR PULS RHUS-T SEP SIL SULPH
, periodic	ACON CALC GRAPH KALI-BI Ars Bry Con Med Sil Sulph
OPTIC NERVE, atrophy	PHOS Nux-v Tab
PAIN: air, cold, agg	HEP SIL Acon Clem Spig
, air, open, agg	HEP SIL Acon Spig
, time, diurnal	KALM SANG Hep
, evening	PULS SEP RUTA ZINC Calc Calc-s Carb-v Carb-s Kalm Petr Staph
, morning	SPIG Ambr Aur Nat-a Nux-v Puls Sep
, night	MERC MERC-S PRUN ZINC Asaf Aur Bry Chin Con Hep Kali-i Plb Spig Staph Symph
, periodic	PRUN Cedr Chin Chin-s Coloc Euphr Gels Nat-m
, right side	ACID-CARB BELL COM SANG Apis Kali-c Kalm Nat-m Prun Ran-b Sil
PARALYSIS: muscles	CAUST GELS NUX-V Con Euphr Nat-m Rhus-t Ruta Seneg
PARASITES: acute	ACON ARN LED SIL Calc Calen Merc-s Puls Staph Sulph
, chronic	ARN SIL Led
, immune mediated reaction	ACON CORTISO Echi
PUPILS	ARG-M ARG-N ARN BELL CALC GELS STRAM THUJ CUPR Chin Hell Hyos Mang Op Tarent
, contracted, both	ACON BELL THUJ Hell Op
, left	ARG-M Tarent
, right	ARG-N
, dilated, both	ARG-N BELL CALC GELS STRAM Hyos
, fit, before	ARG-N Bufo
, during	BELL STRAM Cina
, fever, during	BELL
, irregular / unequal	Op
, lazy reactions	Hell
, light, insensitive to	ARN BELL CUPR Hyos Op
RETINA: detachment	PHOS

UVEITIS / OPHTHALMIA	ACON ALL-C APIS ARN ARS BELL CALC CALC-S EUPHR LYC MERC NAT-M PSOR PULS RHUS-T SEP SIL SULPH
, acute	ACON ARN CALEN HYPER Led Symph
, chronic	ARS CALC GELS LACH MERC-C PHOS SULPH Kalm
, hypopyon	MERC-C THUJ Hep
, surgery, post	CALEN HYPER STAPH
VITREOUS opacity	MERC-I-F Gels Kali-i Phos Seneg Sulph

JAW

CANCER	ANT-T ARS HEKLA Arg -n Aur Calc Graph Merc Phos Rhus-t Sil Symph.
, bone	Ars Ant-c Hekla Symph
, left	Ars Hekla
, right	Ant-c Hekla
DISLOCATION	RHUS-T
EXOSTOSES	CALC-FL CALC-P Ang Hekla
MYOSITIS	ACON CAUST GELS HYPER MERC-S NUX-V RHUS-T Cedr Kali-i Stry
, acute	ACON HYPER Cedr
, chronic	CAUST GELS MERC-C NUX-V RHUS-T Kali-i
, neuralgic	GELS HYPER Stry
PERIOSTITIS	Acid-phos Merc Phos
TMJ: pain	CAUST RHUS-T Arum-t Ign Lach Merc Stry

NOSE

ABSCESS	HEP SIL Bell Calc Lac-c Merc Puls
, bone, osteomyelitis	ASAF AUR SIL Aur-m Hekla Hep Hippoz Phos Phyt
, chronic	CALC SIL
, painful	BELL Hep
CANCER	ARN AUR BELL CALC THUJ Cadm-m Hyos Ip Kali-s Mill Sang Teucr Visc
, chemo, detox	Cadm-m Visc
, hematoma, ethmoid	ARN BELL HYOS IP PHOS Acon Chin Crot-c Dulc Elaps Erig Ferr-p Lach Led Mill Rhus-t Sabin Tub
, secondary problems	ARN CALC Sang
CRACKS	Alum Ant-c Graph Kres
, corners, at	Graph
, nostrils	Alum Ant-c Graph
EXUDATE: acrid	ACID-NIT ALL-C AM-M ARS ARS-I ARUM-T FERR-I GRAPH IOD KRES MERC NUX-V
, colour, brown	SEP Aur Carb-an Lyc Symph
, greenish	KALI-BI KALI-I LAC-C MERC PULS SEP Acid-nit Alum Ars-i Berb Bov Bry Calc-fl Carb-v Ferr-i Nat-c Phos Rhus-t Sil Stict Teucr

269

, red	ACID-NIT ALUM CARB-AN CHIN LACH PHOS SULPH Agar Ars Apis Aur Bell Bor Calc Ferr-p Hep Kali-bi Kali-c Mag-m Nat-a Nat-c Plb Stann Zinc
, pus	ACID-CARB PSOR Elaps Hep
EIPH / Epistaxis	ANT-T ARN BELL HAM LACH LYC MERC PHOS Am-m Bapt Carb-v Cinnm Croc Hyos Ip Kres Mill Meli Sabin Sec
, arterial	BELL PHOS Cinnm Hyos Meli Mill
, colour, brown	SEP Aur Carb-an Lyc Syph
, dark and thin	CROT-H HAM SEC Acid-nit Carb-v Lach Sul
, greenish	KALI-BI KALI-I LAC-C MERC PULS SEP Acid-nit Alum Ars-i Berb Bov Bry Calc-fl Carb-v Ferr-i Nat-c Phos Rhus-t Sil Stict Teucr
, red	ACID-NIT ALUM CARB-AN CHIN LACH PHOS SULPH Agar Ars Apis Aur Bell Bor Calc Ferr-p Hep Kali-bi Kali-c Mag-m Nat-a Nat-c Plb Stann Zinc
, clotted	ANTH BELL LACH NUX-V Chin Croc Sec
, cough, with	ANT-T CINNM DROS IP MELI MILL Epin Ferr-p Ham Led Puls Sulph Tril
, epistaxis	ARN LACH Mill RHUS-T Cinnm
, lower airway disease	ARN LYC Am-m
, persistent	FERR PHOS SULPH Bapt Carb-v Croc Crot-h
, stringy	CUPR LACH MERC Croc Kres
, venous	ARN HAM LACH NUX-V Carb-v Croc Sec
LUPUS	ACID-FL APIS ARG-M ARS CORTISO SEP SULPH Aur-i Alum Echi Eleuth Graph Kres Phyt
OBSTRUCTED	ARN CALC KALI-BI LYC NAT-M NUX-V RHUS-T SIL SULPH Am-c Con Kali-i Rhod Teucr
, air, open in	NAT-M RHUS-T SULPH Rhod
, chronic	CALC SIL THUJ Con
, exudative	KALI-BI LACH THUJ
, foreign body	ARN SIL Hep Myris
, left sided	THUJ Arum-t Mag-m
, right sided	GELS MERC SULPH Sars Teucr
, room, in	PULS THUJ Ant-c Iod Kali-i
, unilateral	LACH NUX-V STAPH SULPH Hep Pyrog Rhod
POLYPS	CALC LYC PHOS Nosodes Teucr
RHINITIS	ACID-FL ACID-NIT ACID-PHOS ANTH APIS ARS BELL BRY CALC CALC-P CAUST DULC FERR-P HEP KALI-BI LACH LYC MERC MERC-S NAT-M NUX-V PHOS PSOR SEP STAPH SULPH
, air, cold agg	ACID-PHOS MERC Kali-ars
, open, agg	ACID-NIT CALC-P DULC KALI-BI PHOS PULS Aeth Graph
, chronic	APIS Canth KALI-BR LYC SIL SULPH Brom Cycl Hippoz Sang Tell

, cough	ACID-NIT ANTH ARS CAUST FERR-P GELS NAT-M PHOS RHUS-T SULPH All-c Colch Euphr Graph Ip Kali-i Spong Tell
, dry and chronic	SIL STICT Carb-v Dulc Nat-m Spong Sulph
, fever	ACON ARS BELL BRY Hep Seneg Tarent
, left sided	All-c Arum-t
, right sided	ARS Calc-s Kali-i Sang
, unilateral	PHOS Phyt Rhod
, violent	ARS BRY CALC Carb-v LYC STAPH All-c Arum-t Carb-v
, watery, air open	ACID-NIT ARS PULS SULPH THUJ Acid-carb Iod
, mornings	ACON NUX-V SEP SULPH THUJ Cycl Euphr
SINUSITIS	HYDR KALI-BI LYC MERC PULS SIL THUJ Acid-fl Ars Calc Cupr Echi Hep Hippoz Kali-chl Kali-i Lem-m Med Nux-v Sang
, frontal	HYDR KALI-BI LYC MERC PULS SIL THUJ Ars Calc Cupr Kali-chl Kali-i Nat-m Nux-v Puls Sang
, infected	ARS CALC CUPR KALI-BI LYC MED MERC NUX-V PULS SIL THUJ Asaf Hydr Kali-i Sang
, sneezing, with	AM-M ARS CARB-S CARB-V COCC MERC NUX-V PULS SULPH
SNUFFLING	NUX-V SAMB Ars Aur Med Thuj. Feline section.

ABDOMEN

ABSCESS	HEP MERC SIL
ASCITES	APIS APOC-C ARS CANN-S DIG LYC TER
, cancer	APIS ARS Apoc
, cardiovascular	APIS Dig Queb
, infection	APIS LYC Ter
, hepatic	ARS LYC
, urogenital	Cann-s Ter
BLANKETING, agg	ARG-N BOV CALC CROT-C LACH LYC NUX-V Apis Carb-v Caust Chin Crot-h Graph Hep Kres Lac-c Nat-s Sars Sep Spong Stann
BLOAT / Tympany	ANTH ARG-N ARS CAUST LACH LYC MAG-P PHOS SULPH Carb-v Chin Cocc Colch Eucal Hyos Kali-c Ter
, prevention	LYC MAG-P
BORBORYGMI	ALOE CROT-T NER PODO PULS SULPH Acid-nit Agar Ars Cocc Gamb Hell Laur Lyc Nat-m Nux-v Phos Psor Raph Sil
DISTENSION	Abies-c Abs Aesc-g Alf All-c Aloe Am-c Am-caust Anac Ant-c
ENLARGED abdomen	CALC SANIC SEP SULPH Bar-c Bar-i Coloc Iod Iris Lyc Psor Thuj
HERNIA	BELL LYC NUX-V Op Plb
, birth, from	AUR NUX-V

, incarcerated	BELL NUX-V OP Acid-sul All-c Carb-v Cocc Coff Dig Plb Sulph Tab
, inguinal	LYC NUX-V Acid-carb Acid-nit Acid-sul All-c Alum Apis Asar Aur Calc Carb-v Cocc Coff Dig Mag-c Op Rhus-t Sil Spig Sulph Verat Zinc
, lymphadenopathy	ACID-NIT BAD CALC CLEM DULC HEP LACH MERC MERC-S SULPH Apis Syph Thuj Tub
, mesenteric	CALC Ars Ars-i Aur Bar-c Bar-i Carb-an Con Form Grat Hep Iod Nat-s Ner Merc
, neonatal	AUR NUX-V
, simple, small	THUJ
, surgical	BELL LACH NUX-V Mill Op Plb
JAUNDICE	ACON ARS BERB CARD CHEL CHINA CROT-H HYDR IRIS JUG LACH LEPT LYC MYRIC NAT-S PHOS PODO SEN THYR
PAIN: acute	COLOC Anth Nux-v Plb
, air, cool, agg	PULS NUX-V
, bending, amel	COLOC KALI-I PULS Bell Bov Caust Chin Colch Cop Iris Lach Mag-p Rheum Stann
, colic, with	ALOE ANTH COLOC DIOS GAMB PODO Arg-n Ars Bell Bry Chin Colch Cop Gran Ip Kali-c Lyc Mag-c Nat-s Rheum Sulph Trom Verat
, defecating, after agg	ACID-NIT SULPH Acid-pic Acid-sul Aloe Carb-v Chin Coloc Merc Nat-m Podo Puls Rheum Zinc
, amel	COLCH COLOC GAMB Calc-p Carb-v Nat-s Rheum Rhus-t
, before	Bry Psor Rumx
, during	BRY SULPH Agar Aran Carb-an Carb-v Con Dulc Graph Kali-c Lil-t Lyc Mag-c, Podo Rheum Rhus-t Rhus-v Sep Tab Zinc
, diarrhoea, before	BRY Psor Rumx
, eating, after	GRAPH STAPH VERAT Acid-phos Acid-sul All-c Alum Anth Ars Carb-v Colch Coloc Gran Kali-c Kali-p Lyc Mag-c Nat-c Nat-m Nux-m Nux-v Phos Puls Rhod Rhus-t Sars Stann Stront-c Sulph Thuj Zinc
, during	MAG-C Coloc Naja Nux-v Ran-b
, excitement, after	IGN Anth Staph
, fever, during	ANT-C ARS CARB-V RHUS-T Anth Cina
, flatulence, with	VERAT Alum Chin Lyc Nat-m Nat-s
, motion, agg	BELL BRY NUX-V Acid-nit Cocc Gels Kalm Rhus-t Sulph
, amel	Con Cycl Puls
, palpation, agg	BELL Carb-s Coff Lac-c Lach Mez Nux-v Ran-b Sulph
, periodical	ANTH CUPR NUX-V Ars Calc Chin Cimic Coloc Cupr-ars Gels Ip
, pregnancy, during	NUX-V Ars Bell Mag-p Nat-s Plb Podo Stann
, time, afternoon	LYC Alum Ars Coloc iris Kali-n
, evening	PULS Bell Calc Chin Dulc Iris Lyc Mag-m Mez Petr Phos Rhus-t Seneg Sep Stront-c Sulph Valer Zinc
, midnight	ARG-N COCC Acid-nit Chin

, air, cold, agg	Puls Nux-v
, amel	Sulph
, vomiting, with	Ars Ip Nux-v
PERITONITIS	ACON ANT-T ARS BELL BRY ECHI LACH LYC PHOS RHUS-T Acid-acet Colch Hyos Pyrog Ter
, chronic	APIS LYC MERC SULPH
, FIP	NOSODE Canth Card Colos Tub
, injury / surgery, from	ACON ARS BELL BRY Colch LACH MERC SULPH ANT-T Myris
, parturient, post	ACON BELL MERC SULPH Myris
, surgery, pre	BRY Colch Echi Myris
TYMPANY	ANTH ARG-N ARS BRY CARB-V CHIN COCC COLCH HYOS LACH LYC PHOS TER URAN
, constipation, with	LACH
, eating, after	CARB-V Nat-m Nux-m Sep Thuj
, during	CARB-V CHIN KALI-C LYC NUX-V SULPH Anth Ant-c Bor Bry Carb-an Colch Graph Kres Lil-t Nat-c Nat-m Nux-m Puls Rhus-t Sep Sil Thuj Zinc
, juveniles	BAR-C CALC CAUST LYC SULPH URAN-N Cina
, painful	ACON ARS BRY CAUST LACH MERC RHUS-T Bar-c Hyos
, time, afternoon	LYC Calc Carb-v Cast-eq Sulph
, morning	Anth Nux-v Sulph
, night	Mag-c Sulph

LIVER

ABSCESS	BELL LACH LYC MERC NUX-V MED Kali-c
CANCER	Nosode LYC PHOS Colos Cadm-s Carc Hydr
CHOLECYSTITIS	BELL LACH LYC Chlol Pyrog
CIRRHOSIS	CUPR HEP LACH LYC NUX-V PHOS Acid-sul Ars-i Aur-m Card-m Chin Hydr Iod Nux-m
FATTY DEGENERATION	CALC LYC MERC PHOS Acid-pic Chel
HEPATITIS	ACON ARS BELL CARD-M CHEL CHIN LYC NUX-V PHOS Acid-nit Anth Bry Calc Carc Hep Hydr Nosodes Kali-c Mag-m Merc Nat-m Podo Psor Tell Apis Bapt Ign Iod Nat-c Staph Sulph
JAUNDICE	ACID-NIT ACON BELL CARD-M CHEL CHIN CHION CON CROT-H IOD LACH LYC MERC NAT-S NUX-V PHOS PLB PODO SEP
, acute	Chel
, blood disorders, from	Chloram Chlorpro. *Anaemia section*
, chronic	Chion Con Phos
, oedema	AUR-M CALC CARD-M LAC-D LACH LYC Acid-fl Apoc Chim Chin Ferr Nat-m Nux-v
, flatulence, with	Anth Carb-v Chin Lyc Nux-v
, liver, primary	ARS LACH LYC NAT-S PHOS BERB Cean Lept Tarax

273

, neonates	ACON ELAT MERC NAT-S NUX-V Bov Chel Chin
OEDEMA	CALC FERR LACH LYC NAT-M NUX-V Acid-fl Apoc Aur-m Card-m Chim Chin
PAIN	ACID-NIT BELL CARD-M CHEL CHIN CHION CON CROT-H IOD LACH LYC MERC NAT-S NUX-V PLB PODO PULS
TONIC: overeating	ANT-C BRY NAT-S NUX-V PULS Carb-v Card-m
VOMITING	MERC NUX-V Iris Podo

PANCREAS

CANCER	Nosode Calc-ars Carb-an Carc Con Hydr Iod Phyt
DIABETES MELLITUS	ACID-PHOS ARG-M LYC PHOS URAN-N Acet-acid Carc Chion Helon Ins Iod Iris Nat-s Nosode Pancr Plb Sulphonam Syzyg Ter
, juvenile type 1	ACID-PHOS PHOS URAN-N Carc Ins Pancr Syzyg Ter
, adult-onset type 2	ARG-M URAN-N Acid-acet Helon Ins Pancr Sulfonam Syzyg Ter
PANCREATIC insufficiency	Ins Pancr
PANCREATITIS	ARS BELL PHOS Acid-bor Bar-c Beryl Bor Carb-an Con Hed Ins Iod Iris Kali-i Nosode Spong
, acute	ACID-BOR BAR BOR CON FLOR IRIS KALI-I MERC-S PANCR Bell Chion Coloc Iod Phos Spong
, chronic	Carb-an Con Iod Pancr Spong

GASTROINTESTINAL TRACT

MOUTH

ABSCESS	HEP MERC SIL
, recurrent	CAUST HEP MERC Bar-c Lyc Nux-v
AEROPHAGY	Allox Aran Arg-m Asar Bell-p Hir Rauw Tell
APPETITE, capricious	BRY CHIN CINA Acid-n Coc-c Cur Hep Ign Iod Ip Mag-m Phos Puls Sang Ther Tub
, good, diarrhoea, with	COCC LACH NAT-M SULPH Acid-sul Agar Alum Ars Bar-c Chin Cycl Crot-c Hell Lyc Phos Rhus-t Sil Sep Tub
, dysentery, with	NUX-V
, weight loss, with	PETR Acid-fl Asaf Calc Iod Lyc Ner Stram Sulph Verat
, great, constantly	Kali-bi Merc Nat-c Nat-m
, pica	ACID-PHOS Arg-m Bry Calc Calc-p Chel Cycl Ferr Hep Lyss Mang Nat-m Sulph
, satiated, easily	CALC CINA IOD NAT-M Abrot Bar-c Calc-p Caust Chin Kali-i Lyc Mag-c Nux-v Sil Sulph
BITING: nails, at	ARUM-T CARC CINA Acon Am-br Ant-t Ars Bar-c Hyos Lyc Nat-m Senec Sil Sulph
BLEEDING	CHIN CROT-H HEP PHOS Acid-sul Acon Arn Ars Arum-t Bell Carb-s Carb-v Chel Ferr Ip Kres Lach Merc Merc-s Nux-v Rhus-t Sec.
, easily	HEP PHOS Merc

, gums	CARB-V CROT-H HEP KRES LACH MERC NAT-M PHOS Acid-phos Acid-sul Am-c Anac Ant-c Arg-n Bov Carb-an Cist Ham Iod Kali-chl Kali-p Mag- m Sep Zinc
, lips	ARUM-T Anth Ars Brom Bry Ign Lach
, oozing	Acid-sul Chel Phos
, palate	Crot-t Lach Phos
, blood, blackish	Carb-v Crot-h Lach
, clotted	Caust
, dental	ARN LACH PHOS Calen Ham Kres
, gums	MERC PHOS Carb-v Crot-h Hep
, injury	ARN LACH PHOS
BOILS: corners, of	ANT-C
CANCER	SEP Colos Con Cund
, epithelial	Cic Con Hydr
, epulis	Acid-nit Borax Calc-fl Calc-s Hekla Hep Merc Rhus-t Sil Staph
, lips	CON CUND Ars Aur-m Carb-an Cic Cist Kres Lach Lyc Sep Sil
, lower	SEP Ars Cist Clem Con Lyc Phos Sil
, ulcerated	CON Ars Aur-m Clem Kali-bi Phos
DISCOLORATION: blue	PLB
, dark	BAPT Aur Bor
, pale	FERR Merc Plb Chel Cycl Staph
, red	KRES MERC Anth Apis Aur Bell Carb-an Dulc Lob Lach Merc-s Nat-s Sep
, white	MERC Acid-nit Acid-phos Crot-h Ferr Kali-bi Staph
DRY: thirst, with	BRY NAT-M Bar-c Camph Carb-s Chin Lach Merc Nat-c Nux-m Phos, Rhus-t Stram
ECZEMA / dermatitis	Mez Nat-m
, corners, of	Arund Graph Hep Rhus-t
, lips, of	Ant-c Mez Rhus-v
ERUPTIONS: corners	ACID-NIT BRY CALC GRAPH MERC Ant-c Bell Cic Cund Hep Ign Kres, Lyc Mang Nat-m Petr Phos Sep Sil
, crusts	ACID-NIT GRAPH Led Merc Mez Nat-m
, pimples	ANTHR ARS KALI-I KALI-C KRES Bar-c Dulc Mag-c
GINGIVITIS	KRES NAT-M SIL Alumn Arg-n Ars Cham Hecla Kres Merc Merc-c Nux-v Calc-s Hep Kali-n Rhus-t
, dental	MERC NAT-M
, offensive	Kres MERC SIL
GUMS: pain	ARS MERC STAPH Agar Anth Arn Ars-i Bell Bov Calc Carb-an Carb-v Caust Crot-h Ham Hep Lach Lyss Sil
, receding	CARB-V KALI-P MERC SIL Acid-phos Am-c Ant-c Arg-n Aur-m-n Bapt Calc Dulc Graph Iod Kali-c Kali-i Kres Merc-s Nat-s Par Phos Staph Sulph Zinc

275

HALITOSIS	ACID-NIT ANTH ARN ARS AUR LACH MERC MERC-S NUX-V PSOR SULPH Ars-i Carb-v Chel Colch Crot-h Eup-per Graph Kali-i Kres Sanic Tub
, mornings	PULS Arg-n Aur Camph Nux-v Sil
, musty	Alum Crot-h Nat-c Rhus-t
, nephritis, with	ARS Colch Iod Kali-i
, smell, cheese	AUR Hep Kali-c
, fish	Sanic
, musty	Alum Crot-h
, offensive	ARN ARS MERC PSOR Carb-ac Eup-per Kres Tub
, sour	NUX-V SULPH Eup-per Graph
, urine	Graph
LIPS	Acid-nit Bor Hep Merc Rhus-t Thuj
, abscess	Hep Merc
, cracked	ACID-NIT BRY CALC MERC NAT-M SEP Graph
, acute	ACID-NIT NAT-M SEP
, chronic	BRY CALC Graph
, infected	ACID-NIT CALC Graph MERC NAT-M Graph
, infection, during	Apis Bell Merc Thuj
PALATE	AUR MERC Acid-nit Acid-phos Apis Aur-m Cinnb Kali-bi Lach Lyc Merc-s Nat-m Phos Phyt Sang
, sloughing	Acid-nit Kali-bi Lach Merc Phos Syph
, vesicles	ARS NAT-M Acid-sul Anac Bar-c Calc Canth Carb-an Chel Kali-ars Mag-c Merc Nat-c Staph Thuj
SALIVA: bloody	BUFO CROT-C MAG-C PHOS Bell Carb-v Crot-h Hyos Kali-i Merc Merc-s Nat-m Nux-v Rhus-t Sec Sulph
, offensive	ACID-NIT MERC Caps Dig Dulc Iod Lach Manc Merc-s Merc-i-r Petr
, viscid	CAPS KALI-BI RHUS-T Arum-t Bar-c Bar-m Bry Carb-v Crot-h Hydr Lach Nat-s Phyt
STOMATITIS	MERC NUX-V SULPH Astac Kali-i
, primary	NUX-V SULPH
, secondary	MERC Astac Kali-i
THIRST: great	ARS BRY NAT-M PHOS SULPH VERAT Acid-acet Acon Chin Cocc Eup-per Ferr-p Lac-d Lycps Merc Podo Stram Thyr
, mornings	ACID-NIT Graph Nux-v Stram Verat
, night	CYCL SIL Acon Ant-c Ars Calc Coff Eup-per Hep Kali-c Lach Mag-c Merc Nat-m Nat-s Phos Rhus-t Spong Sulph Thuj Zinc
, often	ARS Bell Chin Coloc Nat-a Sulph
, small quantities often	ARS LYC Chin Hell Lach Rhus-t Sulph
, thirstless	ACID-PHOS APIS ANT-T CHIN COLCH GELS HELL NUX-M PULS SABAD Acid-hydr Aesc Agn Am-m Ant-c Arg-n Ars Asaf Bell Bov Calen Camph Con Cycl Ferr Ip Kali-c Lyc Mang Ner Op Samb Sep Staph Stram Tarent

, fat, agg	ANG CHIN CYCL PETR PTEL PULS Ars Bell Bry Calc-fl Carb-an Carc Colch Hep Ip Merc Nat-m Sep Sulph
, fish, agg	Acid-fl Kali-s Medus Plb Puls Sep
, meat, agg	Ars Bry Calc Chin Colch Ferr Kali-bi Kali-c Lyss Ptel Puls
, milk, agg	AETH CALC-S CHIN CON LAC-D MAG-M NAT-C SEP STAPH SULPH
, starch, agg	BERB COP NAT-M NAT-S Acid-acet All-c Carb-an Carb-v Kali-c Lach Lyc Plb Puls Pyrog
THRUSH	ACID-SUL BOR MERC NAT-M Allox Kali-chl Nat-hchls Prot Thal
VESICLES	ARS MERC NAT-M Am-m Bor Caps Carb-an Kali-c Kali-i Mag-c
, acute	NAT-M Am-m Bor Caps Mag-c
, chronic	ARS Bor Carb-an Kali-c Kali-i
VOMITING	ANT-T APIS ARG-N ARS BRY CUPR FERR HEP IGN NUX-V PHOS PULS SIL VERAT Acid-carb Aeth Apom Cadm-s Chin Cocc Colch Ip Iris Kres Petr Tab Valer Verat-v Acon Agar Anthr Bell Calc Calc-p Dulc Graph Kali-i Lach Merc Nat-m
WARTS	ACID-NIT ARG-N CAUST THUJ
, lips	ACID-NIT Caust

TONGUE

TONGUE: aphthous	BOR Acid-sul Jug-r Lach Merc Merc-cy Nat-m Phos Sulph
, bleeding	ARUM-T BOR Lach Merc Podo
, burns	CANTH
, cancer	KALI-CY Acid-nit Alumn Apis Ars Aur Aur-m Carb-an Con Hydr Kali-i Lach Phos Phyt Sil
, epithelial	Hydr Kali-c Thuj Ars
, coated	Ant-c Bry Nux-v
, dirty looking	MERC MERC-S MERC-I-F Ars Bapt Kali-chl Lach Mag-c Myric Op Pyrog Sep
, red	ARS CHEL MERC SULPH Bapt Canth Crot-h Gels Iris Kali-bi Lach Merc- i-f Phos Plb Pyrog Rhus-t Sang Tub
, thick	CROT-C DULC GELS Anac Ars Carb-v Glon Lach Mag-p Nat-c
, white	ANT-C Ars Bell Chin Kali-m Puls Sulph
, yellow	MERC-I-F NAT-P Merc Nux-v
, cracked	ACID-FL ACID-NIT AIL ARS ARS-I ARUM-T HYOS PHOS RHUS-T SPIG Bor
, ecchymosis	PHOS Acid sul
, excoriation	SEP Acid-carb Acid-nit Aur Calc Canth Cist Lach Merc Merc-s Nux-v Phos Ran-s Sil
, flabby	CAMPH MERC Acid-phos Hydr Lyss Lycps Mag-m
, glossitis	Bell Kres Lept Merc Phos Rhus-t Sec
, ulcers	Bor Merc-s
, herpes	Nat-m Rhus-t Zinc
, indurate	HYOS NAT-M Arg-n Atro Aur-m Bar-c Carb-v Merc

277

, mapped	NAT-M TARAX Ars Kali-bi Lach Merc Merc-s Ran-s Rhus-t Ter Tub
, motion, difficult	HYOS LACH PHOS Aesc Ars Bell Cic Colch Kali-br Lyc Merc Mygal Nat-c Puls Stram
, nodosites	CARB-AN Sil
, pain	Apis Arum-t Calc Con Ham Kali-c Merc Phyt Plb Puls Thuj Vesp Vip
, paralysis	CAUST GELS LYC OP PLB Acid-hydr Acon Apis Arn Bar-c Bell Cadm-s Cocc Con Crot-c Cupr Dulc Hell Hyos Lach Naja Nux-m Rheum Rhus-t Stram
, geriatric	Bar-c Plb
, left, drawn to	OP Bell Glon Op Plb
, right	OP Cur Nux-m
, protrusion, difficult	LACH Apis Caust Gels Hyos Lyc Mygal
, stiff	BELL RHUS-T Ars Berb Calc-p Carb-v Colch Con Crot-c Crot-h Hell Lach Laur Lyc Merc Nat-c Nat-m Stram
, swollen, huge	*Kali-chl*
, ulcers	LYC SANIC Acid-fl Graph
, vesicles	AM-C APIS ARS LYC NAT-M RHUS-T Am-m Arg-m Bar-c Bor Canth Caps Carb-an Caust Graph Ham Hell Kali-c Lach Mag-c Merc Nat-a Nux- v Sep Staph Thuj
, warts	AUR-M
, withered	Kres
ULCERS: mouth	ACID-NIT ARS AUR LACH MERC-S NAT-M PSOR Bor Iod Kali-i Kres
, cancerous	ARS CON Aur-m Clem Kali-bi Phos
, colour, black	MERC Plb
, grey	MERC
, white	Acid-sul Kali-i
, yellow	Acid-sul Plb
, offensive	ARS Acid-fl Bapt Bor LACH
, painful	ACID-NIT ARS Acid-fl Carb-v

TEETH

ABSCESS: root	HEP SIL Bar-c Calc Hekla Lyc Merc
CRUMBLING: decay	Acid-fl Bor Calc Calc-fl Calc-p Mez Plan
, juveniles	KRES STAPH Acid-fl Calc Calc-fl Calc-p Mez
, rapid	ACID-FL SEP Calc Calc-p Carb-v Merc Syph
DENTISTRY: antibacterial	CALC-P MERC THUJ Kres Mez
, extractions	CALEN Emerald
, haemorrhage	ARN Mill
, pain	ARN HYPER PHOS Coff
DENTITION: delayed	ANTH CALC CALC-P MERC SIL STAPH Acid-fl Chin Kres Tub
, misaligned	CALC-P

, painful	ANTH CALC-P
DISCOLOURED	MERC STAPH Chin
GRIND	APIS BELL Hyos
TARTAR	ACID-PHOS ARS PHOS RHUS-T Acid-fl Ail Bapt Chin Frag Hyos

SALIVARY SYSTEM

SALIVATION: deficient	BELL KALI-Br MERC STRAM
, ducts blocked	BELL MERC STRAM Abel
, infection	ACON APIS BELL Hep Merc-i-f
, parotitis	ACON APIS BELL CALC-FL Phyt
, profuse / excessive	PULS Lyss
, ranula	ACON APIS BELL NAT-M Ambr

THROAT AND PHARYNX

ABSCESS	HEP MERC
CANCER	THUJ Carb-an Carc Colos Led Nosode Tarent
EPIGLOTTIS	ACON APIS CAUST GELS Kali-i Lath Spong
, entrapment	CAUST GELS PHOS Kali-i Lath
, paralysis	CAUST GELS Lath
GUTTURAL POUCH	ARG-M KALI-BI MERC Calc-s Cortico Kali-i Strep-equi nosode
, acute infection	ACON KALI-BI Bapt
PHARYNGITIS	ACID-NIT ARG-M BELL BERB BRY CALC GELS HEP IGN MERC SIL STRAM Acid-fl Aeth Allox Ambr Anthr Astac Caps Carb-s Carb-v Graph Hydr Iod Kali-i Kali-m Lac-c Nosodes Phyt Thymol
, acrid	ACID-NIT CAUST MERC Aesc
, aphthous	BELL BRY GELS IGN Aeth
, cheesy	BELL PSOR Kali-m
, oedema	APIS LACH Crot-h Kali-i
, follicular / lymphoid	NAT-M SEP Anthr Astac Carb-s Carb-v Con Graph Lac-c
, inflamed	ACID-NIT ARG-M ARG-N BERB CALC KALI-BI LACH MERC PHOS SEP SULPH Acid-fl Carb-s Hep Hydr Kali-i Phyt Thymol Wye
, mucous	ARG-M ARS KALI-BI PULS Ambr Phyt
STRANGLES	NOSODE ACON APIS GELS HEP KALI-BI SIL Bapt Strep-equi nosode
, acute	ACON Bapt KALI-BI
, chronic / abscess	Hep SIL
, prophylaxis	Nosode

LARYNX

CONSTRICTED	ACON BELL PHOS Iod Mang

, injury	ACON BELL
, surgery pre / post	ACON PHOS
LARYNGITIS	BELL CALC-FL GELS HEP PHOS SIL Dros Phyt Rumx Thymol
, chronic	CALC-FL Dros Phyt
, follicular, 2-y-o	BELL HEP IGN IOD NAT-M Acid-nit Ail Arg-n Arum-t Hydr Kali-bi Kali-chl Kali-i Lac-c Merc Merc-cy Merc-i-r Phyt Sec Wye
, primary	BELL PHOS SIL
, rhinotracheitis	NOSODE ACON CALC CARB-V CAUST CINNB FERR-P HIPPOZ KALI-BI PHOS SPONG SYPH Dros
PARALYSIS; larynx	ACON ANT-T APIS ARG-N ARN CAUST HEP IGN LACH All-c Beryl Chlorpro Lath Plb Sec
, acute	ARN APIS CAUST LACH All-c Iod Lath
, chronic, LSLH	ARG-N LACH Chlorpro Lath Plb
VOCAL CORDS	APIS ARG-N ARN CAUST LACH PHOS STRAM SULPH Alumn Carb-v Kali-i Mang Mosch Seneg
, acute	APIS LACH STRAM
, chronic	SULPH Alumn Carb-v Kali-i Seneg
, voice lost / aphonia	LACH SULPH Alumn Carb-v Kali-i Seneg

THYROID

, hyperthyroidism	CALC NAT-M Anhal Aqua-m Iod Kali-i Nosode Spong
, hypothyroidism	CALC CORTISO NAT-M Brom Fuc Iod Kali-i Nosode Spong
, thyroiditis	CALC CORTISO ECHI Kali-i Nosode

TONSILS

TONSILLITIS	ACID-NIT CALC-P HEP LACH LYC MERC MERC-S SIL CALC-FL CALC-i Alumn Bapt Bar-c Bar-m Guai Lac-c Tub
, acute	ACID-NIT LACH LYC MERC MERC-C Bapt Hep Lac-c
, chronic	CALC-FL CALC-i CALC-P LYC SIL Alumn Bar-c Bar-m Guai Tub

OESOPHAGUS

BLOCKED	CALC CUPR IGN LACH MERC PULS Alum Cact Carb-v Hyos Kali-c Orni
, geriatric	LACH MERC Alum Cact Carb-v
, juvenile	CUPR IGN PULS Hyos
, traumatic	LACH MERC Alum Cact
OESOPHAGITIS	ACID-NIT ARS CAUST GELS PHOS RHUS-T Alumn
, reflux	ACID-NIT ARS CAUST Alumn
, secondary	ARS CAUST PHOS RHUS-T
MEGAOESOPHAGUS	PHOS Bar-c Bar-m Con
SPIROCERCA	CALC-FL PHOS SIL Carbo-an Con Cund Kali-i Phyt

STOMACH

ABOMASUM	ARG-N AUR BELL LYC NUX-V PULS SIL URAN-N VERAT Chin Colch Raph Tarent
, abomasitis	LYC NUX-V Verat
, dilatation/ displace	ARG-N LYC URAN-N Colch
CANCER	ARS LYC PHOS Acid-carb Bism Cadm-s Carb- Con Cund Hydr
DILATATION	ARG-N LYC NAT-S NUX-V URAN-N Bor Carb-s Carb-v Chin Colch
, chronic	Carb-v
ERUCTATION	ANTH ARG-N ARN FERR NAT-M PLAT PULS SULPH Asaf Carb-v Petr Acid-n Anac Bar-c Caust Chin Colch Hep Kali-c Lach Lyc Nat-c Nat-s Nux-v
, acute	ANTH ARG-N NAT-M Asaf
, chronic	ANTH ARN SULPH Petr
FOREIGN BODY	NAT-M CUPR Ornith
GASTRITIS	ANT-T ARG-N ARS BELL KALI-BI NUX-V PHOS Carb-v Hydr
, acute	ARS KALI-BI PHOS
, chronic	ARG-N ANT-T Carb-v Hydr NUX-V
GASTROENTERITIS	ARG-N ARS CUPR RHUS-T Bapt Colch Mag-s
HICCOUGH	IGN NUX-V STRAM Bism Coloc Hyos Mag-m Nicc
, juveniles	IGN Hyos Mag-m
PYLORIC STENOSIS	BRY CALC LYC NAT-M NUX-V SULPH Alumn Colch Coloc Grat Hydr Op Ornith Raph
TORSION	ARG-N BELL LYC NUX-V SIL URAN-N VERAT Tarent
ULCERATION stomach	ACID-NIT ARG-N KALI-BI LACH LYC NUX-V URAN-N Coloc Mez Paeon
, bile	ANTH ARS NUX-V Chel Ip Verat
, blood	ARN FERR HAM PHOS Carb-v Crot-h
, coughing, with	BRY ANT-T Dros Hep Ip Kali-c
, diarrhoea, with	ARG-N ARS Ip Verat
, drinking, after	ARS BRY Bism Cadm
, paroxysmal	ARS Colch Crot-t Lob PHOS
, projectile	NUX-V Aeth Con Petr Verat
, pyloric stenosis	ANTH ARS NUX-V Chel Ip Ornith Verat
, suckling, when	SIL Aeth Verat
, transport, during	Acid-carb Cocc Petr Tab
, worms	FERR Cina Phyt Sabad Sang

INTESTINES

BLEEDING	CHIN COLCH HAM IP PHOS Acon Ambr Ars Cact Canth Coll Crot-h Erig Eucal Ferr-p Kali-bi Kali-i Kali-p Merc Nux-v Psor Sec Senec Sil Tril Urt-u

BORBORYGMI	LYC NAT-S PULS Aloe Carb-v Hydr Jatr Mag-c
, defecating, before	NAT-M NAT-S SULPH Mag-c
, Diarrhoea, with	Aloe Hydr
, eating, after	PULS SULPH Carb-v Chin
, flatus, amel	LYC NAT-S Carb-v
CANCER	ARS LYC Acid-carb Alum Bism Cadm-s Carb-v Con Cund Hydr
COCCIDIOSIS	Acid-but All-s Hir Ip Merc Nosode
ENTERITIS	ACID-PHOS APIS ARS BELL BRY CUPR LACH LYC MERC NAT-S PHOS SEP STRAM RHUS-T THUJ Calad Camph Card-m Colch Crot-h Nosodes Plb Samb
, acute	ARS CUPR Camph Ip Verat
HAIR BALL	BRY CALC LYC NAT-M NUX-V SULPH Alumn Colch Coloc Grat Hydr Op Ornith Raph
, abdomen enlarged	LYC Alumn Hydr Op Ornith Raph
, painful	BRY NUX-V Colch Coloc Grat Ornith
IBD	APIS BELL CORTISO LACH MERC RHUS-T THUJ Acid-oxal Carb-v Gaert-b Mag-s Op Urt-u
, chronic	APIS BRY CORTISO MERC Acid-oxal Hydr Urt-u
OBSTRUCTION	ACID-NIT AUR ARG-N CHIN COLCH PULS RAPH SIL TARENT VERAT
, acute	Chin Colch Ornith Raph
, chronic	LYC OP Alumn Hydr Ornith Raph
ULCER intestine	ACID-NIT ARS CARB-V Calc Coloc Kali-bi Lyc Ter
, bleeding	TER Caps Merc Phos

COLIC - EQUINE

COLIC: excite, after	ACID-NIT ACON ARG-N ARS BELL GELS
, feeding, after	ACON ANT-T SULPH VERAT All-c Carb-v Colch Graph Nat-c
, acute	ACON SULPH All-c Colch
, develops slowly	SULPH ANT-T Carb-v Graph
, ileocecal entrapment	ACID-NIT ACON BELL BRY MERC PHOS Carb-s Chin Colch Plb
, impaction	BRY CALC LYC NAT-M NUX-V SULPH Alumn Grat Hydr Op Ornith
, acute	BRY LYC NUX-V Ornith Hydr
, chronic	CALC LYC NAT-M OP Alum Grat Ornith
, intussusception	ACON ARS BELL VERAT Chin Coloc Op Plb
, meconium, retention	CALC NUX-V SULPH Ornith Zinc
, prophylaxis	NUX-V Ornith
, recurrent	ACID-NIT ARG-NIT CALC-FL NUX-V URAN-N CALEN Coloc Mez Paeon
, herpes virus	Nosode
, stasis of bowel	PHOS RHUS-T Alum Op Plb

, surgery	ACON ARN BELL RHUS-T STAPH STRAM THUJ VERAT CALEN Bell-p Carb-v Op
, laminitis risk	ACON ARG-N Crot-h
, pre	BELL STAPH Bell-p
, post	ARN STAPH THUJ Bell-p Carb-v Op
, twist	ACON LYC BELL URAN-N VERAT Carb-v Colch
, tympanitic	ACON LYC URAN-N VERAT Am-c Carb-v Colch
, ulceration	ACID-NIT ARG-NIT KALI-BI LACH NUX-V URAN-N Ter
, walking, agg	ACID-NIT BELL BRY NAT-M Cocc Colch Petr
, walking, amel	ACID-NIT BELL BRY LYC PULS SULPH Colch Coloc Ran-b
ENTERITIS: anterior	LACH MERC NAT-M Bar-m Colch Hydr Kali-s

DIARRHOEA

DIARRHOEA; generally,	AGAR ALOE ANTH ANT-T APIS ARG-N ANT-T APIS ARS BAPT BAR-C BRY CALC CANTH CARB-V CHIN CORN CROT-T DULC FERR FERR-ARS FERR-I GAMB HELL HEP IOD IP IRIS KALI-BI LYC MERC MERC-S NAT-M NAT-S PHOS PODO RHEUM SEC SIL SULPH THUJ VERAT
, anticipation, from	ACON ARG-N ARS GELS
, calf	NOSODES Aeth All-s Ang Ars Cadm Camph Chin Crot-t Ip Mag-c Raj Verat
, chronic	ARG-N ARS CALC FERR NAT-S PHOS RHUS-T THUJ Graph Podo Thyr Tub
, constipation, alternates	ACID-NIT NUX-V Ant-c Chel Op Podo Tub
, dentition, during	ATH CALC DULC FERR SIL Rheum
, anxiety, with	CALC SIL
, irritable, with	ANTH Rheum
, eating, after	ARS CALC LYC NAT-P PHOS PULS SEP VERAT Aloe Chin Coloc Crot-t Mag-m Nat-a Podo
, geriatric	ANT-C Phos
, giardia	ACID-PHOS BAPT BOR FERR GELS NAT-M PHOS PODO SQUIL SULPH TUB
, infectious	ACID-PHOS ARS FERR NAT-M NOSODES PHOS SULPH Acid-but Bapt Bor Chin Hyos Podo Squil Tub
, bacterial	FERR NAT-M Bapt Nosode
, helminthiasis	ACID-PHOS Acid-but Bapt Chin Nosode
, parvovirus	ACID-PHOS BAPT BOR FERR GELS NAT-M PHOS PODO SQUIL STROPH SULPH THYR TUB NOSODE.
, protozoal	ACID-PHOS Acid-but Bapt Chin Nosode
, viral	ACID-PHOS BAPT BOR FERR GELS NAT-M PHOS PODO SQUIL SULPH TUB VERAT NOSODE.
, juveniles	ANTH ATS CALC MERC PHOS PSOR SEP SIL STRAM SULPH Aeth Calc-s Ip Mag-m Nat-a Nat-c
, neonates	SEP Aeth Nat-a Nat-c
, offensive	MERC-C Kres Lac-c Merc-i-f Merc-i-r
, time, diurnal	NAT-M CUPR Ornith

283

, evening	MERC-C Kres Lac-c Merc-i-f Merc-i-r
, midnight, after	ARS Ferr-ars SULPH Kali-ars
, morning	SULPH Aloe Podo
DYSENTERY	ARS MERC NUX-V PHOS RHUS-T SULPH Carb-s Carb-v Chin

ANUS AND RECTUM

ABSCESS	Hep Calc-s
ANAL SACS	SIL Calc-s Hep Ornith Sanic
, impaction	Ornith Sanic SIL
, infection	Calc-s Hep
BLEEDING	ACID-NIT HAM NAT-M PHOS Acid-fl Kali-c Ornith
, constipation, with	NAT-M Acid-fl Kali-c Ornith
, foreign body, with	ACID-NIT PHOS
, surgery, post	ACID-NIT
CANCER	ACID-NIT ARS PHOS THUJ Hydr
CONSTIPATION	ACID-NIT ANTH APIS ARS BRY CALC CAUST LYC MERC-C NAT-M NUX-V PHOS PLAT PLB RUTA SEP SIL STAPH STRAM SULPH THUJ VERAT Op
, bleeding	ACID-NIT NUX-V
, chronic	NAT-M NUX-V OP SULPH Alum
, Faeces, retract	NAT-M SIL THUJ Op
, soft	PULS SIL SULPH Alum Carb-s Nux-m
, juveniles	BRY CALC LYC NAT-M NUX-V Plb SEP SIL Alum Hydr
, neonates	CALC NUX-V SULPH Op
, pain, great	ACID-NIT SULPH Tub
ERUPTIONS	ACID-NIT NAT-M Petr
EXCORIATION	CAUST LYC MERC-C PULS SULPH Carb-s Graph Kres Petr
, Faeces, from	APIS MERC-C NUX-V SULPH Aloe Kres
, raw	CAUST LYC MERC-C PULS SULPH Carb-v Graph Petr
ELIMINATION: inappropriate	ACON ARS BELL NAT-M PHOS PSOR RHUS-T STAPH SULPH VERAT Aloe Con Hyos Nat-p Op Podo
, anus, wide open	APIS PHOS
, behavioural problem	ARG-N ARS FERR PHOS SULPH Hyos
, coughing, during	PHOS SULPH
, excitement, from	Hyos
, fear, from	PHOS Op Verat
, paralysis	NUX-V Alum
, sleep	ARS BRY PHOS PSOR PULS RHUS-T SULPH Con Hyos Podo
FISSURE / FISTULA	ACID-NIT ANTH ARG-N AUR BERB CALC CALC-FL CALC-P LYC SEP SIL THUJ Bcg Carb-v Graph Hir Kali-c Paeon Paro-i Prot Rat Trios

, acute	ANTH BERB Calc-s
, pain, severe	ACID-NIT LYC THUJ Paeon Rat
, rectum involved	ACID-NIT
FLATUS	ANTH ARG-NIT HEP LYC NAT-S NUX-V PLB SIL STAPH SULPH URAN-N All-c Aloe Asar Carb-v Chin Cocc Coloc Con Graph Ner Op Raph Tell
, diarrhoea, with	LYC NAT-S Aloe Carb-v Ner
, food, after	IGN SEP Aloe
, noisy	ARG-N CAUST NAT-S Aloe Mez
, odourless	PHOS SULPH THUJ Agar
, offensive	ANTH ARN PSOR STAPH SULPH Hep
INCONTINENCE: faecal	ACID-PHOS APIS ARN BELL HYOS NAT-M PHOS PSOR RHUS-T SULPH VERAT Acid-oxal Aloe Coloc Con Hyos Podo Tub
, anus, wide open	APIS PHOS
, excitement, from	Hyos
, Faeces, formed	BELL Aloe Coloc
, lying down	Acid-oxal
, sleep, during	ACID-PHOS ARN ARS PHOS PSOR Con Hyos Podo Tub
INJURY	ACID-NIT APIS CALC CROT-H HAM LYC NAT-M PHOS RUTA Aloe Am-c Mill Rat
, haemorrhage	ACID-NIT HAM Crot-h Mill
, painfully swollen	ACID-NIT APIS NAT-M Aloe
PARALYSIS: anus	PHOS SIL Aloe Alum Kali-p Sec
, surgery, after	Kali-p
PROLAPSE	DULC FERR FERR-P IGN LYC MERC-C SEP Bell-p Podo
, Diarrhoea	CALC DULC MERC-C Podo
, parturition, post	FERR FERR-P NUX-V Hydr Podo
STRICTURE	NAT-M RUTA SIL Aesc Calc-s
SWELLING	APIS HEP RUTA SULPH Aesc Coll Graph Paeon Podo
TENESMUS	ACID-NIT APIS ARS MERC MERC-C NUX-V Alum Caps Colch Coloc
, Diarrhoea	ARS MERC-C SULPH Alum Colch Coloc
, Faeces, after	MERC-C MERC NAT-M PULS SULPH Agar Colch Mag-c
, before	MERC-C NUX-V SULPH Agar Coloc
ULCERATION	ACID-NIT ANTH Alumn Kali-i

CARDIOVASCULAR SYSTEM

BLOOD

ANAEMIA	ACID-NIT ACID-PHOS ARS BELL CALC CALC-P FERR LACH MED MERC MERC-S NAT-M PHOS PULS SEP SULPH THUJ

285

, aplastic	ARS Chin Tnt
, debility, great	ACID-PHOS Acid-acet Chin
, homolytic	ACID-NIT ARS CALC FERR LYC MERC NAT-M PHOS Ferr-ars Mang
, haemorrhage	ARS FERR LACH Acid-acet Chin Crot-h Fic
, nutritional	CALC-PHOS FERR SIL
, parasitism	ARS MERC THUJ
, babesiosis	ARS MERC THUJ Nosode Acid-but Bapt Chin-s Chlorpro Thal Tnt
, thrombocytopenia	X-ray
BLEEDING	ACID-NIT ACID-PHOS ARS BELL CALC CALC-P FERR LACH MED MERC MERC-S NAT-M PHOS PULS SEP SULPH THUJ Chin Cinnm Cor-r Crot-h Hydr Lat-m Mill Sabin Stront-c
, recovery	Chin
, clots	ANTH PLAT RHUS-T Sabin
, dark	Croc
, fluid, serum-like	Sabin
, coagulation, poor	ACID-NIT FERR LACH PHOS Both Crot-c Lat-m
, coloured, black	FERR PULS Chin
, brownish	Carb-v
, dark	LACH Croc
, red	ACON Ip Mill
, exertion, after	ACID-NIT BELL Cinnm Mill
, injury	Mill
, internally	BELL Chin
, orifices, from	PHOS Both Crot-h
, passive	Chin
, prolonged	Chin
, ropy	Cor-r
, slight	ARN Hydr
, surgery, collapse	CALEN Stront-c
BLOOD PRESSURE	CRAT LACH NAT-M PHOS SEP Verat
, high	CRAT LACH NAT-M Verat
, low	PHOS SEP Carb-v
CANCER	ARS NAT-S Cean Colos Nat-a Phyt X-ray

BLOOD VESSELS

CIRCULATION: weak	ACON BELL CALC-FL CALC-P CROT-H LACH PHOS SEP Aesc Sec Tab
, acute	ACON BELL Aesc
, chronic	CALC-P Aesc Sec

PHLEBITIS / Phleg-leg	ACON APIS BELL BRY CALC CALC-FL HAM KALI-BI LACH RHUS-T All-c Bufo Clem Kali-c Prot Vip
, acute	ACON APIS BELL LACH Vip
, chronic	BRY CALC-FL RHUS-T
PURPURA haemorrhagica	LACH LED PHOS Nosode of Strep-equi Ter
SEPTICEMIA	ARN ARS BRY CROT-H ECHI LACH LYC PHOS SULPH Anthr Bapt Crot-c Kali-p Pyrog Tarent-c
THROMBOSIS	APIS ARS CROT-H LACH Both Clem Sec Vip
, acute	APIS ARS LACH Both
, chronic	Sec Snake venoms
VARICOSITIES	ACON BRY CALC FERR LACH PULS RHUS-T Acid-fl Carb-v Clem Vip

HEART

ARRHYTHMIA	ACID-PHOS MERC NAT-M Chin Dig Sec Verat-v
BRADYCARDIA	GELS Adon Dig Kalm Lycps
CONGESTIVE: failure	ACON APIS CRAT Apoc Beryl Chlorpro Glon Kres Mand
DILATATION	CRAT LAUR Cact Dig Spig
ENDOCARDITIS	ACON ARS AUR ECHI Kalm Myris Spig Spong
, pre-dentistry	Myris Echi
FIBRILLATION	Acon Aur Dig Chin-s Kalm Staph
HYPERTROPHY	ACON ARN AUR CRAT PHOS RHUS-T Aur-i Cact Kali-c
MURMURS	CRAT FERR RHUS-T Cact Coll Dig Kalm Naja Spig Spong
, disease, with	CRAT FERR Dig Naja Spig
, exercise, amel	CRAT RHUS-T
OEDEMA	APIS ARS AUR CRAT LACH LYC Apoc Coll
, heart disease, with	AUR CRAT LYC
, primary	APIS CRAT Apoc
VALVE: disorders	FERR RHUS-T Adon Cact Coll Dig Kalm Lycps Naja Spig Spong

PULSE

FAST	ACON APIS ARN BELL DIG FERR-P GELS MERC NAT-M NUX-V PHOS RHUS-T SULPH Bapt Crot-c Dig Spig
FREMITUS	ANT-T CALC Spig
FULL	ACON ANT-T BELL BRY STRAM Alum BERB Chel Dig Graph Hyos Kali-i
IMPERCEPTIBLE	ACON GELS SIL Camph Carb-v Colch
SLOW	BERB GELS STRAM Cann-i Dig Op Verat Verat-v

RESPIRATORY SYSTEM

COUGHING

287

AIR: cold, agg	ARS CAUST HEP NUX-V PHOS All-c Hyos Kali-i Rumx
, amel	Cocc
, damp and cold, agg	CALC DULC Iod
, dry and cold, agg	ACON HEP PHOS Spong
, open, agg	ARS HEP PHOS Coff Kali-i Rumx
, amel	ARG-M ARG-N BRY MAG-P NAT-S PHOS All-c Brom Coc-c Iod Kali-s Lil-t
, walk in, agg	ARS PHOS Rumx
, amel	BRY MAG-P PULS Brom Iod Kali-s
COLD: on becoming	ARS HEP NUX-V PHOS PSOR RHUS-T Kali-c Rumx Tub
CONSTANT	CAUST LYC Alum Chin Rumx Spong
DEEP	Dros Spong Stann Verat
DENTITION: during	ANTH CALC CALC-P
DRINKING: after	ARS BRY PSOR Dros
DRY	ACON ARS BELL CALC IGN LACH NAT-M NUX-V PHOS PULS SULPH Alum Brom Carb-an Chin Hyos Iod Kali-c Mang Petr Rumx Spong Tub
, diurnal	Alum Spong
, evening	HEP IGN LYC PULS SULPH Brom
, fever, during	ACON BRY NAT-M NUX-V PHOS RHUS-T Con Hyos Ip Kali-c Sabad
EATING: agg	ARS BRY CUPR KALI-BI NUX-V Rumx
EVENING	ACID-NIT ARS CALC HEP IGN LYC MERC PULS Caps Carb-v Stann
EXCITEMENT: agg	ANTH Cist Spong
EXERCISE: after	BRY CALC FERR NAT-M PULS Acid-oxal Brom Kali-i
FEVER: during	ACON ARS CALC NAT-M NUX-V PHOS Con Ip Kali-c Sabad
GERIATRIC	ANT-T CRAT PHOS SIL Bar-c
HACKING	ACON ARS BRY LACH NAT-M PHOS SEP Alum Dros Nat-a Nosodes Sang Tub
, acute	ACON
, chronic	Polycrest plus Dros
LOOSE	ARS BRY CALC HEP PULS SEP SULPH Acid-sul Carb-v Kali-i Stann
LYING down: agg	APIS CAUST PULS Con Hyos Kres Rumx Sang
, amel	FERR THUJ Euphr Mang
PAINFUL	BRY All-c Caps
SUFFOCATIVE	ANT-T CUPR HEP NUX-V SULPH Alum Apoc Carb-v Chin Cina Dros Hyos Ip Samb

LUNGS

ABSCESS	CALC HEP PHOS SIL

AFRICAN horse sickness	ANT-T APIS ARS BELL GELS NAT-M PHOS All-c Am-c Apoc Carb-v Crot-h CUPR Nosodes Queb Spong Verat
ASPHYXIA	ANT-T CUPR LAUR Carb-v Camph Op
ASTHMA	ANTH ARS CUPR DULC MED NAT-S NUX-V PHOS PULS SIL THUJ All-c Blatta Camph Carc Chel Cina Dros Iod Ip Kali-i Kali-s Lob Samb Spong Tub
, bronchial mucous	ANT-T ARS BRY Blatta Ip Lob
, coughing severe	ANT-T ARS CUPR NUX-V Cina Dros Ip
, cyanosis	ARS CUPR Carb-v Samb
, evening and night	ARS PULS Carbo-v Chel Samb
, excitement, agg	CUPR NUX-V PHOS Carc Ip Lob Mosch Valer
, geriatric	ANT-T ARS SIL Bar-c Carb-v Con
, juvenile	ANTH ANT-T ARS MED NAT-S PHOS PULS Carc Ip Kali-s Samb Tub
, vaccination, agg	ANT-T SIL THUJ
, wheezing	ARS LYC NAT-M NAT-S Carb-v Kali-c Lob Samb
BLEEDING	ACID-NIT ACON ANTH ARN ARS FERR HAM PHOS Cact Chel Ferr-ars Mill Sec Stann Urt-u
, clots	ANTH ARN PULS RHUS-T Chin Elaps Ip Sabin
, exertion, agg	ARN RHUS-T Mill Urt-u
, frothy	ARN PHOS SIL Led
BRONCHIECTASIS	ANT-T HEP KALI-BI Nosodes Tub-a
BRONCHITIS	ANT-T ARS BRY FERR-P HEP LYC NAT-S PHOS PULS SIL Aesc Bar-m Dig Dros Hippoz Hydr Ip Sang Senec Spong Stann Tub
, chronic	ANT-T CALC DULC Hep Hydr KALI-BI LYC PULS SULPH Aesc Am-c Carb-v Seneg Stann
, geriatric	ACON BELL BRY LACH NUX-V PHOS RHUS-T SEP SULPH Cact Camph Dig Ip Spong Ter
, juvenile	ACON ANT-T BRY CALC-FL CORTISO HEP LACH LED LYC PHOS SIL SULPH Am-c Beryl Carb-v Coc-c Hist Ip Led Lob Nosodes Queb
CONGESTED	Am-c Beryl Coc-c Lob Nosodes Queb
COPD / emphysema	ANT-T BRY PHOS SULPH Ip Led Nosodes
, allergic	SULPH LYC
, multifactorial	APIS CORTISO CRAT NAT-S Abrot Apoc Queb Verat
, resistant cases	BRY CALC RHUS-T Carb-v
EXPECTORATE: bloody	DULC LYC MERC NAT-S PHOS PSOR PULS SULPH THUJ Calc-s Carb-s Carb-v Kaliums Par Stann
, colon, brownish	DULC LYC MERC NAT-S PHOS PSOR PULS SULPH THUJ Calc-s Carb-s Carb-v Kaliums Par Stann
, grey	ANT-T LYC NAT-M PHOS SEP Kali-chl Seneg
, greenish	CALC CALC-P PHOS PULS SEP SIL Blatta Calc-s Hep Hydr Kaliums Stann Tub
, white	ACON APIS ARN ARS FERR PHOS PULS Kali-i
, yellowish	ARG-M ARG-N FERR KALI-BI SIL Alumn Apoc Cact Samb

, frothy	ARN KALI-BI SIL Calc-s Hep Hydr Kali-c Sel
, gelatinous	CALC LYC PHOS SEP SIL SULPH Nat-a Blatta Con Kali-c Stann
, lumpy	ANT-T KALI-BI LACH NAT-S Apoc Hydr Seneg
, purulent	ACON CUPR GELS PSOR Am-m Bapt Eup-per Lob Nosodes
, ropy	ACON GELS Eup-per
INFLUENZA	CRAT FERR Dig Naja Spig
, acute	Nosodes
, heart, strain after	Am-c Bapt Lob PSOR
, prophylaxis	ACON ARN BRY HEP SULPH Apoc Carb-an Iod Kali-c Seneg
, secondary infection	APIS CORTISO Apoc Queb
OEDEMA	Queb
, acute	ACID-NIT ACON ANTH ARN ARS FERR HAM PHOS Cact Chel Ferr-ars Mill Sec Stann Urt-u
, neonate / juvenile	ACON BRY SULPH Kali-c
PLEURISY	Hep Iod Kali-c
, acute	ACON ANT-T ARS BRY FERR-P HEP LYC MERC PHOS PULS RHUS-T SEP SULPH Carb-v Lob Seneg Verat-v
, chronic	LYC PHOS SULPH Carc
, pneumonia, with	ANT-T BRY Dig FERR-P NAT-S NUX-V Lob Op Seneg
, chronic	PHOS
, geriatric	BRY LYC PHOS SULPH
, left	ANT-T BRY FERR-P LYC MERC NUX-V PHOS SULPH Ip Kali-c Lob

RIBS

FRACTURE / injury	ACON ARN BRY CALC-P RUTA Am-c Echi Kali-c Ran-b Symph
, pain, acute	ACON BRY CALC RUTA
, chronic	BELL BRY CALC Kalm Spig
, intercostal strain	BRY PHOS RHUS-T Echi Ran-b

RETICULOENDOTHELIAL SYSTEM

LYMPH GLANDS	BELL CALC HEP MERC RHUS-T SIL SULPH
, abscess	CALC Calc-s MERC SIL SULPH Hep Kali-i
, cancer	ARS DULC MERC PHOS Phyt SIL SULPH Aur-m-n Aster Carb-an Carc Cist Con Echi Kaliums Tub
, lymphadenitis, 'phleg'	BELL CALC DULC MERC PHOS SULPH Bar-m Carc Cist Con Echi Kaliums Phyt SIL Tub
IMMUNODEFICIENCY	ACID-PHOS NAT-M SULPH THUJ Cadm-m Colos Echi Eleuth Gins. Potencies 6X – 12X.
, geriatric	NAT-M THUJ Colos Echi Eleuth Gins

, juvenile	ACID-PHOS Cadm-m Colos Echi Eleuth
IMMUNE MEDIATED	ACID-PHOS ARS CORTISO NAT-M SULPH THUJ Echi Eleuth Gins Herpvir Hist. Potencies 200CH.

SPLEEN

SPLEEN	ARS CALC CORTISO NAT-M NUX-V PHOS SULPH Anthr Aur-m-n Cadm-m Calc-ars Cean Chin Colos Con Cortico Ferr-i Hippoz Iod Urt-u Visc
, cancer	CALC-ARS Aur-m-n Cean Colos Cortico Iod Visc
, splenitis	APIS ARN BRY NAT-M NUX-V Cean Chin
, splenomegaly	ARS CALC FERR LACH NAT-M NUX-V PHOS SULPH Ars-i Aur-m-n Calc-ars Anthr Cean Chin Con Cortico Hippoz Iod Urt-u

URO-GENITAL SYSTEM

BLADDER

CALCULI	ACID-NIT APIS ARS BERB CALC LYC MERC RHUS-T STAPH Acid-benz Acid-oxal Acid-uric Lith Nosodes Pareir Sars Ter Urt-u
, casts	APIS ARS PHOS Canth Nosodes Ter
, crystalluria, oxalates	ACID-NIT BERB CAUST Acid-oxal Ter
, phosphates	ACID-PHOS CALC PHOS Acid-benz Nosodes Solid
, struvite	ACID-PHOS BERB Acid-benz Canth Nosodes Ter
CANCER	CALC THUJ Teucr
CYSTITIS / FLUTD	ACID-BENZ ACON ARIS BERB CANTH COLOC DULC HIST LYC NUX-V RAUW STAPH SULPH THLAS UVA Berb Caust Chim Coc-c Cop Cub Eup-per Equis Lith-carb Helon Oci Pop Sulfon Terebe Trit-p Urea
, acute	BELL BERB DULC LYC PULS SEP Acid-benz Canth Coloc Hist Sars Ter
, catheterisation after	CALEN STAPH
, chronic	ARG-M STAPH Equis Eup-pur Pareir
, painful	BELL Canth Equis
, tenesmus	BELL MERC NUX-V Canth Lil-t Pareir Ter
PARALYSIS	ARN ARS CAUST DULC GELS NUX-V SULPH Op Zinc
, geriatric	ARS Equis
, parturition, after	ARS CAUST
RETENTION: urine	ACON APIS ARG-N ARN ARS BELL CAUST GELS LYC NUX-V RHUS-T Am-c Canth Caps Con Op Pareir Tarent
, ataxia, with	ARG-N
, exertion, after	ARN RHUS-T Caps
, juvenile / neonates	APIS ACON
, painful	CAUST NUX-V Canth
, parturition, post	ARS CAUST

291

, prostatomegaly, with	APIS STAPH Dig
, tenesmus	BELL Canth Equis

KIDNEY

NEPHRITIS	APIS ARN ARS BELL BERB BERB-A CALC-P LYC MERC MERC-S NAT-M NAT-S SULPH Acid-benz Am-c Bapt Calc-s Canth Gink-b Kali-chl Kali-i Kres Oci Plb Sulfa Ter Urt-u
, acute	APIS ARS BERB MERC MERC-C NAT-M NAT-S PHOS Am-c Gink-b Kali-chl Ter
, chronic	ARS MERC MERC-C Dig Kali-i Kres
PKD	BERB NAT-M PSOR Colch Kali-chl
SHARPEI FEVER	APIS BERB NAT-M PHOS Kali-chl
URAEMIA	BELL CUPR Am-c Dig Kali-s Ter

URINATION

DRIBBLING, involuntary	ARN CAUST HEP NUX-V
, injury	ARN CAUST
, morning	SEP Alum
, rising, on	LYC
, prostate disease	BERB NUX-V PULS Aloe Dig Sabal
, retention	CAUST NUX-V
, sitting, during	PULS Sars
, urination, after	BERB Cann-i Clem Hep
FREQUENT	BELL CALC LYC MED MERC PHOS SEP SULPH Bar-c Bor Carb-an Kres Sars Ter
, daytime	PSOR RHUS-T Mag-m
, exposure from	CALC PULS Sars
, geriatric	Bar-c
INFREQUENT	ARG-N Canth Cycl Laur Op
TENESMUS	BELL Canth Equis

URINE

ACRID	ARN HEP MERC MERC-S SULPH Acid-benz Laur
ADDISONS DISEASE	CALC CORTISO NAT-M PHOS SEP Iod
ALBUMINURIA	APIS AUR HEP LYC MERC NAT-P RHUS-T Cedr Glon Hell Nat-a Nat-c Plb Ter
, chronic	Cedr Petr Plb
, heart disease, with	AUR CUPR LACH Calc-ars Colch Crot-h Dig Kalm Ter
, pregnancy, during	APIS ARS GELS LYC MERC NAT-M SEP Canth Chin Kali-ars Ter
, viral infections	APIS ARS LACH LYC PHOS NAT Canth Colch Hell Hep Kali-chl Kali-s Ter
ANURIA	ACON APIS ARN ARS LACH LYC PHOS STRAM Canth Carb-v Laur Verat

CASTS	APIS ARS HEP MERC PHOS PLB Canth Cimic Ter
COLOUR: black	LACH Acid-carb Chel Colch Ter
, bloody and chronic	Erig
, bloody and clotted	ACID-PHOS LYC PLAT Alumn Cact Chim Ip Mill
, cloudy or milky	ANTH APIS AUR BERB BRY Canth LYC MERC PHOS SEP Carb-s Carb-v Chel Chin Cina Con Graph Hep Sabad
, collarless	CAUST GELS NAT-M PHOS SEP SULPH Agar Apoc Cann-i Coff Dig Equis
, reddish	ACID-PHOS BERB BRY SEP STRAM Acid-benz Chel Canth
INCONTINENCE	ACID-NIT APIS ARG-N ARN ARS BELL CAUST FERR MAG-P MED NAT-M PULS RHUS-T SEP SIL SULPH Acid-benz All-c Apoc Buffo Equis Foll Graph Hyos Kres Lac-c Nosode Oena Sanic Tub
, cough, during	APIS CAUST LYC NAT-M PHOS PULS Colch
, excitement, during	CAUST NAT-M NUX-V PULS SEP
, fits, during	Bufo Hyos Oena Plb Zinc
, geriatric	ARS THUJ All-c Aur-m Cic Iod Sec
, HRT	CAUST PULS SEP Foll Oest Test
, juvenile	BELL CAUST LYC Cina Equis Kres Lac-c Tub
, walking, while	ARG-N BRY CALC CAUST FERR NAT-M PULS Lac-d Mag-c Sel Zinc
ODOUR	ACID-NIT ACID-PHOS AUR DULC FERR LACH Asaf Bor Carb-v Daph Iod Juni Mosch Pareir Petr Ter Tub
, ammonia, of	ACID-NIT AUR DULC FERR LACH MERC PHOS Carb-v Asaf Iod Mosch Pareir Petr Tub
, eggs, rotten of	Daph
, horse, of	ACID-NIT Acid-benz Nat-c
, putrid	ACID-PHOS CALC SEP Acid-benz Aur-m Calad
, sour	CALC MERC SEP Ambr Graph Nat-c
, sweet	ARG-M PHOS Cop Cub Ter
, violets	PHOS Clem Cop Cub Ter
POLYURIA	CALC LYC MED MERC SEP SULPH Bar-c All-c Bor Carb-an Kali-c Kres Mez Sabal Ter
, time, afternoon	All-c
, diurnal	SULPH
, evening	LYC Acid-fl Kali-chl Laur
, nocturnal	Many
, exhaustion, with	CALC-P LYC MED Acid-acet Chin-s Cimic

FEMALE SYSTEM

HRT: generally,	CAUST PULS SEP Foll Oest

MAMMAE

ABSCESS	BELL BRY HEP LACH MERC PHOS SIL SULPH Crot-h Phyt
CANCER	LACH MERC SIL Aster Bell-p Brom Carb-an Carc Con Iod Kres Lac-c Phyt Plb Sang Scroph-n Thyr
, exudate, bloody	LACH PHOS THUJ Aster Kres Sang
, offensive	Cund
, epithelial	ARG-N ARS LACH PHOS SEP SIL Ars-i Bufo Clem Con Hydr Kres Phyt
, oestrous, enlarge	PULS SEP Con Kres
, hard	Con Phyt
, injury, from	HYPER Bell-p Con Phyt
, invasive	PHOS Aster Carb-an Cund
, painful	LACH PHOS Aster Chim Clem Hydr
, scarred	Graph SIL
, ulcerated	CALC PHOS SIL SULPH Phyt Hep
LACTATION	ACON PULS Agn Alf Hyos Urt-u Yohim
, drying off	APIS Urt-u 200CH
, eclampsia	ACON BELL CALC-P MAG-P Hyos Agar
, excessive	Lac-c Urt-u
, inadequate	Agn Alf Colos Urt-u 4X. Alfalfa ø – 2X
, inappropriate	MERC PULS Asaf Cycl Tub Urt-u 200CH
MASTITIS: acute	ACON APIS BELL BRY LACH SULPH Carb-v Hep Nosode Phyt Pyrog Urt-u
, chronic	BRY CALC-FL SIL SULPH Carb-v Hep Lac-c Nosodes Phyt
, herd problem	Nosodes
, injury from	ARN Bell-p Con
, pre-partum	SIL SULPH Carb-v
ULCERATED	HEP MERC SIL Aster Phyt

OVARY

ANOESTROUS	LYC PHOS PULS SEP Foll Iod Nat-c Oest Tub
, juvenile, onset delayed	Tub
, postpartum	SEP
, species, all	LYC PHOS PULS SEP Foll Iod Nat-c Oest Tub.
CYSTS	APIS LACH LYC THUJ
, left	LACH THUJ
, right	APIS LYC
NYMPHOMANIA	Anh Grat Lil-t Orig Murx
OOPHORITIS	ACID-NIT ACON APIS ARS BELL LYC MERC PALL PHOS PLAT PULS RHUS-T Cimic Coloc Lil-t Sabin
, acute	ACON APIS BELL BRY HAM LACH MERC PLAT PULS Canth Cimic Coloc Iod
, left	LACH THUJ

| , right | APIS ARG-M BELL BRY LYC PALL Podo |
| **SPRING HEAT:** mare | APIS LACH LYC MED PLAT SEP STRAM |

TEATS

TEATS: generally,	ANTH CAUST SIL Acid-fl Cast-eq Crot-t Graph Petr Phyt Rat Sars
, bleeding	HAM LYC MERC SEP SULPH
, cracked	ANTH ARN HAM LYC MERC PULS SEP Acid-fl Cast-eq Graph Hydr Mill Phyt Rat
, painful	ANTH ARN CALC-P HAM LYC MERC PULS SEP Cast-eq Graph Helon Hydr Lac-c Mill Phyt Rat

UTERUS

ATONY	PULS SEP Am-m Caul Helon Thlas
, oestrous abnormal	PULS SEP Carb-v Thlas
, postpartum	PULS SEP Am-m Helon
ENLARGED	APIS CALC LACH LYC PULS SEP THUJ Con Hell Kali-i
, endometrial cysts	CALC PULS Sars
, oestrous abnormal	LYC SEP Kali-i
, postpartum	APIS LACH Hell
FLUID filled	APIS ARS LACH LIL-T PALL Agn Brom Bufo Iod Kali-Br Lyss
HAEMORRHAGE	ACID-NIT ANTH ARG-N BELL CALC HAM PHOS Croc Crot-h Erig Ip Kali-c Kres Sabin Tril Ust Vib
, atony, with	HAM Carb-v Chin
, caesar, after	ACON PHOS Erig Ip Sabin
, clotted	ANTH BELL Ust
, colour, black	ANTH PULS Acid-sul Kres
, pale	FERR
, red	BELL PHOS Erig Ip Sabin
, clots, with	BELL Sabin
, copious	PHOS Erig Ip Tril
, motion, agg	BELL PHOS Ip Mill Sec Tril
, foetal loss, after	PLAT Croc Kali-c Sabin Sec
, intermittent	PHOS
, mating, at	ARG-N Kres
, parturient	HAM Erig Ip Sabin Sec
, passive	Carb-v Erig Tril Ust
, pregnancy, during	PHOS Kres
PROLAPSE	ARG-M ARG-N AUR CALC NAT-P PLAT PULS SEP Bor Lil-t Nat-a Pall
PSEUDOPREGNANCY	CALC PULS SEP Cycl
PYOMETRA	PULS SEP Alet Caul Echi Hydr Pyrog

VAGINA & VULVA

FLATUS: vagina / vulva	ACID-PHOS CALC LYC NUX-V PHOS SEP Brom Lac-c Mag-c Nat-c
, juveniles	ACID-PHOS CALC NUX-V SEP PHOS
, matures	NUX-V SEP PHOS Mag-c Nat-c
HYPERPLASIA: vulva	ACID-NIT APIS MERC PHOS Agar Cur Ferr-i Graph Iod Kres Lil-t Urt-u
RAPE	ACON ARN IGN NAT-M PLAT STAPH Carc Op
VAGINITIS	ACID-NIT APIS ARS HAM MED PULS SEP THUJ Aesc Ant-c Bor Calc-s Canth Hydr Kali-s Kres
, acute	APIS ARS MED PULS THUJ Canth Kres
, exudate, acrid, with	CALC PULS SEP SULPH Bor Calc-s Kali-p Kres
, pruritus	ACID-NIT CALC SEP SULPH Brom Calad Calc-s Canth Kres
WARTS: vulva	ACID-NIT NAT-S THUJ

PREGNANCY

BEHAVIOUR, changes	ACON CUPR NAT-M SEP STAPH PALL PLAT Cimic
BLEEDING, uterus	ACID-NIT SEP Cann-i Erig Ip Kres Sabin
, labour-like pains	ANTH
, overexertion, from	ACID-NIT Cinnm Erig
, second trimester, in	SEP Cann-i Erig
DIARRHOEA: during	ACID-PHOS PULS SULPH Caps Mez Nux-m
, chronic	Nux-m
, mucous	Caps
, prolapse rectum	Mez
FOETAL LOSS	ACON ANTH ARN BELL GELS NUX-M PHOS SEP SIL STAPH Alet All-c Caul Cimic Cob-n Erig Goss Hydr Ip Kali-c Nosode Sabin Sec Thyr Vib
, anaemia, from	FERR SEP
, bleeding, threatens	ACID-NIT CALC HAM LYC PHOS PULS Croc Ip Kres Sabin Thlas Tril Ust
, exertion, from	ARN RHUS-T Erig
, fear, from	ACON GELS IGN Op
, infection, from	GELS Bapt Camph Colos
, injury, from	ARN Cinnm RHUS-T
, placental insufficiency	NUX-V PHOS SEP SIL Alet Caul Cimic Helon Plac Sabin Verat-v
, time, first trimester	APIS SEP Caul Cob-n Kali-c Vib
, second trimester	APIS RUTA Eup-pur
, third trimester	PULS RUTA
HAIR loss	LACH SEP
LABOUR; inadequate	Calc Puls Caul
, premature	ANTH BELL CALC PULS Caul Cina Dios
URINATION: involuntary	ARS NAT-M PULS SEP Oest Symph
VARICOSITIES	CALC-FL LACH Aesc Sec

PARTURITION

BEHAVIOUR, difficult	ACON ANTH CUPR Op
, dam	ACON ANTH CUPR Op
, neonate	ACON

CAESAREAN	ACON ANT-T ARN HAM PHOS PULS Cal Caul Echi Erig Ip Sabin Sec Vib
, dam, haemorrhage	ACON PHOS Erig Ip Sabin Sec
, metritis	Cal Caul Echi
, pain	PULS STAPH RHUS-T Pareir Vib
, neonate	ACON PHOS
, placental retention	CAUST GELS Caul Cimic Kali-c LYC
, shock	ACON
DYSTOCIA	ANTH BELL CALEN CAUST NUX-V PHOS PULS SEP Bell-p Caul Cinnb Coff Kali-i Sabin Sec
, cervix, ringwomb	GELS Cimic Caul Con Lob Verat-v
, contractions weak	PULS CAUST Caul Kali-i
, haemorrhage	HAM PHOS Erig Ip Sabin Sec
, malpresentation	PULS Caul
, manipulation, great	CALEN Bell-p
, painful	ANTH BELL Coff NUX-V SEP
, prolonged	Sec Cinnb
ECLAMPSIA / milk fever	APIS BELL CALC CALC-P MAG-P MERC Parathyr
, prophylaxis	CALC CALC-P
FEVER	ECHI LACH LYC PULS RHUS-T SULPH Carb-s Pyrog
FLATUS: vagina / vulva	ACID-PHOS CALC LYC NUX-V PHOS SEP Brom Lac-c Mag-c Nat-c
, juveniles	ACID-PHOS CALC NUX-V SEP PHOS
, matures	NUX-V SEP PHOS Mag-c Nat-c
HYPERPLASIA vulva	ACID-NIT APIS MERC PHOS Agar Cur Ferr-i Graph Iod Kres Lil-t Urt-u
RAPE	ACON ARN IGN NAT-M PLAT STAPH Carc Op
VAGINITIS	ACID-NIT APIS ARS HAM MED PULS SEP THUJ Aesc Ant-c Bor Calc-s Canth Hydr Kali-s Kres
, acute	APIS ARS MED PULS THUJ Canth Kres
, exudate, acrid	CALC PULS SEP SULPH Bor Calc-s Kali-p Kres
, pruritus	ACID-NIT CALC SEP SULPH Brom Calad Calc-s Canth Kres
WARTS: vulva	ACID-NIT NAT-S THUJ

POSTPARTUM

INJURY, torn tissues	ACON ARN CALEN STAPH Led
METRITIS	ARN ARS BELL BRY IGN PULS VERAT Bart Cantz Hydr Sabin Sec.
RETAINED PLACENTA	CAUST GELS Caul Cimic Kali-c LYC
WOUNDS	ACON APIS BELL HYPER LACH LED Canth Hep Myris Urt-u

MALE

EJACULATION: problem	ARG-N CAUST KALI-BI MERC-C NAT-M PHOS PSOR Calad Camph Cop Graph Hydr Nosodes Petr Sabal
, bloody	Canth CAUST MERC Petr Sars
, incomplete	LACH LYC PHOS PSOR Agar Calad Camph Eug Graph Lyss Nosodes
, milky	KALI-BI NAT-M Cann-s Hydr
, painful	BERB CALC SEP SULPH Agar Cann-s Canth Con Kali-c Kres Sabal
, purulent	ARG-N MERC-C NAT-S PULS THUJ Cann-c Cop Cub Hep Hydr Kali-s
, watery	NAT-M SEP Cann-s Nat-p Orchi-e (c) Sel
IMPOTENCE	ARG-M CALC IGN LYC MED NUX-V SEP SIL STAPH SULPH Agar Agn Anac Bar-c Calad Calc-s Chin Clem Coff Con Graph Halo Rauw Rhod Sel Visc
, desire: soon lost	ACID-PHOS NUX-V
, erection, weak	LYC SULPH Agn Bar-c Orchi-e (c)
, lacking libido	ARG-M IGN LYC PSOR PLAT SEP SIL STAPH Agn Anac Bar-c Calad Clem Coff Graph Orchi-e (c) Rhod
, present	PHOS
, geriatric	LYC
MATING: aggressive	Acid-fl Acid-pic Anac Cann-i Canth Graph Tub Zinc
SEMEN; deficiencies	ACID-PHOS ARG-N LYC Agn Ana Cal Con Sel

PENIS PREPUCE SCROTUM
SPERMATIC CORD

PENIS: abscess	MERC-C Hippoz
, bleeding	ARN ARS Cinnm Mill
, cancer	ACID-NIT ARG-N ARS MERC NAT-S PHOS THUJ Con Hep Sabin
, excoriation	ACID-NIT ARS CAUST MERC NAT-M SULPH THUJ Nat-c
, herpes	ACID-NIT ACID-PHOS Crot-t DULC MERC NAT-M RHUS-T SEP THUJ Sars Graph Hep Nat-c Petr
, injury	Bell-p Calad Con
, painful	ARS MERC IGN Cann-i Cann-s Lith
, phimosis	ARN ARS CALC HAM LYC MERC RHUS-T Cann-s Canth Dig Hep
, prepuce, prolapse	ARS IGN MERC Bell-p Calad Cann-i Cann-s Con Lith
, sarcoid	ACID-NIT AUR LACH SIL THUJ Ant-c Cast-eq
, spermatic cord, scirrhous	BERB PHOS PULS Calen Kali-c Spong
, torsion	ARS BERB IGN MERC Cann-i Cann-s Clem Lith
, ulcerated	ACID-NIT KALI-BI MERC SULPH THUJ Ars-i Hep

PROSTATE

PROSTATE	ACID-NIT CALC MERC PULS SIL STAPH THUJ All-c Alum Bar-c Caps Chim Con Cub Cycl Dig Sabal Sel
, painful	BELL CAUST LYC PHOS PULS RHUS-T STAPH THUJ All-c Alum Caps Chim Con Cub Cycl Sabal Sel

, prostatitis, acute	ACID-NIT MERC PULS SIL STAPH THUJ Sabal Verat-v
, chronic	AUR LYC MERC MERC-C SEP STAPH THUJ Con Ferr-Pic Sabal Sel
, prostatomegaly	PULS THUJ Bar-c Chim Con Dig Iod Sabal

TESTES

TESTES: atrophy	ARG-N AUR GELS Caps Carb-an Iod Kali-i Rhod Sabal
, cancer	PULS STAPH THUJ Carb-an Con
, Cryptorchid	Bar-c CALC-FL Clem NUX-V
, injury	ARN BELL-P CALEN HYPER RHUS-T STAPH
, Orchitis, bilateral	ARG-M ARS BERB HAM MERC-C PULS Bar-c Con Iod Nosodes
, left	Alum Nosodes Spong
, right	ARG-N AUR
, painful, bilateral	ARG-M AUR BERB MERC-C PULS SEP STAPH Clem Rhod Spong
, left	PULS STAPH
, right	ARG-M AUR Clem Rhod
, spermatogenesis, weak	LYC Bar-c Nosodes

MUSCULOSKELETAL

ARTHRITIS

BURSITIS: acute	APIS BELL BRY FERR-P LACH RHUS-T Cimic Rhod
, athletic	BRY RHUS-T Acid-form Cimic Kalm Led
, chronic	ACID-PHOS BRY CAUST DULC LACH RHUS-T SULPH Acid-fl Led
, intra-articular	Apis Arg-m Bry Colch Echi Rhus-t Sal-ac
IMMUNE MEDIATED	ACID-PHOS APIS ARS CORTISO FERR NAT-M SULPH THUJ Bapt Chin Colos Echi Eleuth Gins Herpvir Hist
, acute	APIS ARS CORTISO Echi
, chronic	ARS CORTISO Colos Bapt Echi
LUPUS	ACON APIS BRY DULC RHUS-T RHOD RUTA
NODOSITES: bony	AUR CALC LYC Acid-benz Ant-c Colch Kali-c Kalm Led
, fibrous	CALC-FL RUTA Graph Guai Kalm Rhod Thiosin
SEPTIC	CALEN ECHI LACH LED MED MERC Bapt Bufo Cimic Colos Myris

BACK

Azoturia / MUR	ACON ARN BELL BERB BERB-A BRY RHUS-T BELL-P Cimic Helon Thal
, acute	ACON BELL BERB-A
, chronic	ACON ARN BELL BERB-A

, prophylaxis	BERB BERB-A Bell-p Cimic Helon
CRAMPING	BELL CAUST CUPR MAG-P PHOS Berb Chin Cina Crot-h
, acute	BELL CUPR Chin
, recurrent	CAUST CUPR MAG-P PHOS Chin Cina
DISC SYNDROME	APIS ARN BRY CALC-FL CAUST GELS GUAI HYPER NUX-V PHOS RHUS-T RUTA SIL SULPH Acid-oxal Acid-pic Aesc Agar Bell-p Crot-h Kali-c Op Thiosin
, acute	APIS BRY HYPER PHOS Aesc Crot-h
, chronic	Acid-pic Aesc Agar Bell-p Thiosin
INJURY	ARN BRY HYPER RHUS-T RUTA Bell-p Cimic Ran-b
MOVEMENT: poor	BELL BRY CALC FERR GRAPH LYC LED NUX-V RHUS-T SULPH Aesc Agar Bell-p Caps Con Ran-b
, asymmetrical	RHUS-T Bell-p
, weak	RHUS-T Bell-p Con
, painful	BERB CALC LYC RHUS-T Bell-p Colch Guai
NECK	ACID-PHOS ARS BELL CAUST CIMIC CUPR FERR GELS GUAI LACH LYC NAT-M PHOS RHUS-T THUJ Brom Chel Cic Cimic Graph Lac-c Op Pareir Rhod
, flexion reduced	CAUST LACH RHUS-T Cimic Lac-c
PAIN: neck	ARG-M BELL BRY CALC DULC FERR GELS GUAI LACH LYC NUX-V PHOS PULS RHUS-T SEP SULPH Aesc Agar Chin Colch Con Kali-c Led Lil-t Naja Ust
, acute	APIS BRY HYPER PHOS Aesc Crot-h Kali-c
, chronic	GELS SIL Chel
, poll	GELS SIL Chel
SACROILIAC disease	ACID-NIT ANT-T BERB BRY CALC FERR GELS GUAI HYPER LYC NUX-V LYC NUX-V PULS SEP Aesc Agar Chin Dna Flav Mand Stry Sulfa Tell Vario Visc
, chronic	GELS GUAI Hyper SIL Chel
, acute	ACID-NIT BERB GELS HYPER NUX-V SEP
VERTEBRAE	ARN BRY CALC HYPER NAT-S RHUS-T RUTA SEP SIL Aesc Agar Cimic Ran-b
WITHERS	ACID-NIT ARN ARS CALC CALC-P CUPR GUAI HYPER LYC NAT-S NUX-V PHOS RHUS-T SEP Chel Clem Mez Tell
, fistulous	ARS Clem Mez
, kissing spines	ACID-NIT CALC HYPER Chen Tell
, muscular	ARN HYPER RHUS-T Chel Tell
, scoliosis, left	LYC NUX-V PHOS
, right	CUPR LYC

BONE

CYSTS	ARG-M CALC CALC-P Kali-c
DYSPLASIA and physis	ARG-M CALC CALC-FL HEP LYC MERC SIL STAPH Asaf Astrag
EPIPHYSITIS	ACID-NIT ARN AUR CALC CALC-FL

	CALC-P RUTA SIL Cart Hekla Symph
FRACTURES	ARN BRY CALC-P RUTA Acid-carb Symph
, initially	ARN BRY Symph
, later	CALC-P RUTA Acid-carb
, non-union	CALC-P Dna Symph
OSTEOMYELITIS	CALC CALC-FL CALC-P SIL Cart Echi Hekla Myris Nosodes
OSTEOPOROSIS	ACID-NIT ARG-M CALC-P LYC MERC SIL Asaf Parathyr Oest Orchi-e (c) ACID-NIT CALC-P RUTA SIL Acid-fl
, non-surgical	CALC-P RUTA SIL
, surgical	RUTA Acid-fl
SEQUESTRUM	ACID-NIT ARN AUR CALC CALC-FL CALC-P RUTA SIL Cart Hekla Symph
SPLINT BONE	ACID-PHOS ARN AUR BRY CALC CALC-P RUTA Acid-carb Mez Symph
, acute	BRY CALC-P RUTA Acid-carb
, chronic	AUR CALC RUTA Mez
, prophylaxis	CALC-P RUTA SIL
, topical	ARN RUTA Symph

FRONT LIMB

SHOULDER

ABSCESS	ACID-NIT HEP MERC RHUS-T SIL
BURSITIS	CAUST FERR RHUS-T SULPH Ambr Chel Cimic Sang Sars
, acute	CAUST FERR RHUS-T Cimic
, chronic	FERR SULPH Chel Cimic
PAIN	FERR LED RHUS-T SULPH Chel Sang
PARALYSIS, 'sweeny'	CAUST RHUS-T Ferr-i

ELBOW

BURSITIS	ACON APIS ARS BRY CALC-P HYPER MERC Guai Rat
, acute	ACON APIS BRY
, anconeal process	CALC-P RUTA SIL
, arthritis, with	BRY MERC Rat
, chronic	ARS CALC-P Guai
, trauma	BRY HYPER RUTA

CARPUS

BURSITIS	ACON APIS ARS BRY CALC-P HYPER MERC Guai Rat

CARPITIS	ARN BRY CALC CALC-P HEP LYC MERC RHUS-T RUTA SIL STAPH Acid-carb Acid-form All-c Asaf Aur-m-n Carb-an Cart Echi Eup-per Kali-i Stict Symph
, acute	CALC-P LYC RUTA Cart
, chronic	MERC SIL STAPH Acid-carb Ang Cart
, intra-articular	Apis Arg-m Bry Colch Echi Rhus-t Sal-ac
DEVIATION	CALC CALC-P RUTA Cart Symph
FRACTURE	ARN BRY CALC-P RUTA Acid-carb Symph
INJURY	BRY HYPER RHUS-T RUTA
PARALYSIS	Plb

FETLOCK AND PASTERN

BURSITIS	ARN ARS CALEN CAUST HYPER LACH LED RHUS-T SIL SULPH Am-c Chel
, acute	ARN ARS CALEN
, chronic	ARS CAUST Am-c Chel Led
, DJD	ARG-M ARN BRY CALC-P RUTA Acid-carb Cart Eup-per Symph
, intra-articular	Apis Arg-m Bry Colch Echi Rhus-t Sal-ac
ECZEMA: periarticular	CALEN CARB-V GRAPH NAT-M SULPH Ant-c Canth Carb-v Kres Mez Petr
, chronic	CALEN NAT-M SULPH Ant-c Graph Kres Mez Petr
, topical	CALEN Graph Kres
INJURY	ARN ARS CALEN HYPER LACH
, surgery	CAUST Echi Led
LIGAMENTS	APIS CALC-FL CAUST RUTA Dna Thiosin
RINGBONE	APIS CALC-FL CAUST LED LYC RUTA SIL Acid-benz Cart Graph Lith
, acute	APIS CALC-FL RUTA SIL Acid-benz Cart Lith
, chronic	CAUST LYC RUTA Cart Led
SESAMOIDS	APIS ARS CALC-FL CALC-P CALEN CAUST HYPER LACH MAG-P Cart Thiosin
, acute	APIS ARS CALC-FL HYPER Cart
SIDEBONE	APIS CALC-FL CAUST LED LYC RUTA SIL Acid-benz Cart Graph Lith
, quittor	ARN ARS CALEN HYPER LACH
, chronic	CALC-P CAUST MAG-P Cart Thiosin
SUBLUXATION	ARN ARS CALEN

HOOF and NAILS

COFFIN JOINT	APIS ARN BRY CALC-FL CALEN LED LYC RUTA SIL Acid-benz Acid-carb Eup-Per Graph Lith Symph
, bursitis, acute	ARN APIS ARS BRY CALEN
, chronic	ARS CAUST Am-c Chel Led
CORNS	NAT-M SIL THUJ Aesc Ant-c Cast-eq

CORONARY BAND	HYPER MAG-P SIL Graph Teucr
, injury	HYPER MAG-P Graph
DIGITAL CUSHION	ARN ARS CALEN HEP HYPER LACH LED Calc-s
, acute	ARN HYPER Led
, chronic	LACH Calc-s
HORN	HEP NAT-M SIL THUJ Aesc Ant-c Calc-s Cast-eq Graph Sec
, brittle	Aesc Ant-c Cast-eq SIL
, disease, during	Calc-s Graph Hep Sec THUJ
, *seedy toe*	CALC-FL THUJ Aesc Ant-c Cast-eq Crot-h
LAMINITIS	ACON ARG-N BELL CALC-FL NUX-V THUJ Aesc Ant-c Cast-eq Crot-h Jug-r Myris Zea
, acute	ACON BELL THUJ Aesc Jug-r Zea
, chronic	CALC-FL THUJ Aesc Ant-c Cast-eq Crot-h
, latent	ACON BELL NUX-V Aesc Jug-r Thuj Zea
NAVICULAR DISEASE	ARG-M CAUST LED LYC RHUS-T RUTA SIL Acid-benz Cart Crot-h Graph Lith Vip
NAILS	ARN CALC-FL CAUST HYPER PSOR SIL THUJ Ant-c Cast-eq Caul Cimic Graph Kres Rhod
, working dogs	CALC-FL Ant-c Cast-eq
PEDAL BONE	ACID-NIT APIS ARG-M AUR CALC-FL CAUST LED LYC MERC RUTA SIL Asaf Graph Lith
PYRAMIDAL DISEASE	APIS CALC-FL CAUST LED LYC RUTA SIL Acid-benz Cart Graph Lith

HIND LIMB

ATAXIA	ARG-N GELS PHOS ZINC Alum Agar Cocc Con Hell Ner Plb Zinc
, acute	ARG-N PHOS Alum Con
, chronic	GELS Alum Agar Con Zinc
ATROPHY	ARG-N NUX-V RHUS-T Abrot Plb
CRAMP	ANTH ARG-N BERB CUPR CALC-P CAUST COLOC GELS MAG-P NUX-V RHUS-T RUTA SULPH Am-c Anac Guai Plb Sec Thiosin
, contracted, permanent	CAUST NUX-V RUTA Am-c Guai Plb Thiosin
, prophylaxis	ARG-N BERB CUPR NUX-V Anac Sec
OEDEMA	APIS ARS LYC Aesc Chin Samb Ter
PHLEBITIS hind limb	ACON BELL BRY CALC CALC-FL CALEN LACH RHUS-T Aesc Clem Myris Sec Vip
, acute	ACON BELL BRY Aesc Sec Vip
, chronic, 'phleg-leg'	CALC-FL LACH Aesc Sec
, prophylaxis	CALC-FL Aesc Sec

HIPS

ARTHRITIS	ARG-M ARS AUR CALC-FL CALC-P CAUST COLOC LED RHUS-T SIL STRAM SULPH Aesc Am-c Card-m Cart Chel Chin Colch Kali-c Kali-s Mang Tub

303

, bursitis	ARS CALC-FL CAUST RHUS-T SULPH Aesc Am-c Chel Led
, osteoarthritis	ARG-M CALC-P Cart Kali-c Mang
DISLOCATION	ARN CALC CALC-FL Aesc Dna
JUVENILE: laxity	CALC-FL CALC-P RUTA Aesc

STIFLE

ARTHRITIS	ARN BELL BRY CALC-FL CALC-P ECHI NAT-M PULS RHUS-T SIL SULPH Cart Mang Stict Verat-v
, bursitis	CALC-FL CAUST Chel Led Stict
, osteoarthritis	ARG-M CALC-P Cart Mang
CRUCIATE ligaments	CALC-FL CAUST NAT-M RHUS-T RUTA Cart Thiosin
INJURY	BRY CALC-FL RHUS-T RUTA Cart Guai Thiosin
, intra-articular	Apis Arg-m Bry Colch Echi Rhus-t Sal-ac
PATELLA	BRY CALC-FL RHUS-T RUTA Cart Chel Guai Thiosin

HOCK

ACHILLES tendon, strain	ARN BRY CALC-FL LED PULS RHUS-T RUTA SEP Cart Guai Stront-c Thiosin Valer
, acute	ARN BRY CALC-FL RHUS-T RUTA
, chronic	CALC-FL RUTA Cart Guai Thiosin
ARTHRITIS	APIS ARG-M BRY CAUST LED MED MERC RHUS-T SIL SULPH Acid-form All-c Cart Chel Mang Stict
, bursitis	APIS BRY CALC-FL CAUST MERC RHUS-T SULPH Chel Led
, capped hock, I/A	APIS BRY MERC
, intra-articular	Apis Arg-m Bry Colch Echi Rhus-t Sal-ac
, osteoarthritis	ARG-M CALC-P Cart Kali-c Mang
CURB	ARN BRY CALC-FL LED PULS RHUS-T RUTA SEP Guai Thiosin Valer
, acute	ARN BRY CALC-FL RHUS-T RUTA
, chronic	CALC-FL RUTA Guai Thiosin
, topical	RHUS-T RUTA Thiosin
SPAVIN; bone	ARG-M CALC-P Cart Kali-c Mang
, bursitis	APIS BRY CALC-FL CAUST MERC RHUS-T SULPH Chel Led
STRINGHALT: physical	CALEN CAUST GELS NAT-M NUX-V RUTA STRAM SULPH Agar Cic Coff Colch Dna Mygale Op Passi Stry Valer Zinc
, toxic	CORTISO HYPER Anth Led Ros-d Urt-u
THOROUGHPIN	APIS BRY CALC-FL CAUST MERC RHUS-T SULPH Chel Led

MUSCLE

MUSCLE; generally	ACON ANTH ARG-M ARN BELL BERB BRY CALC CAUST CUPR HYPER LYC MAG-P MERC NAT-M

	NAT-S NUX-V PULS RHUS-T SEP THUJ Acid-sul Anac Bell-p BERB-A Canth Chel Chin Chin-s Cimic Cina Coloc Con Iris Rhod Valer
, azoturia: myositis, acute	ACON ARN BELL BERB BRY NUX-V BERB-A Rhod
, recurrent	ARG-M BERB MAG-P SEP Bell-p Cimic
, cramp, lumbar	ANTH ARG-N BELL BERB CALC CAUST CUPR NAT-M Anac BERB-A Iris Rhod
, shoulders	PHOS Chel
, injury	ARN BERB Acid-sul Bell-p

TENDONS and LIGAMENTS

TENDON: contraction	ARG-M ARN ARS BELL CALC CALC-FL CALEN CAUST DULC LYC MERC NAT-C NAT-M NUX-V PHOS PULS RHUS-T RUTA SEP SIL SULPH THUJ ACID-NIT Guai Kali-i Mang Plb Ran-b Thiosin
, joints, at	CAUST NAT-M Anac Graph Thiosin
, neonates	CALC-FL CAUST NAT-M Thiosin
, tendonitis, acute	ARN CALEN RHUS-T THUJ Con Dna Rhod
, chronic	CALC-P CAUST RUTA Con Dna Guai Plb Thiosin
, bone, attachment, at	ARN BRY CALC-P CALEN RUTA Acid-carb Con
, chronic	CALC-P CAUST RUTA Con Guai Plb Thiosin
, ossification, with	CALC-FL CALC-P RUTA SIL Thiosin

SKIN: GENERAL

ACNE-LIKE	ECHI HEP LACH NUX-V SEP SIL Calc-s Colos Kali-br
, juvenile	NUX-V SEP SIL Calc-s Echi
ACANTHOSIS	Sep Sulfa Thuj
ACTINOMYCOSIS	Acid-nit Hekla Hippoz Kali-i
ALOPECIA	ACID-PHOS ARS LYC NAT-M PHOS SEP STAPH Alumn Bov Graph Kali-ars Kali-c Sel Thal Thyr Zinc
, body	ACID-PHOS Bov Graph Kali-ars Kali-c STAPH Zinc
, head	PHOS SEP SIL Zinc Acid-fl Bar-c Graph Kali-ars
ATOPY	Consider all remedies associated with pruritis and infection, especially: ARS CAL CORTISO HEP KALI-BI LACH PSOR PULS SIL THUJ Colos Cortico Hist Thal Acid-bor
BED SORES	ARS HYPER LACH LED SEP SIL Chin Graph Petr
, dry	HYPER Chin
, moist	Chin Graph
BITE WOUNDS	ACON APIS BELL HYPER LACH LED Canth Hep Myris Urt-u
, first aid	LACH HYPER Led
, pain	BELL HYPER Led
, shock	ACON
, swelling	APIS Urt-u

BLEEDING	ACON ARG-M ARS MED PSOR SULPH Alum Bar-c Bov Graph Petr
, eczema	ARG-M MED PSOR
, self-inflicted	ACON ARS
BRUISING	ACID-PHOS ARN HAM LED PHOS Acid-sul Bell-p Sec Symph
, first aid	ARN HAM Sec
, later	ARN Acid-sul Bell-p
BURNS / SUNBURN	BELL PULS Canth Sol Urt-u
, acute	BELL PULS Canth Urt-u
, chronic	All topical skin treatments
CANCER: benign	ACID-NIT ACID-PHOS CALC CAUST MED MERC MERC-C NAT-S Petr THUJ Graph Hep
, angleberry	LACH SIL THUJ Ant-c Nosodes
, bleeding	ACID-NIT THUJ
, cauliflower-like	LACH SIL Ant-c
, fibroma	Con Iod.
, growth, rapid	THUJ
, horny	Ant-c
, moist	ACID-NIT THUJ
, polyp-like	CALC CALC-P Con PHOS STAPH THUJ Teucr
, bleed easily	PHOS Sabin
, fleshy	Carb-an
, nasal	Teucr
, vaccination, post	CARC MALAND MEZ THUJ VAC Ant-t Echi Kali-m Psor Sil
CANCER: malignant	ACID-NIT ARS BELL LACH LYC MERC PHOS SIL Sol SULPH THUJ URAN-N Ars-i Calc-s Carc Con Cund Hydr Hydrc Kali-s Kres Lap-a Ran-b X-ray
, epithelial	ACID-NIT LYC Ars-i Con Nosodes X-ray
, sun induced	ACID-PHOS ARG-N ARS LACH Carc Card-m Sol
, sarcoid	ACID NIT ANT-C ANT-T ARS AUR CALC CAUST DULC GRAPH LACH NAT-M NAT-S RUTA THUJA Cast-eq Sabin Sec SIL Vacc
, begin with	CORTISO Ferr-ars Carc Colos Echi Vac
, follow on	Carc
CELLULITIS	HEP KALI-BI LACH SIL Acid-bor
CORTISONE toxicity	ARS CORTISO PSOR PULS THUJ Colos Cortico Hist Thal
, pruritus	study that sections
CRACKS	ACID-NIT CALC SEP SULPH Ant-c Carb-s Graph Petr Sars
, mucocutaneous	ACID-NIT Petr
, periarticular	CALC
CYST: interdigital	CALC-S GRAPH HEP-S LACH SIL

, sebaceous	CALC-FL KALI-BR Bar-c Calc-sil Con Kali-i Dermatitis: staphylococcal NOSODE CALC-S HEP-S LACH Graph Kali-s Sil
DISCOLOURED	ACID-NIT APIS ARS BELL CALC FERR LACH LYC MERC NUX-V PLAT PULS RHUS-T SEP SIL SULPH THUJ Carb-v Dig Op Plb Sec Verat-v
, darker	Carb-v Plb Sec Verat-v
, HRT required	see that section
, lighter	ACID-PHOS ARS LYC SIL STAPH SULPH Kali-i
DRY	ARS BRY CALC DULC LED LYC MED NAT-M SIL THUJ Alum Ambr Chin Kali-ars Kali-i Plb Sec Teucr

ECZEMA / DERMATITIS

ECZEMA: acute	Chin-s Crot-t Rhus-v
, chronic	Polycrest first
, anal sac disease	See Rectum
, bleeding, with	ACID-NIT MERC SULPH
, coloured, blackish	LACH NUX-V Ant-c Asaf Crot-h
, coppery	ARS BERB LACH
, mealy	ARS CALC PHOS SIL
, red	MERC PHOS SULPH Acid-sul Am-c Kali-c
, whitish	ARS NAT-M Alum Mez
, yellow	ACID-NIT DULC MERC Bar-c
, cracked	Ant-c Cist
, crusty, allergic	Graph Led
, desquamating	AM-C BELL KALI-S MEZ NER PSOR SEP Ars Ars-i Aur Bov Clem Dulc Graph Kali-ars Kali-s Lach Merc Phos Rhus-t
, dry	ARS AUR CALC PHOS SEP SIL Ars-i Aur-m Bar-c Calc-s Led Mez Verat
, hard	Ran-b
, horny	Ant-c Ran-b
, moist	ARS CALC LYC MERC RHUS-T STAPH SULPH Carb-s Graph Mez Rhus-v
, offensive	SULPH
, patches	ACID-NIT MERC
, scratching, after	Con LYC SULPH Rhus-v
, periarticular	Aeth Am-c Ant-c Graph Kali-ars
ECZEMA:	BELL PHOS SEP Am-c Ars-i Kali-s Mez
, excoriated	MERC NAT-M SULPH Petr
, face	DULC Ant-c Bor Cic Graph
, limbs, periarticular	GRAPH Ant-c Kali-ars
, miliary	DULC Mez Nosodes Thyr
, painful	ACID-PHOS ARN BELL NUX-V SIL SULPH

307

, periorbital	PSOR SULPH Chrysar
, petechiation	BRY PHOS Aran Rhus-v
, pimples, bleed	Cist
, hard	Bov
, pruritic	DULC KALI-BI Crot-t
, pustules, black	Anthr LACH
, red	ACID-NIT Cic
, white	Ant-c
, yellow	MERC
, pustules, pruritic	DULC KALI-BI Crot-t
, ulcerated	ARS DULC MERC
, scaly	ARS PHOS SEP BERB-A Clem Phyt
, seasonal, spring	PSOR
, summer	KALI-BI
, winter	Petr Rhus-v
GRANULATION	ARS CALC LACH SIL Alum Kali-m
GRANULOMA: lick	CALC-FL ECHI IGN SIL THUJ Tarent
HAIR: brittle	PSOR THUJ
, dry	CALC NAT-M SEP THUJ
, falling, disease, after	ACID-PHOS Aloe Thyr
, handfuls	PHOS Mez
, juvenile	Bar-c SIL
, neutered, females	Nosodes Thyr Thal Ust
, males	Nosodes Thyr Iod Thal Ust
, parturition, after	LYC NAT-M SULPH
, patches in	APIS PSOR Acid-fl
, pregnancy, during	LACH SEP
, hard	RHUS-T SEP Ant-c Graph
, tangle, easily	NAT-M PSOR Acid-fl Mez
HRT	PULS SEP Agn Nosodes Thyr
KIDNEY: disease	ARS BERB KALI-CHL NAT-M PHOS Am-c Merc Urt-u
LIVER: disease	BERB CHEL LYC NUX-V Aesc Hydr Merc-s
LUPUS	ACID-FL ACID-NIT APIS ARG-M ARS AUR KALI-BI SEP SULPH CORTISO Ars-i Cund Hydr Hydrc Mand Sol Tell Tub
, cortisone toxicity	CORTISO Cortico Thal
, erythematosus	ARS CORTISO Acid-sul Carb-v Hydrc Mand Tell
, immune mediated	Colos Echi Eleuth
, nasal	ARG-M Sol
MANGE	ARS HEP LYC MERC PSOR SEP SIL SULPH THUJ Calc-s Hydrc Ichth Kali-ars Mez Thal

, generally,	THUJ Polycrest Colos Echi Eleuth Gins Hydrc Mez
, chronic	ARS CALC LYS MERC RHUS-T STAPH SULPH CALEN Carb-s Graph Mez Petr Staphyloc
MUD FEVER	CALEN Graph Petr
, barrier cream	ARS CALC LYC MERC RHUS-T STAPH SULPH Carb-s Graph Mez Petr Rhus-v
, eruptions	ARS CALC CUPR FERR NAT-M PHOS SIL Ars-i Bapt Chin Ferr-ars Mang Zinc
NUTRITION, poor	ACID-NIT ARS DULC LYC MERC NAT-M NAT-S RHUS-T SIL Anac Nosode
PEMPHIGUS	CORTISO Colos Nosodes
, desensitization	CALC DULC NAT-M SEP THUJ Bac Chrysar Nosodes Phyt Tell Tub
RINGWORM	ACID-NIT KALI-BI SULPH Acid-fl Aster Cund Echi Hydr
RODENT ULCER	See CANCER section on sarcoid
SARCOID	ACID-NIT CALEN PHOS SIL Acid-fl Cast-eq Graph Thiosin
SCARS	CALC-FL Hydrc Kali-ars Sulfa Tarent-c
STUD TAIL	ARS Nosodes Kali-ars Maland Vario
SWEET-ITCH / 'mange'	ANTH CALC FERR SEP Acid-fl Chin Mang
SWEATING: anxiety	ACON ARS Ars-i NAT-M SIL
, anhidrosis	CAUST FERR Hep Samb
, long lasting	BRY MERC STRAM THUJ Chin Mag-c
, oily	PSOR STAPH Carb-v
, offensive	Carc PULS
, side, left	PHOS PULS
, right	ARN ARS CALC CAUST HEP KALI-BI LACH LYC MERC PULS RHUS-T SIL SULPH Ars-i Calc-s Con
ULCERS	Acid-carb Acid-nit Anan Anthr Calen Carb-v Echi Ger Hep Merc Mez Thuj
, exudate, pus	ARS BELL PULS Acid-fl Acid-nit Asaf Carb-an Carb-v Caust Graph Hep Kali-bi Kres Led Lyc Merc Nux-v Phyt Sil
, painful	ACID-PHOS CON LYC OP Ars Bapt Bell Bry Calc Carb-v Cocc Dulc Hell Hyos Lach Ner Phos Puls Sec Sep Stram.
, painless	APIS CORTISO NAT-M RHUS-T Bov Cortico Hist Nosode Urt-u Vac
URTICARIA	ACID-NIT BELL CALC CAUST DULC MERC NAT-S SULPH THUJ Ant-c Bar-c Calc-s Nosodes
WARTS	Ant-c Cast-eq THUJ
, hard	Ant-c Cast-eq CAUST
, horny	ACID-NIT THUJ
, inflamed	ACID-NIT THUJ
, jagged	ACID-NIT THUJ
, large	ACID-NIT THUJ
, moist	ACID-NIT CAUST

, pedunculated	CALC THUJ
, smell of cheese	Ant-c DULC
, smooth	CAUST Hydr THUJ
, topical treatment	ACID-NIT CALC CAUST DULC LACH SIL SULPH
WOUNDS	ACID-NIT LACH SIL
, chronic	ARS CALC LACH SIL Alum Kali-m
, granulation, excess	CALC-FL CAL CAUST SIL Acid-fl Graph Kali-br Thiosin

CANCER / NEOPLASIA

HAEMORRHAGE	HAM PHOS Cinnm Cist
IMMUNE modulation	Cadm Colos Echi Eleuth Gins Visc
METASTASES: reduce	NOSODES CALC-FL Plb
, liver	NOSODES Hir RNA
, lymphoid	NOSODES BRY Absin Scroph-n Stan
PAIN: control	ACON APIS ARN Absin Acid-form
, swelling	Phyt
, infection	Led
REDUCE: drug dose	ANT-T Caul THUJ
TOXICITY: cachexia	Alf Ferr-ars
, chemotherapy	Cad-s
, Diarrhoea	Aloe
, radiation	CALEN X-ray
, vomiting	Coca
ULCERATION: digestive	ACID-NIT ARG-N LYC NUX-V Hydr
, topical	CALEN

CANCER: SPECIFIC AREAS

ANUS / RECTUM	ACID-NIT CALC-FL RUTA THUJ Colos Hydr Kali-cy Visc
BENIGN	ACID-NIT ACID-PHOS AUR HEP MED MERC NAT-S THUJ Thyr Ust
BLOOD: anaemia	ARS CALC CALC-P NAT-M NAT-S THUJ Acid-pic Ars-i Benz Carb-an Cean Chin Ferr-ars Kali-p Nat-a Nosodes Visc
, debility	Cean Chin Kali-p
BONE	CALC-FL SIL Acid-fl AUR-i AUR-m Cadm Colos Con Hekla Visc
BRAIN	PHOS Bar-c Colos Con Kali-i
CHEMOTHERAPY	NUX-V THUJ Cadm-s Colos Ip Visc
DEATH: prepare for	ANT-T ARS LYC PHOS Carb-v Chim Euph-re Tarent
EPITHELIAL	LYC Ars-i Carc Colos Con Hydr Phyt Sol Visc
EYES	CALC LACH LYC PHOS Colos SEP Sol Visc

FACE	ARS DULC HEP LACH PHOS SIL Carb-an Colos Hydrc Kali-ars Kali-s Visc
LIPOMA	BELL Am-m Bar-c Beryl Cadm-s Nosode Phyt Scroph-n
LIVER	LYC PHOS Cadm-s Calc-ars Carc Chel Chlol Colos Hydr Mag-m Nosodes Visc
LYMPHOID	ARS CALC-FL NAT-M PHOS THUJ Absin Ars-i Aster Aur-m Carb-an Carc Colos Con Iod Kali-m Nosodes Phyt Raja-s Scroph-n Sol Tub Visc
MAMMARY CANCER	HEP LACH MERC PHOS SEP SIL THUJ Acid-carb Aster Bell-p Bufo Carb-an Colos Con Graph Hydr Kres Nosode Phyt
, bleeding	PHOS
, exudate, bloody	Aster
, astral enlargement	Con
, injury, after	Bell-p Con
, large	Con Phyt
, painful	ARS PHOS Chim Clem Hydr
, scarred	PHOS Graph
, stone hard	Con Phyt
, ulcerated	CALC PHOS Phyt SIL Hep
MELANOMA: horses	NOSODE LYC Ars-i Carc Colos Con Hydr Phyt Sol Visc
MOUTH: lips	ARS DULC LACH LYC PHOS SEP SIL Aur-m Carb-an Cic Cist Clem Con Cund Hydr Kres Visc
, epithelial	ARS PHOS Cic Merc-i-f
, palate	AUR Hydr
, throat	ARS Carb-an
, tongue	ACID-NIT APIS ARS LACH PHOS Aur-m Alumn Carb-an Con Hydr Kali-cy Kali-i Phyt SIL
, ulcerated	ARS KALI-BI PHOS Aur-m Clem Con
NOSE	ARS AUR CALC SEP Acid-carb Aur-m Carb-an Colos Kali-i Kres Phyt Visc
RADIOTHERAPY: detox	CALC-FL Acid-fl Cadm-s Chel Colos Rad Visc X-ray
SKIN	ARG-N LYC THUJ Acid-acet Ars-i BELL Beryl Colos Con Cund Hydr Hydrc Kali-ars Kali-s Kres Lap-a Nosodes Phyt Ran-b Sol Visc
STOMACH	LACH LYC MERC PH OS SEP SIL STAPH SULPH Absin Acid-acet Acid-carb Ars-i Bism Cadm-s Caps Carb-an Colos Con Crot-h Cund Hydr Iris Kres Mez Ornith Visc

FELINE SPECIAL

BREEDING: failure, female	CAUST NAT-M SEP PLAT PHOS PULS Agn Alet AUR Bell-p Calc-s Foll Nat-p Oest Thyr
, anaemia	FERR-P SEP
, foetal loss: early	APIS PULS SEP Am-m Caul Cob-n Helon Kali-c Kali-i Thlas Vib
, second trimester	APIS RUTA Eup-pur
, third trimester	PULS RUTA

311

, bleeding, with	ACID-NIT CALC HAM LYC SEP PULS Chin Cinnm Croc Erig Ip Kres Sabin Thlas Tril Ust
, infection, from	GELS Bapt Camph
, injury, after	ACID-NIT ARN RHUS-T SEP Cinnm
, placenta weak	NUX-V SEP Sabin Verat-v
, neonatal mortality	ACID-PHOS ACON ARS CALC CALC-P FERR SIL Bapt Chin-s
, infection	ANTH ANT-T ARS BRY CALC PHOS PULS SIL SULPH Aeth Ip Mag-s Podo Rheum Tub
CHLAMYDIA felis	ACON APIS ARG-N CALEN NAT-M RHUS-T SULPH All-c Calc-s Euphr
, acute	ACON APIS All-c Euphr
, chronic	Polycrest but often SULPH
, exudate, bland	All-c Euphr
, clear	ACON BELL
, mucopurulent	ARG-N RHUS-T Calc-s
, neonatal	ACON APIS ARG-N Colos RHUS-T. Actual Colostrum
FELINE calici herpes	ACID-NIT ACON CALC CALC-FL KALI-BI LYC MERC NAT-M PHOS PULS RHUS-T RUTA SEP SIL SULPH THUJ Bor Can-s Colos Con Led Pareir Samb
, acute	Polycrest Samb
, chronic	Polycrest Can-s Colos Hippoz Samb
, prophylaxis	Nosode Colos
FELINE L V	Nosodes Polycrest ARS NAT-M Carc Card-m Cean Colos Phyt
FIV	ACID-PHOS ARS CALC FERR NAT-M PHOS SULPH Chin Echi Eleuth Gins
FIP: ascites with	APIS BRY LYC Apoc Phyt

FEVER

FEVER: generally,	ACID-NIT ACON APIS ARN ARS BELL CALC ECHI FERR-P GELS LACH LYC NAT-M NAT-S PSOR RHUS-T SULPH Anthr Bapt Cadm-s Cedr Chin Kali-s Myris Nosodes Op Pyrog Tarent Tub
, acute, bacterial	ACON ARN ARS BELL Echi Myris
, other	PSOR Bapt Cedr Chin Eup Led
, viral	ACON ARS BELL GELS
, chronic	ACID-NIT CALC GELS NAT-S Chin Echi Op Verat
, CNS involvement	APIS BELL GELS NAT-S Echi Op Verat

GAME / WILDLIFE

GAME: generally,	ACON ANTH ARG-N ARN BELL BERB CALC CRAT IGN NAT-M NAT-S NUX-V RUTA STAPH Carb-v China Echi Led Myris Uran Verat
CAPTURE: confinement	ANTH GELS NUX-V STAPH
, darting	CRAT NAT-S Carb-v Verat
, fear	ACON ARN BELL BERB NAT-M China

, recovery, stress	ANTH GELS NUX-V STAPH
, separation anxiety	STAPH
INFECTION / INJURY	ARG-N CALEN IGN NAT-S NUX-V Carb-v Led Myris Uran Verat
TRANSPORT	ACON ANTH GELS

GENERAL

ABSCESS	ACID-NIT ARN BELL HEP LACH MERC RHUS-T SIL SULPH Acid-carb Calc-s Myris Tarent-c
, acute	MERC SIL Hep
, chronic	Hep
, colour, green	MERC-C PULS
, white	CALC LYC
, yellow	LYC Calc-s Hep
, exudate, bloody	Asaf Hep
, offensive	Carb-v Hep Kres
, thick	PULS Calc-s
, thin	CAUST LYC MERC-C SIL SULPH Asaf
, watery	Asaf
, recurrent	ARN Pyr
BITE WOUNDS	ACON APIS BELL HEP HYPER LACH LED Canth Myris Urt-u.
CONVALESCENCE	ACID-PHOS CALC CORTISO GELS PHOS PSOR Caul Carc Graph Kali-c
, fever, after	Hell
, infection	GELS Carc
, parturition	SEP Caul
, pneumonia	PHOS Kali-c
DEHYDRATION	ARS CALC-P CARB-V CROT-H FERR GRAPH MERC NAT-M NAT-P NUX-V PHOS PULS SEP SIL STAPH VERAT Calad Carb-an Chin Chin-s Con Iod Kali-c Kali-p Nux-m
, fluid loss, from	CALC NAT-M Chin
, prophylaxis	NAT-M Chin
OEDEMA: generally,	APIS ARG-N ARN BRY CALC CALC-P LACH LYC PHOS SIL SULPH VERAT Acid-fl Agar Agn Aloe Alum Am-c Am-m Ambr Anac Bar-c Carb-an Colch Con Graph Hydr Hyos Iod Iris Kali-c Op Sec Sel Seneg Teucr Thiosin Tnt
, albuminuria	APIS Aur-m
, anaemia	FERR PHOS Ter Tnt
, heart disease	ARS LACH LYC Aur-m Lac-c
, kidney	DULC Colch Ter
, liver	Aur-m Card-m

313

, pregnancy, during	APIS
, splenic	LACH Aur-m Cean
OBESITY: generally,	ARS AUR BELL CALC FERR GRAPH KALI-BI LYC PHOS PULS SULPH Am-br Am-c Ang Calc-ars Caps Coc-c Croc Fuc Ins Kali-c Lac-c Phyt Thyr
, HRT	Nosodes
, juveniles	CALC Caps

GERIATRIC

GERIATRIC heart	CRAT Apoc Beryl Chlorpro Dig Mand
, HRT	Oest Orchi-e (c) Plac
, joints	BERB LYC NUX-V RHUS-T Aesc Con Symph
, kidney	BERB Acid-benz Bapt Gink-b Ter
, liver	ARS NAT-S NUX-V PHOS Card-m Chel Ins
, mind	ACID-PHOS Anac Bar-s Con Hell Zinc
, skin	ARS BERB PHOS THUJ

JUVENILE

ANAEMIA: aplastic	ARS Chin Tnt
, haemolytic	ACID-NIT ARS CALC FERR LYC MERC NAT-M PHOS Ferr-ars
, nutritional	CALC-P FERR SIL
, parasitism	ARS MERC THUJ
, babesiosis	ARS MERC THUJ Bapt Chin-s Nosode Tnt
ASTHMA	ACON ANTH ANT-T ARS BELL BRY LACH PHOS PULS Am-c Bcg Bac Coc-c Dig Ip Kali-c Laur Led Lob Samb
BACKWARD	CALC-P Bar-c Carc
CONFIDENCE: lack of	ACON ARG-N ARS BRY CALC-FL GELS LYC NAT-M PHOS SIL STAPH Bar-c Carc
CONSTIPATION	BRY CALC LYC NUX-V Alum Coloc Mand Op Ornith
, bowel inactive	Op
, generally,	Alum Ornith
, meconium	CALC NUX-V Alum Ornith
CRYPTORCHID	AUR CALC-P NUX-V PHOS SIL THUJ Bar-c Carc Clem Nosode Thyr
DESTRUCTIVE	AUR NUX-V PHOS SIL THUJ Cina Tub
DIARRHOEA	ANTH ARS CALC PHOS PULS SIL SULPH Aeth Ip Mag-s Podo Rheum Tub
ECZEMA	NAT-M PSOR RHUS-T SULPH THUJ Mez
GASTRO-ENTERITIS	ACID-PHOS ANT-T ARS BRY PULS
GROWING PAINS	ACID-PHOS CALC CALC-P Guai
INCOORDINATION	Alum Con
INSOMNIA	ANTH CARC PULS Bcg Coff Kali-br Passi Scut
, dentition	ANTH Scut

, habitual	Coff Passi
INTUSSUSCEPTION	ARS Op Plb Verat
JOINT-ILL	APIS BRY CALEN DULC ECHI HYPER LED Colos Myris Nosode
, treatment	BRY Colos Echi Led
, prophylaxis	Echi Myris
RESPIRATORY	ANT-T KALI-BI NAT-M PHOS PULS Bar-c Beryl Bor Colos Lob Maj Nosodes Queb
SKELETAL	ACID-PHOS CALC CALC-P PHOS RUTA SIL Ang Euph-r Kalm
, dysplasia / physis	ACID-PHOS CALC-P RUTA
, epiphysitis	ACID-PHOS CALC-P RUTA Ang
TONSILITIS	BELL HEP MERC Bar-c Hir Gink-b
VACCINOSIS	APIS THUJ Colos Eleuth Nosodes Syc-co Vac
, prophylaxis	THUJ Nosode Colos Syc-co Vac

METABOLIC SYNDROMES

METABOLIC; generally,	CALC CALC-P MAG-P STRAM Agar Alf Apoc Bar-m Cann-i Cortico Eup-per Iris Pancr Sel Syzyg
, acetonemia	LYC Card-m Cortico
, acidosis	Nat-p
, Cushing's disease	ARN CALC CORTISO HYPER LYC NUX-V PHOS Colos Cortico Chlorpro Ins Querc Syzyg Tarax ACID-PHOS
, diabetes mellitus	ARG-M LYC PHOS URAN-N Acet-acid Carc Chion Helon Ins Iod Iris Nat-s Nosode Pancr Plb Sulphonam Syzyg Ter. Also, see appropriate sections.
, dysplasias / physis , eclampsia	CALC CALC-P STRAM Bell-p Parathyr
, exertional myopathies All recommendations in association with expert nutritional advice.	Hyperkalaemic periodic paralysis: ACON BELL PHOS Acid-oxal Con Kali-p Nat-m **Malignant hyperthermia**: ACON BELL PHOS Acid-oxal Con Ins Kali-p Nat-m **Myofibrillar myopathy**: ARN NAT-M PHOS Cact Conv Crat Admit this is a rare condition. Remedies offered in the hope of stimulating debate and research. **PSSM1**: ACON ARN BELL BERB BERB-A BRY RHUS-T BELL-P Cimic Helon Ins Sel Thal. Admit this is a rare condition and offer suggested remedies in the hope of stimulating debate and research. **PSSM2**: ACON ARN BELL BERB BERB-A BRY RHUS-T BELL-P Cimic Helon Sel Thal. Admit this is a rare condition and offer suggested remedies in the hope of stimulating debate and research. **EM Type1:** ACON ARN BELL BERB BERB-A BRY RHUS-T BELL-P Cimic Helon Ins Sel Thal. Admit this is a rare condition and offer suggested remedies in the hope of stimulating debate and research. **EM Type2:** ACON ARN BELL BERB BERB-A BRY RHUS-T BELL-P Cimic Helon Sel Thal. Admit this is a rare condition and offer suggested remedies in the hope of stimulating debate and research.
, hypocalcaemia	BELL CALC CALC-P CUPR STRAM Agar

, hypomagnesemia	GELS MAG-P STRAM Mygal
, insulin resistance	ACID-PHOS ACON ARG-M BELL LYC NUX-V PHOS SULPH URAN-N Acet-acid Carc Chion Helon Ins Iod Iris Nat-s Nosode Pancr Plb Sulphonam Syzyg Ter
, laminitis	ACON ARG-N BELL CALC-FL NUX-V THUJ Aesc Ant-c Cast-eq Crot-h Jug-r Myris Zea.
, obesity	ARS AUR BELL CALC FERR GRAPH KALI-BI LYC PHOS PULS SULPH Am-br Am-c Ang Calc-ars Caps Coc-c Croc Fuc Ins Kali-c Lac-c Phyt Thyr

POISONING

ANAEMIA	ARS PHOS Clem Phyt Sulfa
CARDIAC	ACON ARN LACH CRAT Cact Dig Lat-m
CNS	ARG-M ARG-N BELL CALC CAUST CUPR IGN SIL SULPH Alum Bar-m Bufo Cic Hyos Kali-br Oena Plb Thyr Visc
GASTROENTERITIS	ANT-T ARS NUX-V PHOS Carb-v Hir Verat
HYPERKERATOSIS	ARS PHOS Cast-eq Clem Phyt
LIVER	CUPR HEP LYC MERC PHOS SULPH Acid-sul Ars-i Aur-m Card-m Chin Hydr Iod Senec
NEPHRITIS	ARS MERC NAT-M PHOS Am-c Kali-chl Plb
RESPIRATORY	ANT-T CUPR LACH All-s Carb-v Dig Laur Verat
STOMATITIS	DULC KALI-BI MERC-C SIL DULC KALI-BI MERC SIL

POISONING; SPECIFIC

ACARICIDES	NOSODE ARG-N CALC CAUST GELS LACH NUX-V Plb SIL STRAM Agar Alum Hell Helon Kali-br Lil-t Zinc
ACIDS	NOSODE DULC FERR KALI-BI LACH MERC NAT-M SEP SIL STAPH Astac Acid-sul Kali-chl Podo
ACORN	NOSODE ARG-N CALC CAUST GELS LACH NUX-V SIL STRAM Agar Alum Hell Helon Kali-br Lil-t Plb Zinc
AFLATOXINS	NOSODE BERB PHOS Plb SEP Agar Chel Chion Cur
ALKALOIDS	NOSODE ARG-N CALC CAUST GELS LACH NUX-V Plb SIL STRAM Agar Alum Cocc Graph Hell Helon Kali-br Lil-t Zinc
, digitoxin	NOSODE ACID-NIT CRAT Chin Dig.
, morphine, codeine	NOSODE Agar Alum ARG-N CALC CAUST GELS LACH Lil-t NUX-V Plb SIL STRAM Cocc Graph Hell Helon Kali-br Zinc
ANAESTHETIC: overdose	**NOSODE** PHOS Acid-acet Carb-v Chlf
ASPIRIN	ACID-NIT KALI-BI NUX-V PHOS URAN-N **Acid-sal** Ger
AVOCADO	NOSODE ACON ARN CACT LACH LAT-M Dig Glon Kalm Laur Naja Spig Tarent
BHC	NOSODE ARG-N CALC CAUST GELS LACH NUX-V Plb SIL STRAM Agar Alum Cocc Graph Hell Helon Kali-br Lil-t Zinc
CARBON MONOXIDE	NOSODE Acid-acet
CORTISONE	NOSODE ARG-N CALC CAUST GELS LACH NUX-V SIL STRAM Agar Alum Plb Cocc Graph Hell Helon Kali-br Lil-t Zinc

FOOD POISONING: fats	NOSODE PULS Carb-v Ip
, fish	NOSODE PULS Carb-v
, fruit	NOSODE ACID-PHOS PSOR Nat-p
, shellfish	NOSODE LYC Acid-sal Aloe Brom Podo Urt-u
, water, polluted	NOSODE ARS Bapt
FLUNIXIN	NOSODE ACID-NIT KALI-BI NUX-V PHOS URAN-N Acid-sal
IVERMECTIN	NOSODE ARG-N CALC CAUST GELS LACH Lil-t NUX-V Plb SIL STRAM Agar Alum Cocc Graph Hell Helon Kali-br Zinc
KIMBERLEY disease	NOSODE ARG-N CALC CAUST GELS LACH Lil-t NUX-V Plb SIL STRAM Cocc Graph Hell Helon Kali-br Zinc
LEAD	NOSODE BELL CAUST Coloc Kali-i NAT-S Op PLAT Plb SULPH Acid-sul Alum Alumn
MEGESTROL acetate	NOSODE PLAT PULS SEP
MONENSIN	NOSODE ARN BELL LACH CALC FERR HAM PHOS SULPH Acid-sul Both Carb-v Chin \Crot-h Erig Ip Meli Mill Sabin
MUSHROOM	NOSODE ARG-N CALC CAUST GELS LACH Lil-t NUX-V Plb SIL STRAM Agar Alum Cocc Graph Hell Helon Kali-br Zinc
OLEANDER	NOSODE ACON ARN LACH CACT Chin-s Lat-m Dig Glon Kalm Laur Naja Spig Tarent.
ONION	NOSODE ACID-NIT
ORGANOPHOSPHORUS	NOSODE ALUM ARS ARG-N CALC CAUST CUPR GELS Carb-v Bapt Bism Cocc Coloc Graph Hell Helon
PARAQUAT	NOSODE ACON BELL CUPR LACH Camph Carb-v Dig Laur Op Verat
PHOTOSENSITISATION	NOSODE APIS ARS DULC LYC SULPH NAT-M RHUS-T URT-U Anac Astac Bov Cop
POTATO: green	NOSODE ARG-N ARS CUPR MAG-P RHUS-T SIL Verat Bapt Bism Carb-v Coloc
SCORPION	NOSODE Guai.
SNAKE bite: coagulopathic	ACON BELL CALC HAM PULS Cinnm Cocc Mill Nosodes
, cytotoxic	ARG-N ARS SIL STRAM Alum Graph Lil-t Nosodes Plb
, keratitis	ACON CALEN STAPH Euphr
, neurotoxic	ARG-N BELL IGN Agar Cic Hyos Kali-br
SPIDER BITE	NOSODE ARG-N CALC CAUST GELS LACH Lil-t NUX-V Plb SIL STRAM Agar Alum Cocc Graph Hell Helon Kali-br Zinc
SUGAR	NOSODE ARG-N CALC LYC MERC SULPH
VACCINOSIS	NOSODE CALC HYPER MERC SULPH THUJ Carc Kali-m Malan Mez Per Sars SIL Tub Vac
, acute reaction	NOSODE CORTISO HYPER Led
, eczema	NOSODE APIS CORTISO THUJ Crot-h Mez
, fits	NOSODE CORTISO SIL
, prophylaxis	NOSODE HYPER THUJ Led
, sleeplessness after	NOSODE THUJ
X-Ray toxicity	CADM-S X-RAY

Xylitol	NOSODE ARG-N CALC CAUST GELS LACH Lil-t NUX-V Plb SIL STRAM Agar Alum Cocc Graph Hell Helon Kali-br Zinc

SURGERY

AMPUTATION	HYPER PHOS CALEN Coff
ANAESTHETIC	Overdose. PHOS Acid-acet Carb-v Nosode
, bleeding	ARN HAM Cinnm Mill
, hernia	NUX-V Bell-p
, infection	ARN Echi Hep Pyrog
, pain	ANTH BRY HYPER
, shock	ARN ACON Camph Carb-v Op Stront Verat
CONVALESCENCE	ACID-PHOS ACON BRY PHOS Alf Chin Cina Coloc Kali-p Kali-s
COLIC	ARN HYPER RUTA STAPH Nosodes
, appetite, stimulate	BRY Alf Chin Cina
, weight loss	Alf Chin
DENTAL: bleeding / pain	ARN HYPER RUTA STAPH Mill
OCULAR	LED STAPH Seneg Symph
SURGERY: preparation	ARN HYPER RUTA STAPH Nosodes
, recovery from	ACID-PHOS ACON BRY PHOS Alf Chin Cina Coloc Kali-p Kali-s

AVIAN GENERAL

INFECTION: bacterial	**NOSODES** ARG-N ARS BERB LYC PHOS Bapt Carb-v
, viruses	**NOSODES** ACID-PHOS FERR NAT-M THUJ Echi Eleuth
CANCER	CALC LYC MERC PHOS Acid-pic Card-m Chel
AVITAMINOSIS etc	Nosodes.
BEHAVIOUR	MIND section
DIARRHOEA	ACID-PHOS ARS DULC NAT-S Aloe Podo
EYE DROPS	CALC Am-c Euphr Hydr Samb Sang
IMMUNE: enhance	GELS NAT-M Am-c Cinch Echi Gins
NEBULIZATION	ANT-T CRAT PULS Cocc Lob Rumx
PRE-RACE	ARN Coc Kali-p Acid-lact Nat-c Sel
RECOVERY	CALC FERR MAG-P SULPH Bell-p Carb-v

TISSUE SALTS

1 CALC FLUOR. Found in earth and rock.
In connective tissue to maintain elasticity.
Dental defects: enamel and poor development. Tissue weakness including weak vasculature.
2 CALC PHOS. Found in soil.
In bone, teeth, soft tissues, cell structure. Blood proteins. New cell production.

Weak immune system prone to virus infection. Juvenile: delayed dentition and bone maturation. Poor healing following injury, fractures, and disease. Anaemia. Unfit from poor muscle response.

3 CALC SULPH. Found as 'Plaster of Paris.'

Connective tissue: particularly the blood.

Chronic, superficial bacterial skin infections. Poor skin and hair quality. Slow healing wounds. Liver and pancreatic support.

4 KALI MUR. Potassium chloride.

Constituent of fibrin.

Chronic bacterial, inflammatory processes. Respiratory and skin.

Slow healing skin injuries: burns. Diarrhoea from fatty foods. Constipation during pregnancy.

5 FERRUM PHOS. Found in all body tissues except nerves. Abundant in blood.

Major anti-inflammatory effects. Recent physical and viral problems associated with throbbing pains. Minor respiratory and gastrointestinal disorders.

6 KALI PHOS. Major constituent of brain and nerve tissue. Role in blood cells and muscle tissue. A major influence in body metabolism by slowing tissue degeneration. End stages of inflammation. Derangement of nervous system including anxiety, depression, hysteria. Lead to debilitating conditions of the bowel, bladder, and infertility.

7 KALI SULPH. Found in epithelial tissues. End stages of inflammatory process. Tissue oxygenation. Catarrhal conditions of mouth: halitosis. Asthma, and bronchitis.

8 MAG PHOS. Cellular systems including blood, bone, brain, muscle, **nerves,** and teeth.

The 'anti-spasmodic' salt for its relationship with painful conditions including colic, cramps and spasm of gut muscle, ovaries, urinary tract, and respiratory system.

9 NAT MUR. As 'Common Salt' a vital role in water regulation. Control of cellular fluid balances and sodium transport.

Influences under and over production of fluids including Diarrhoea, constipation, hay fever, exudation, milk production, tears, and salivation. Any inflammatory process with fluid including insect bites, and early arthritis.

10 NAT PHOS. The 'Acid Neutraliser' reduces intra-cellular acid build.

Appetite loss, indigestion, and catarrh. Peri-articular thickened tissues.

11 NAT SULPH. 'Glauber's salts' in intracellular tissues. Regulates fluid contents. Stimulates local metabolism. Chronic, intermittent, inflammatory changes in excretory organs, including kidney, liver, pancreas, and lungs. Chronic tympanitic colic.

12 SILICA. Cellular connective tissues of hair, nails, nerves, and skin. Detoxification and elimination of waste and toxins. Slows aging. Chronic asthma and bronchitis. Delayed healing of skin. Defects of hair, horn, and nails. Brittleness and excessive shedding.

Others: Certain companies produce a wide range of tissue salts than those originally described by the founder. Tissue salt **combinations.** It is now customary practice for these salts to be commercially available in related groups for ease of administration and to give a wider cover of related needs. Some complexes with indications:

Anaemia	Calc phos Ferr phos Nat mur Kali phos.
Asthma	Kali phos Mag phos Nat mur Nat sulph.
Hair Ball / Impaction	Calc fluor Kali mur Nat mur Silicea.
Diarrhoea	Calc phos Ferr phos Kali phos Kali sulph Nat sulph.
Nervous exhaustion	Calc phos Ferr phos Kali phos Mag phos Nat mur.
Tonic: Nerves & brain	Calc phos Ferr phos Kali phos Mag phos Nat phos.
Gastritis & flatulence	Nat phos Nat sulph Silicea.
Pregnancy: during	Mag phos Calc phos Kali phos Calc fluor.
Lack of Vitality	Nat mur Kali phos Calc phos.

RECOMMENDED READING

Despite the vast amount of useful material readily available on the internet, the following books are the author's favourites.

W. **Boericke**,1994, *Pocket Manual of Homoeopathic Materia Medica and Repertory*, B. Jain Publishers Pvt. Ltd., India.

Christopher **Day**,1996, *The Homoeopathic Treatment of Small Animals Principles and Practice*, The C.W. Daniel Company Ltd., England.

Jacques **Jouanny**, *The Essentials of Homoeopathic Materia Medica,* Boiron SA 1984.

Dr. O.A. **Julian**, 1990, *Materia Medica of New Homoeopathic Remedies*, Beaconsfield Publishers Ltd., U.K.

James Tyler **Kent**, 1994, *Lectures on Materia Medica*, B. Jain Publishers Pvt., Ltd. India

George **Macleod**,1990, *The Treatment of Horses by Homoeopathy*, The C.W. Daniel Company Ltd., England.

George **Macleod**, MRCVS, 1991, *The Treatment of Cattle by Homoeopathy*, The C.W. Daniel Company Ltd., England.

George **Macleod**, MRCVS, 1992, *A Veterinary Materia Medica and Clinical Repertory with a Materia Medica of the Nosodes*, The C.W. Daniel Company Ltd., England.

George **Macleod**, MRCVS, 1994, *Dogs: Homoeopathic Remedies*, The C.W. Daniel Company Ltd., England.

George **Macleod**, MRCVS, 1995, *Cats: Homoeopathic Remedies*, The C.W. Daniel Company Ltd., England.

Robin **Murphy**, N.D., 1993, *Homoeopathic Medical Repertory – 1st Edition*, Hahnemann Academy of North America (HANA), USA.

J **Saxton** and P **Gregory.** *A Textbook of Veterinary Homeopathy*, Beaconsfield 2005.

George **Vithoulkas**, 1986, *The Science of Homoeopathy*, Thorsons Publishers Ltd., England.

ACKNOWLEDGEMENTS

Author admits support of The Lord Jesus Christ whose Death and Resurrection brought the world hope.

This work succeeded because of advice, encouragement, and support of fellow creatures:

Barbara Sanne *Royal Malta*	Alexecovet (Pty) Ltd.
Melissa and Andrew	Barclay Digby
Buddy Maroun	*Bubbles*
Chia	*Coco*
Frostwing	*Follow the Falcon*
Golden Man	*Golden Man*
Munschkin	John and Jill Wileman
Jean Hemming	*Lady Theresa*
Shannon	Linda Engelbrecht
Karen van de Venter and *Myvin*	Maverick
Stewie Pettigrew	*Papillon*
Michael Levien Natura labs	Peter and Jane Fitchet
David Lilley	Sheba
Louis Goosen and Lauren Watt	*Smurf*
Just do it Joey	

DR ALEX NIVEN: THE AUTHOR

Website, **dralexniven.com**

As his prolific writing career fruits, Dr Alex Niven presents for your interest, education and hopefully enjoyment his complete portfolio.

As an approachable character, he enjoys the individualised touch.

Please email him on alex@dralexniven.com

Grouped as,
Memoir Stories
The **Overtoun** Novels
Veterinary **Textbooks**.

THE MEMOIR STORIES

VETERINARY MEMOIRS is an absorbing, five volume series reflecting on the varied Cases touching VET DR ALEX Niven's life, and his family, during a fifty-year adventure with animals as diverse as cattle, dogs and horses to elephant, rhino, and lions during a career taking them from Scotland through England onto South Africa.

In Volume One, **THE BENT BULL**, gasp with him when facing a charging lion, thrill over Hansie's cancer cure and share Alex' adventure with Lady Nordic who saved his life.

The nutcase Jack Russell, Charlie always draws laughter. Mind you... that is the nature of the breed but what he did with the newspaper, well... that had even Niven shaking his head. Did he really use superglue to repair a fractured leg?

Then there was the police officers mentally disturbed and baldy bird and her tale of naughty goings-on in Drofter which got local tongues wagging.

When taking the rejected Red Heaven to win a group one race, success illustrated value of homoeopathy. A perfect example of how he often employed his mantra, they are only dead when the heart stops!

In Vol Two, **OUR CALF TESSA** they share the hysterical tale of the lollipop which stuck to Chang's.... and made him lame.

Rachael's death is a tearjerker illustrating vets do more than wrap bandages on puppies' paws. From disaster came one their favourite animals.

When teaching Simon how to unblock a cat's penis jampacked full of crystals, flighty urine illustrated how young vets learn from taking advice.

An abused lady is a human-interest story illustrating vets always have at least two patients to consider. Human guardians deserve respect.

While Theresa's bed warmer illustrates Alex's dedication to saving lives, exercising of his vocation depended on the fabulous girl sharing his life.

Slug bait poisoning in Vol Three, **GOATS AND GIRLS,** illustrates Niven's concern for the environment by highlighting dangers associated with careless use of poisonous chemicals. He illustrates the desirability of teamwork among colleagues.

For him, a sad story reflects on how tractors destroyed romance of the heavy horse, the fabulous Clydesdales who made Scotland famous.

Settled impossible Grumble Guts with a diagnosis of partial sight enforcing management changes setting him off on the road to success.

In **TURKEY TALES,** Vol four introduces a remarkable animal lover who funded her hobby from jewellery theft although it was her bird's egg-bound plight which first created interest. Extraordinary truth of the British governments approach to anthrax as a weapon in WWII highlights the horrid disease and causes shivers as did his first ever visit to a dead cow. No! Never brought it back to life!

An overturned horsebox not only describes plight of injured horses, but also the attitude of the owner declared he deserved the same fate. Horrid human greed illustrates why selected people should never own animals.

In a similar theme, an American vet described his farmer's method of catching a pregnant cow. If successful, unbelievable.

His first experience of dehorning an adult cow led to plastic surgery.

Even wondered at where the expression *shit* came from. Alex describes its derivation amid another absorbing tale of the link between human and animal distress. When involving social services to help Mrs Woods, dying from neglect, his effort triggered powerful emotions.

As a youngster, family adventures with a collection of wild things from frogs to hedgehogs kept them entertained in days before TV and computers.

FAMILY MATTERS in Vol five, illustrates happy moments including the best day of his life when marrying the gorgeous Dumbarton girl, Theresa.

The vet's first day almost never made it into print as it still evokes powerful and unpleasant memories. Everything went wrong on what he hoped must be a fabulous introduction to his longed-for career.

Theresa's first visit to a calving cow provided exceptional insight into farming, including how to reflect on a bull's massive equipment when deciding... male or female. Experience of birthing triggered hormones.

Juliet, a silly fantailed pigeon added different dimension to animal welfare.

And, when kneeling beside a sick pony to listen for signs of pneumonia, were connections entitled to believe Christianity cured its bronchitis?

A case of Siamese twins began as an extraordinarily difficult birthing,

Alex describes where the greatest success of his life began over fifty years earlier when God blessed him with marriage to Theresa Mulvenna, justifiably described as the catch of Dumbarton.

WORKS OF FICTION

OVERTOUN
A five-volume novel.

OVERTOUN
VOLUME ONE:
OVERTOUN

Story line. August 1982. Medic Henderson, when attending a road traffic accident, treats concussed Gerry, an old nemesis he fought with over a girl. Henderson's aberrant personality unfolds when killing Gerry by blocking the oxygen tube.

Celine, a trainee medic under his wing, witnesses enough of Henderson's malpractice to raise suspicions Gerry's death is needless, criminal. Unable to cope, she leaves the Vale Hospital and joins Overtoun Maternity Hospital. Haunted by memories, she, encouraged by colleagues digs into the murder.

June 1981. Fiona, rejoicing at the success of her engagement party, drives her fiancée Tom to a special layby on Loch Lomond where they first consummated their relationship. Reckless after drink, she crashes the car and kills Tom.

Maurice and Alice witness the accident. She supports Fiona while he attends to Tom. Finding him dead; he removes him from the passenger seat and lays him out on the beach beside the driver's door.

To prevent Fiona from a drunk driving charge, he persuades his girlfriend to lie to the police, convincing them Tom drove the car.

Medic Henderson captivates Fiona when transporting her to the hospital. Later, she enters an abusive marriage with him. Treating her as a surrogate mother, she delivers a weak infant, whom Matron, her own sister, fearing his death may have desperate consequences for Fiona's life, swaps him for one of the Stewart's twin boys born at the same time.

When both boys become ill, that introduces us to neonatal ICU specialist, Sr Holly. She determines to romance and later marry the brilliant, perfect specimen, but hopelessly shy Dr Patrick Cairns.

His concern for Fiona results in him suggesting they swap twins, although Deirdre changes his opinion. Protecting her brother from repercussions, she convinces him it a bad idea, then orchestrates the swap by herself.

Sr Angela, as Matron Cairn's deputy, develops increasing concerns around matron's management of infants. When on the point of uncovering this, Deirdre in a masterstroke of perfect timing, promotes her to assistant matron. A move suppressing further investigation.

Nurse Ingrid earns well for illegally collecting tissue samples from infant girls. On behalf of a North Korean company, unknown to her they hope to develop a biological weapon against Caucasian women. When this goes wrong, the volume ends...

OVERTOUN
VOLUME TWO:
OVERTOUN TWINS

Story line. Overtoun's Matron Deirdre Cairns believing him dying earlier swapped her sisters infant, for a Stewart infant, one of twins. Did this to protect her sister Fiona from Henderson, her deranged husband.

Elder of the three siblings while Matron of Overtoun Hospital intrigue and innuendo cause her to despair authorities must uncover her crime. Her only solution, as she considers, is to prepare for suicide.

News of Nurse Ingrid's death brings hope, but mental instability worsens.

Deirdre hates Henderson. Rejoices when Celine divulges how other medics, intent on mounting investigation around Gerry's death reveal fresh information.

Midwife Sr Catherine's investigations increase tension throughout the hospital. After establishing twins have birthmarks, she uncovers the swap. Before unmasking crime, a road accident results in her sustaining a debilitating, chronic, head injury. Her diary uncovers the truth around her dislike of the Cairns family.

While enraptured with her child, the swapped Stewart twin, Fiona's remarkable sense of smell, alerts Deirdre to the possibility she recognises the child as not hers.

The infant becomes ill.

Henderson's distorted personality worsens when appreciating medics may uncover, he murdered Gerry. Tremendous mood swings lead to impotence and increasing dependence on his alter ego, the equally deranged Mirror Man who decides Henderson must murder Deirdre to prevent her uncovering their crime.

Patrick Cairns, middle of the siblings is a doctor at Overtoun Hospital. His medical skill saves infants lives. Patrick and Henderson fight, during which the latter sustains a head injury.

In time, this leads to serious altercation between him and Mirror Man.

Massive fight between them results in them breaking the mirror. Henderson slashes at Mirror Man with a piece of broken glass. Henderson collapses from a severed jugular vein. When in danger of dying Deirdre arrives on the scene intent on convincing him not to divulge her secret but finds him lying in a bloody pool. Although she summons ambulance, does she work hard enough to save his life?

Their black Labrador, Afrika, continues to support Patrick.

Sr Holly is midwife and ICU specialist. An effervescent, dedicated character, she works hard with Patrick to save infants. At last, wearing down his resistance he proposes.

Margaret Stewart, the twins mother copes with swap until one child, the swapped one, takes ill. Angus, her husband's support helps her through a tough time.

Francesca Cormie is born at Overtoun at same time as the subject children. Clarice, her mother, disguised her pregnancy, maintaining she adopted the girl. With no intention of having a permanent man, but wishing to get pregnant, she selected Angus Stewart as sperm donor and seduced him for that purpose.

Three infants play significant parts in later volumes.

Sr Samantha from the Vale Hospital plays a role when during an emergency power failure at that hospital, she leads a team of staff and pregnant mums to Overtoun. Tiredness causes her to make a medical error. This opens the way for Deidre to promote Angela to matron, thereby allaying her interest in the crime.

Ends with Deirdre, convinced her crime exposed by Sr Catherine, secludes herself at home awaiting police.

OVERTOUN
VOLUME THREE:
OVERTOUN, HORSES

Story line. Police visit Deirdre's home and ask her to accompany them. At first, relieved for she expected their visit, surprise followed when they advised they were taking her to Overtoun hospital to attend a medical emergency.

A massive train crash in Dumbarton Central Station meant they drafted in all available medical personnel to assist with disaster management.

Eight years later. Holly and Patrick, now married with two children host a Cairn's family lunch. Still ravaged by guilt and loss, Deirdre, mental health regularly deteriorating almost reveals how she swapped infants. Life progresses to stage of children as teenagers then adults as we follow their careers into vet medicine and the police force.

Vet and twin Niall's involvement with best friend Evan when researching homoeopathy in HIV research at Glasgow University promise wonderful things. Niall becomes engaged with Francesca; ignorant they share a father. Twin Calder meets bogus vet, Georgiou Houdalakis, and together enter the hideous life of killing horses to claim insurance payouts.

In parallel, the Commissioner of Police instructs Alroy; Niall's unknown twin, to run a secret investigation into that business.

We follow this through twists and turns between Britain and Kentucky, where it involves Paulo Grizelli, horse breeder and drug distributor.

OVERTOUN
VOLUME FOUR:
OVERTOUN, KENTUCKY

Story line. Niall and Evan's research on HIV promises success.

As his first patient he treats Alroy; not yet introduced as his twin, and on death's door from HIV. Only after saving his life learns their happy relationship. Introduce Yvette and Louis, American horse vets who engage in fraud in parallel with Calder and Georgiou. They link up with Chinese agents to create a novel method for diamond smuggling by transporting gems inside the horses. This takes them on trips to Europe.

Patrick Cairns establishes Deirdre had swapped the twins, that Calder is Fiona's natural son, while Niall and Alroy are true twins.

Corrupt racehorse trainers collaborate with bogus vet Georgiou and Calder to kill horses. Alroy and the FBI sniff the prospect of a major takedown, including American and Chinese drug dealers. The vets travel to Kentucky to kill Senor Angelo, a fabulously valuable racehorse, now a stallion at stud.

In a smart takedown, the FBI rescue the horse and make arrests as Senor Angelo has the last laugh.

OVERTOUN
VOLUME FIVE:
OVERTOUN, RHINO

When Glasgow University sells off Niall and Evan's HIV project to a multinational company, they horrify on learning they mothball what should have been a fabulous effort proving homoeopathy is real, lifesaving medicine. They sacrifice it for a less effective but more lucrative product. This leads to Niall and fellow vet and friend Evan leaving the world of research and while undecided about their future, Niall received a potentially fatal hammer blow leading to his split from fiancé Francesca. Her mother reveals devastating truth around her parentage and how mum Clarice selected a sperm donor.

After a disastrous attempt to enter farming practice in Dumfries, Niall heads off to join Glasgow University friend Gugu on her family farm in South Africa. He, hoping for an extended holiday to recharge his sagging mental state lands in a situation where Gugu and her family have other intentions. While they work hard to ensure she captures her dream man, problems with animals bring her intentions to fruition. Introduce Sarah Kelly, a Dumbarton girl, and another vet. Her tempestuous life with a would-be suitor which never gets beyond a simple kiss, leads to her visiting South Africa to work on Gugu's second family farm.

There, amid a gun battle she saves Evan's life from a deranged poacher and killer which by awakening deep seated neurochemicals controlling love, confirms it time for Sarah to get involved in affairs of the heart.

Rhino poaching takes centre stage where the hideous reality of a Nigerian and Chinese partnership threatens to wreak havoc on Ipulazi.

In a masterly stroke, they invite the recovering Alroy to visit to continue convalescing from his near-death experience with HIV.

But in practical terms, commission him to lead the investigation against the poachers.

Gugu's aunt leads the team who interrogate two Nigerian embassy workers. Via a brutal but effective session of intense questioning, a scalpel opens tongues.

A fitting final finds poacher and their informants receiving suitable, tribal punishment with Gugu at last claiming her man.

DR ALEX NIVEN

NON-FICTION
HOMOEOPATHY TEXTBOOKS

VOLUME ONE
VETERINARY HOMOEOPATHY:
REPERTORY AND MATERIA MEDICA

The Repertory includes a detailed discourse on 480 remedies and their interactions. This includes detailed clinical indications and the signs of disease and the conditions to which they relate.

The Materia Medica highlights various disease parameters, their signs and offers pointers towards selecting appropriate remedies.

As an example, consider the remedy Berb-a, of proven value in the management of lameness conditions in horses. indications alongside the various organs, help in confirming clinical conditions where this remedy may assist.

Reflects role aggravating conditions play in mediating disease.

MODALITIES, Agg; evening and night.

Amel; cold washing.

Also significant is it relationship and similarity with other remedies including Aloe Ars Berb Psor Sulph which offer alternative selections.

Berb-a
BERBERIS AQUIFOLIUM
Mahonia aquifolium Plant
UROGENITAL, Azoturia. Lithiasis with proteinuria and tenesmus. PU.
LAMENESS, Azoturia; profound muscle pain and stiffness.
SKIN, Widespread blisters and papules.
COMPETITION, Azoturia and high muscle enzymes in sport horses.
MODALITIES, Agg; evening and night. Amel; cold washing.
COMPARE, Aloe Ars Berb Psor Sulph.
CONSIDER, Acute allergic eczemas including flea bite and veld mange.
For Azoturia, is better than Berb.
Cystitis and lithiasis.
POTENCY, 6X. 30CH.

Worth pointing out where the author highlights Berberis aquifolium as being more useful than the similar Berberis vulgaris. An indication of where his extensive clinical experience and willingness to experiment allow him to make such a confident claim.

VOLUME TWO:
THEORY AND CLINICAL APPLICATION

While authors have written extensively and well on homoeopathic theory, Niven's basic introduction highlights the main points with a twist.

For here he discusses a detailed approach to an individual case, and how experience with various species revealed different cure rates and reaction responses. His introduction to management of cancer with nosodes because it includes cure in live cases offer groundbreaking research for the future.

Collection of samples using specialised PRP syringes, and their further preparation under the NIVEN KORSAKOVIAN system is a first, as it recognises the necessity of succussing samples one thousand times during nosode and sarcode preparation. Far more than standard practice, by reporting clinical success, this offers hope for future workers to refine and achieve success. Because space prevents the description of an extensive number of conditions, here the author highlights IBD, a nuisance of a disease which causes marked distress in animals and owners.

Also, as this is one which responds especially well to homoeopathy, it illustrates where cure is possible. Thus, it includes secondary, and concomitant conditions, with the ever-present threat of serious, chronic gastric ulceration with cases restored to full function.

IBD. INFLAMMATORY BOWEL DISORDER must not be confused with rarer IBS; irritable bowel disease, which although it plagues humans causes us less headaches... should that be gut aches!

A challenging condition, around a dozen dog breeds are at greater risk of contracting the condition. Maybe related to bacterial imbalance, worsened by food intolerance and as this may involve a single ingredient makes diagnosis time consuming. Another condition where an abnormal, personal immune response complicates the issue. Associated with chronic diarrhoea, flatus, and colic. Can develop secondary liver disease and often is associated with skin problems. Treatment considers toxaemia from standard drug therapy. Gastric ulceration possible.

Widespread use of cortisone results in a partial improvement but is toxic.

Reduce such treatments slow. Aim for complete resolution.

Good news. A spectacular disorder for VH as it frequently responds well to management.

Remedies, APIS BELL CORTISO LACH MERC RHUS-T THUJ Acid-oxal Carb-v Gaert-b Mags Op Urt-u.

Chronic, Cortiso Gaert-b or Merc 30CH. Hydr or Acid-oxal 12X. Apis Bry or Urt-u 6X. TD. Months. SD.

VOLUME THREE:
EQUINE HOMOEOPATHY

This specialised work focuses on conditions plaguing horses including the big ones.

- Lameness
- Colic
- Coughing
- Behaviour

Practicalities of training horses, irrespective of which discipline, depends on attitude of horse and owner. While it does not fall within the author's remit to treat people... well, he presents situations where a slight modification in the trainer's approach resulted in improving horse's behaviour.

A sad fact is obvious. In the author's practice he often faced difficult horses, either because they are either inherently problematic or reached a state whereby faulty or imperfect human interaction creates barriers.

It was due to the fact of these cases becoming terminal, which drove Niven into researching the topic to establish which mental conditions respond to homoeopathic adjustment.

Important to state this, although it can be spectacularly successful, this can at best be only likely with good owner management. Remembering always that horse, rider, and trainer work best when as a team they act in synch.

Niven's skill becomes apparent when considering his management of difficult cases and how when illustrating them he engenders confidence.

VOLUME FOUR:
MATERIA MEDICA

Present the materia medica section as described in the main work as a standalone work.

VOLUME FIVE;
CLINICAL APPLICATION

Present clinical application as described in the main work as a standalone work.

VOLUME SIX:
COMPANION ANIMAL HOMOEOPATHY
By popular request, Dr Alex presents this stand-alone work containing basics need for clinicians to treat even advanced diseases in pets including the Small Furry things, Amphibians, Reptiles and Birds, and other non-equine animals.

INDEX

Chelone Glabra 107
Chemosis 265
Cherry Eye 265
Chimaphila Umbellata 107
Chininum Arsenicosum 107
Chininum Sulphuricum 107
Chionanthus Virginicum 108
Chlamydia Felis 319
Chloralum Hydratum 108
Chloramphenicolum 108
Chloroformium 109
Chlorpromazinum 109
Chlorum 109
Cholesterinum 110
Chorea 259
Chrysarobinum 110
Cicuta Virosa 110
Cimex Lectularius 111
Cimicifuga Racemosa 111
Cinchona Succirubra 111
Cinnamomum Ceylanicum 112
Circulation 286
Cirrhosis 272
Cistus Canadensis 112
Citrullus Colocynthis 113
Clematis Erecta 113
Cobaltum Nitricum 114
Cocainum Hydrochloricum 114
Coccidiosis 281
Cocculus Indicus 114
Coccus Cacti 115
Coffea Cruda 115
Coffea Tosta 115
Coffin Joint 302
Colchicum Autumnale 117
Colic – Equine 281
Colics: Impacted
Colics: Impacted
Collinsonia Canadensis 117
Collinsonia Canadensis 117
Colostrum Bovis 117
Colostrum Bovis 117
Coma 259
Coma 259
Company: Averse to 252
Company: Averse to 252
Company: Needs 252
Company: Needs 252
Concentration: Poor 252
Concentration: Poor 252
Concussion 260
Concussion 260
Confidence: Low 252
Confidence: Low 252
Confused 252
Confused 252
Congestive Heart Failure 286
Congestive Heart Failure 286
Conium Maculatum 117
Conium Maculatum 117
Conjunctivitis 265
Conjunctivitis 265

Conjunctivitis; Exudate 265
Conjunctivitis; Exudate 265
Consolation Aggravates 252
Consolation Aggravates 252
Consolation: Agg
Consolation: Agg
Constipation 283
Constipation 283
Convalescence
Convalescence
Convallaria Majalis 118
Convallaria Majalis 118
Copaiva 118
Copaiva 118
COPD 289
Coprophagia 252
Corallium Rubrum 119
Cornea 265
Corns
Corns 302
Cornus Circinata 119
Coronary Band 302
Corticotrophinum 119
Cortisone Toxicity 306
Cortisonum 120
Corylus Avellana 121
Corynanthe Yohimbe 121
Coughing 287
Cramp 299 302
Crataegus Oxyacantha 121
Cresolum 121
Crocus Sativus 122
Crotalus Horridus 122
Croton Tiglium 123
Cruciate Ligaments 303
Cryptorchid
Cubeba Officinalis 123
Cucurbita Pepo 124
Cundurango 124
Cuprum Aceticum 125
Cuprum Arsenicosum 124
Cuprum Metallicum 125
Cuprum Oxydatum 125
Curare 125
Curb 303
Curcuma Longa 126
Cushing's Disease 260
Cusparia Febrifuga 126
Cyclamen Europaeum 126
Cystitis 290
Cytisus Laburnum 127
Dandruff 262
Dangerous
Daphne Indica 127
Daphne Mezereum 127
Daphne Mezereum 127
Datura Stramonium 128
Datura Stramonium 128
Deafness 263
Deafness 263
Defiant 252
Defiant 252

331

335

337

www.ingramcontent.com/pod-product-compliance
Lightning Source LLC
Chambersburg PA
CBHW082208290526
45794CB00009B/3467